ADVANCES IN PSYCHOLOGY

92

Editors:

G. E. STELMACH

P. A. VROON

NORTH-HOLLAND
AMSTERDAM • LONDON • NEW YORK • TOKYO

PSYCHOPHYSICAL APPROACHES TO COGNITION

PSYCHOPHYSICAL APPROACHES TO COGNITION

Edited by

Daniel ALGOM
Department of Psychology
Bar-Ilan University
Ramat-Gan, Israel

1992

NORTH-HOLLAND
AMSTERDAM • LONDON • NEW YORK • TOKYO

NORTH-HOLLAND
ELSEVIER SCIENCE PUBLISHERS B.V.
Sara Burgerhartstraat 25
P.O. Box 211, 1000 AE Amsterdam, The Netherlands

ISBN: 0 444 88978 7

Transferred to digital printing 2007

PREFACE

It was as great an honor as it was a challenge for me to be asked to edit a book on a topic of my choice for North Holland -- within the framework of the Advances of Psychology series. The relationship between psychophysics (conceived in its broadest sense) and cognitive psychology has concerned me for some time and I was fortunate to detect a similar preoccupation with the subject on the part of the other contributors. Thus, the overriding theme of these chapters concerns the question of how we reconcile at a fundamental level the inconsistencies, if not the chasm, that seem to separate these two branches of experimental psychology. I was equally fortunate to enjoy the full cooperation of my contributors who gave generously of their time, their other extensive scientific commitments notwithstanding. I learned a great deal reading their chapters and my sincere hope is that the reader will share at least some of my experience and enthusiasm.

An edited volume enjoys a rarely acknowledged advantage: It lets the proper authors speak for themselves rather than through the commentary of another individual. The present authors did so with clarity and depth, each addressing the main theme in a different, self-contained way. Nevertheless, at the same time, each contributed to a fairly unified whole, providing an almost narrative account of the major issues pertaining to a possible "interface" between sensation and cognition. If the reader appreciates our concerns and continues to wonder and worry about them, then we justify our title.

It is a pleasure to acknowledge the help of the many people who contributed to this project -- primarily, of course, the authors. I wish to thank Dr. K. Michielsen, of North-Holland Publishing Company, who initiated and followed the project with encouragement, grace, and patience. Malka Shemesh was more than an extremely competent typist -- her sundry ideas, suggestions, and friendship made my editing chores that much more manageable. The making of the book was greatly aided by the work of Amnon Dekel, Ainat Pansky, and Vered Shakuf who read large portions of the book and helped with other aspects of preparing the manuscript.

Substantially, many colleagues and students provided valuable thoughts about the issues surrounding a book like this, but I will not present a list now. I must, however, acknowledge the inspiration I have gained from Professor Harvey Babkoff who besides being my mentor, served as a close collaborator on many of my research projects.

We like to portray science as that human endeavor dealing with the general rather than with particulars. Regardless of the merit of this viewpoint, it certainly does not apply to the making or writing of science. Preparing this volume coincided with the tumult caused by the Gulf War in which my family and I were unwitting participants. The difficult times highlighted the help and understanding my wife and children provided me throughout. I dedicate this book to them.

CONTENTS

CONTRIBUTORS

Daniel Algom

Department of Psychology, Bar-Ilan University, Ramat-Gan

Norman H. Anderson

Department of Psychology, University of California, San Diego

John C. Baird

Department of Psychology, Dartmouth College, Hanover NH

Stanley J. Bolanowski, Jr.

Institute for Sensory Research, Syracuse University

Eugene Galanter

Department of Psychology, Columbia University

George A. Gescheider

Department of Psychology, Hamilton College and Institute for Sensory Research, Syracuse University

Timothy L. Hubbard

Department of Psychology, Eastern Oregon State College

Lawrence E. Marks

John B. Pierce Laboratory and Yale University

Robert D. Melara

Department of Psychological Sciences, Purdue University

Gary B. Rollman

Department of Psychology, University of Western Ontario

Ronald T. Verrillo

Institute for Sensory Research, Syracuse University

Lawrence M. Ward

Department of Psychology, University of British Columbia

Psychophysical Approaches to Cognition
D. Algom (Editor)

1

INTRODUCTION TO PSYCHOPHYSICAL APPROACHES TO COGNITION

Daniel Algom
Bar-Ilan University
Ramat-Gan, Israel

Psychology, regardless of whether one deems it to be a full-grown *Naturwissenschaft* or a gargantuan undertaking in hermeneutics, a *Geisteswissenschaft* trying to make sense of human life -- a field set out to interpret or impart meaning to a manifold human condition -- carries its distinctive set of dichotomies. Reviewing the member dimensions of such a set may support a panoramic, yet in-depth appraisal of the current state of our science. A further gain may be reaped from such an examination. It may assist to disentangle those dichotomies that are fairly recent, perhaps the products of the prevailing paradigm or *Zeitgeist*, from earlier classifications that may prove to be more fundamental.

Pitting the sensory against the cognitive comes naturally to most contemporary psychologists. The terms denote a pair of polar processes, a contradistinction that permeates the gamut of psychological discourse from informal discussion to textbook organization. Sensory and cognitive usually carry the adjectives low-level or early and high-level or late, respectively. The classification also seems to carry an unmistakably modern ring. Most uninitiated observers and some seasoned psychologists surmise that the chasm between psychophysics and cognitive psychology is a byproduct (fortunate or unfortunate as the case may be) of the particular course of development traversed by modern experimental psychology.

Many trace the disparate development of the two fields, or rather their "incommensurability," to the advent of behaviorism. "Two opposed points of view," John B. Watson wrote in 1925, "are still dominant in American psychological thinking -- introspective or subjective psychology, and behaviorism or objective psychology." And, sure enough, fifty years after the publication of Behaviorism, the publisher succinctly avers on the back cover: "His statement is still true today" (Watson, 1925/1970). Watson's "subjective psychology" included the systems of Wundt, Titchener, and James, as well as Gestalt psychology. Concerning the latter, Watson correctly recognized its conceptual origin in Kant's philosophy --

outwitting in that respect the creators of Gestalt psychology themselves (who tantalizingly were unaware of the intellectual underpinning of their own endeavor). Although, today, Watson's is a minority voice vis-a-vis the relative merits of the two psychologies, the gap separating them apparently has not narrowed.

Others believe the divorce of sensation and cognition to be even more recent. Foremost among those are many of today's cognitive psychologists, who "Like the citizens of the United States, France, and the Soviet Union ... share a myth of revolutionary origin" (Leahy, 1987, p.454). Moreover, they claim that the revolution occurred fairly late such that their "subject seems so new that you might well think cognitive science erupted into the world complete, a few years back, like Athena springing fully adult from Zeus' head ... Even the field's practitioners can fall into this view" (Lieber, 1991, p.viii). Indeed, many proponents of information processing or cognitive science believe that "in 1960 a Kuhnian scientific revolution occurred during which information processing overthrew behaviorism" (Leahey, 1987, p.454). An objective review (if that is at all possible), however, concludes that" ... it is reasonable to doubt if there was a revolution" (Leahy, 1987, p.454), a well founded skepticism that I fully share (Algom, 1991). Nevertheless, even if the talk about the revolution of "information processing" really is tantamount to mythinformation processing, it might well have served to exacerbate the divide between sensation and cognition. For every revolution needs its nemesis, if only to justify its uniqueness; and sensory processes seem an ideal candidate for just that role. Hence, whereas sensation and cognition evolved independently in the first century BCE (Before the Cognitive Era, cf. Marks, 1991), the two became incommensurably distinct since. Or so the story goes.

Given psychology's young age as a science, it was perhaps inevitable that someone or another would propose that the separation of the cognitive and the sensory is provisional, but an accidental consequence of psychology's peculiar development. Hence, depending on one's vantage, the chasm comprises either a childhood disease or part of psychology's rites of passage. The only problem with all such viewpoints is that they are wrong. Far from being a recent tentative development, the disassociation of sensation and cognition is as old as the first systematic inquiry of mind. The disjunction has its roots in antiquity, notably in the Platonic theory of knowledge; as such, it pervaded layers of Western culture, reaching well beyond the confines of psychology. My aim at this point is to make explicit the extent to which Plato's core notions about mind inform our contemporary discourse about perception and cognition.

The most famous of Plato's schemes for subdividing the "mind" or "psyche" is their tripartition in the Republic into rational, affective, and appetitive systems. A great divide, indeed a constitutional conflict is said to pit the rational against the appetitive portion (the affective system is not involved in that fundamental psychological contrast as Plato repeatedly notes). In this schema, the appetitive apparatus "apprehends sensory perceptions, sensual demands, and concrete, particular, mortal objects," whereas the rational part deals with the "claims of the higher mental functions" (Simon, 1972, p.396). One can hardly avoid imparting value(s) to the conflict, "contrasting ... *higher* and *lower* forms of mental activity" (Simon, 1972, p. 396; emphases added) as the contrast is repeatedly couched in terms of a division between earth-bound bodily processes and heavenly mental processes. Summarized in Table 1.1 are the contrasting attributes of (what Simon characteristically enough depicts) "baser parts of mind" and "higher parts of mind."

I tried to summarize -- without claiming exhaustiveness or even representativeness -- some of the attributes popular in current usage of sensory and cognitive processes. They are listed in Table 1.2. Shedding the veneer of modishness from our current nomenclature, one cannot fail to notice how much the portrayals of sensory and cognitive on the one hand, and appetitive and rational on the other, are interdependent. The Platonian split between bodily and mental processes continues to inform the modern partition of psychological processes into perceptual and cognitive. So does the inferior status of empirically derived or sensory information in Plato's theory of knowledge. The spontaneous allocation of the terms "high-level" and "low-level" to cognitive and sensory processes, respectively, betrays a deep-rooted metaphor in Western thought.

Table 1.1: Plato's division of the mind. The contrasting attributes of "higher" and "lower" forms of mental activity (After Simon, 1972).

Lower Portion	**Higher Portion**
Appetitive	Rational
Somatic	Psychic
Being born and perishing	True being
Opinion (doxa)	True knowledge (episteme)
Pictorial, illusory	Ideational
Shadow	Sun
Asleep, dreaming	Awake
Childish	Adult
Imitation	Abstract understanding
Flux	Stability
Conflict	Harmony
Heterosexual	Homosexual and asexual
Mortal	Immortal, timeless
Particular	General

Table 1.2: The contrasting attributes of sensation and cognition commonly used in current experimental psychology

Sensory	**Cognitive**
Peripheral	Central
Mechanistic	Decisional
Low-level	High-level
Simple	Complex
Front-end	Back-end
Automatic	Inferential, heuristic
Involuntary	Voluntary, creative
Early	Late
Impenetrable	Penetrable
Primitive, primary	Sophisticated, secondary
Physiologically constrained	Semantic, symbolic

Ironically perhaps the sensory-cognitive duality entered psychophysics itself, influencing the *Weltanschanuung* of several of its key figures. Again, the roots are early indeed. Democritus, who some 2500 years ago wrote, "Sweet exists by convention, bitter by convention, color by convention; atoms and void [alone] exist in reality," espoused a psychophysics that comprises (at least) two structures or processes: a sensory system that reacts to impinging energy and a cognitive system that acts on the input of the former (Marks & Algom, 1990; see the chapter by *Marks* for a fuller discussion of the implications for a psychophysics based on Democritus ideas). The attributes perforce follow naturally: the sensory apparatus is early and mechanistic, the cognitive apparatus is late and symbolic. The last term is noteworthy; for the basic notion conveyed by Democritus seems to be that perceptual experiences exist as representations of the world. As *Marks* demonstrates convincingly in his chapter, this view traces a venerable tradition through Galileo, Locke, and Newton, to contemporary cognitive psychology.

Fechner also proposed a dual-track psychophysics with "inner psychophysics" far outweighing "outer psychophysics". Wundt borrowed Leibniz's distinction between *perception* and *apperception* to mark activities that we now would label sensation and cognition. Under the rubric of perception Wundt included the processes by which the sensory system modulates and responds to incoming stimulus energies and information. Subsumed under apperception were attentive processes by which people focus selectively on various aspects or elements of perception. Hence, perception has been said to be automatic, mechanical, even "thoughtless" (cf. Fancher, 1990), whereas apperception, by way of contrast, is voluntary, conscious, even creative. However, unlike many of their predecessors, Fechner and Wundt eschewed explicit value judgments. No one psychological component was deemed superior; rather, both (all) portions were considered indispensable for the proper functioning of a unitary mind.

Let me pose now the question of real import, regardless of the dating of the split between sensation and cognition in contemporary psychology. Does that partition serve a useful purpose? I think not; nor is the division tenable on any substantive ground. Therefore, the unification of these two branches of experimental psychology is highly desirable -- theoretically as well as methodologically. That is the premise on which the present volume was motivated.

I should probably issue a caveat before proceeding. We can and must, of course, separate "sensory" and "cognitive" factors in empirical research. One can manipulate them independently in a research protocol, and yet conceptually integrate both in the overall model of response to stimuli. This integration, I argue, is sine qua non for meaningful psychological theorizing. One should construe psychological phenomena in terms of *both* sensory and cognitive contributions. Signal Detection Theory (SDT) is a good example for first providing explicitly for both sensory and cognitive influences, and then integrating them within the framework of a comprehensive model (see the chapters by *Melara* and *Ward* for discussions of the role of SDT in psychological analysis). Again, a few remarks, mainly of historical savor, may help highlight the principal issue.

Plato's partition of the mind, and particularly his denigration of sensory knowledge did not leave room for the development of good *psychological* theories of perception, learning or memory. As the chapter by *Algom* attempts to show, Aristotle did succeed in creating such theories precisely because he discarded much of the Platonian dualism, especially as far as psychology is concerned. Amongst his other contributions, Aristotle largely anticipated the modern discipline of *memory psychophysics* (note the coalescence of the sensory and the cognitive), coming close to proposing a (re)perceptual, analogous account of memory. That perception and cognition tap but different aspects of an otherwise inseparable psychological whole was grasped by additional Greek precursors of our subject. Epicharmus, for instance, living approximately 2500 years ago, said, "The mind sees and the mind hears. The rest is blind and deaf" (cited in Coren & Ward, 1989). Which is an excellent way of saying that "mental experience" (i.e., the only experience available to us) is composed of elements that by themselves do not reflect the integrated reality that they sample.

My point, of course, is not to refute the existence per se of perceptual and cognitive processes. What I do refute is the possibility to conceive them independently. We simply lack differential access to one process free of influence from the other. Both phenomena are products of processing by the entire mind. Sensation is as fully psychological as cognition; it is neither less nor more direct, simple, or early. Not is it easier to observe. Introspection does not provide a window to sensation, that is to say to sensation *only*. If it is a window, then it affords a look (blurred, to be sure) at the end-product of an entire psychological process. That is what the students of the Wurzburg school so painstakingly demonstrated (and what Wundt failed to accept). Indeed, the assumption that introspection provides an exclusive opening to sensation precipitated its demise as an experimental method as well as the downfall of structuralism. And, as *Marks'* chapter makes it clear, any such Window Hypothesis is doomed to fail regardless of the vista facing the window.

The crucial point is to recognize the need to provide for (a) mind in any serious psychophysical undertaking. Our most influential theories have indeed provided for one, as the chapter by *Ward* demonstrates. At times, though, the role of the mind has been implicit, but searching for it is well worth the effort, because many long-standing psychophysical issues could be resolved if only we knew more about the nature of its influence. Thus, contrary to common impression, S.S. Stevens did provide a critical function for conscious, cognitive processes in his psychophysics. Any sensory judgment presupposes an intentional process of abstracting the judged dimension from the totality of the stimulus. The operation of *matching* requires the abstraction of a commensurate dimension on the basis of which the sensory analysis is prosecuted. And the dimension of choice is dictated by a goal-directed organism. As *Ward* points out, the "goal" in Stevens' system corresponds to the elaborated machinery of "cognitive algebra" in *Anderson's integration psychophysics*. The hegemony of psychological (as opposed to merely sensory or conscious) operations is the hallmark of *Anderson's* refreshing approach. *Galanter*, too, explores the links between *intentions* and behavior, and shows how a comprehensive psychophysics must start with the former to model the latter. All of which revives the integrated nature of Wundt's notions of apperception and perception, if not Fechner's metaphysics.

The sensory should not be at war with the cognitive; their genuine ɜoretical integration -- however fuzzily sketched at first -- should yield deeper understanding and practical progress. That it does is demonstrated by a new and ambitious expressive theory proposed in the chapter by *Galanter*. His approach comprises the potential to resurrect psychophysics from the laboratory and apply it to real-life situations. Moreover, the confluence of the sensory and the cognitive should not be construed too parochially, because it surfaces at all levels of psychophysical inquiry. *Gescheider, Bolanowski, and Verrillo* elucidate in their chapter the sensory-cognitive interplay present at the level of the psychophysical magnitude judgment. And *Rollman* does the same in his chapter on pain, at several levels of analysis. Pain has posed a puzzle for laymen and scientists alike largely because of the virtually intractable interweaving of its sensory and cognitive components. This feature may account for the designation of pain as a "passion of the mind" (rather than as a perceptual system) by Plato and Aristotle.

I believe the case is compelling for cognitive effects to be considered seriously by psychophysicists. By the same token, cognitive theory should be informed by sensations or what we profess to know about them. Unfortunately, for many a cognitive psychologist, sensation still appears to be the last bastion of fixed mechanistic (i.e., psychologically trivial) properties, best left to those unprepared or uninterested enough to deal with real psychology. That an "interface" between models of cognitive psychology and psychophysics is not only possible but badly needed is shown in the chapter by *Melara* on the psychology of similarity and categorization. There, unifying models from the two domains led to several important insights. A variety of interesting cognitive issues can be couched in terms of sensory processing, or modelled by techniques borrowed from modern combinational or multidimensional psychophysics. It seems no accident that several contributors to this volume independently use the term *cognitive psychophysics*.

The approaches to Cognitive Psychophysics attempts to legitimize cognitive influences in psychological theorizing (and, conversely, to provide for the sensory in cognitive theory). Moreover, it attempts to change the traditional approach of classical psychophysics to explore the pathway between sensation and cognition unidirectionally, from the periphery to the center only (*Anderson*), depicting an organism whose behavior is essentially reactive (*Galanter*). A satisfactory theory should rather start from the person says *Galanter*; it should shift the conceptual base of classical psychophysics and work from the center outward, says *Anderson*. These ideas surface in virtually every chapter in this volume and capture the essence of the approach dubbed here Cognitive Psychophysics.

The legend has it that Hermann Ebbinghaus, while in Paris, came across a copy of Fechner's Elemente der Psychophysik, which inspired him to study memory in the same manner as Fechner examined sensation. It took a century, though, after the establishment of psychophysics and the modern field of memory for a discipline of *memory psychophysics* to emerge. The chapter by *Algom* traces that development and assesses the prospects of that young offspring domain. In a similar vein, mental imagery has been considered for decades a cognitive subject unrelated to psychophysics. No more. Modern research has shown that mental images display visual characteristics in common with perceived objects. They exhibit constraints that, in various respects, correspond to those in visual perception (cf. Finke, 1989). The chapter by *Baird* and *Hubbard* examines this fascinating subject, reinforcing again the usefulness of psychophysical approaches to cognition.

A final remark on the organization of chapters. Although all contain data and theory, some are primarily theoretical in outlook, others are primarily empirical, examining special modalities, domains, or issues. The former four appear next. However, as the demarcation is fairly vague in the present case no formal division to sections is warranted.

References

Algom, D. (1991). *Perakim betoldot hapszichologia* [Issues in the history of psychology]. Tel-Aviv: Ministry of Defense Publishing House.

Coren, S., & Ward, L.M. (1989). *Sensation & Perception* (3rd ed.). New York: Harcourt Brace Jovanovich.

Fancher, R.E. (1990). *Pioneers of psychology* (2nd ed.). New York: Norton.

Finke, R.E. (1989). *Principles of mental imagery*. Cambridge, MA: MIT.

Leahey, T.H. (1987). *A history of psychology* (2nd ed.). Englewood Cliffs, NJ: Prentice-Hall.

Lieber, J. (1991). *An invitation to cognitive science*. Cambridge, MA: Blackwell.

Marks, L.E. (1991). The dynamics of ratio scaling. In S.J. Bolanowski, Jr., & G.A. Gescheider (Ed.), *Ratio scaling of psychological magnitude* (pp. 27-42). Hillsdale, NJ: Erlbaum.

Marks, L.E., & Algom, D. (1990). Context effects and loudness scales: Ghosts in the auditory machine? In F. Muller (Ed.), *Fechner Day '90*. Wurzburg, Germany: International Society for Psychophysics.

Simon, B. (1972). Models of mind and mental illness in ancient Greece: II. The Platonic model. *Journal of the History of the Behavioral Sciences*, **9**, 3-17.

Watson, J.B. (1925/1970). *Behaviorism*. New York: Norton.

Psychophysical Approaches to Cognition
D. Algom (Editor)

2

INTEGRATION PSYCHOPHYSICS AND COGNITION

Norman H. Anderson
University of California, San Diego

Table of Contents

I. Introduction

Integration psychophysics is concerned primarily with relations among sensations or perceptions. Its conceptual base is primarily cognitive, within the mental realm. Classical psychophysics has a different conceptual base, in the relations between the physical stimulus and sensation. This difference in conceptual base leads to fundamental differences at every level of investigation. These differences derive mainly from the two kinds of laws that epitomize these two approaches to psychophysics: psychophysical law and psychocognitive law.

II. Psychophysical Law and Psychocognitive Law[1]

The basic difference between classical psychophysics and integration psychophysics concerns where order and law are sought: *psychophysical law* in one case; *psychocognitive law* in the other.[1] Classical psychophysics seeks order at the psycho-physical interface, that is, in the relations between physical stimulus energy and psychological sensation. The study of these relations was a natural focus of sensory psychology, and the idea that they obeyed an exact

[1] The term *psychocognitive law* is used in place of the previous *psychological law* (Anderson, 1970) because some readers had difficulty distinguishing psychological from psychophysical. The integration diagram, however, allows for sensory integration at peripheral levels. Although the proposed new term may be misleading in this respect, it seems to eliminate the previous confusability and it emphasizes the importance of cognitive determinants of sensation. Marks (1974) has suggested the term *psychosensory law* in place of *psychological law*, but that neglects the cognitive determinants. The main point is that the integration function is typically a function of two or more variables, which may be sensory, perceptual, and cognitive. Because of this many-variable form, integration psychophysics can work entirely within the organism, without necessary reliance on physical metrics.

mathematical form became imprinted through Fechner's argument that the psycho-physical relation was logarithmic. Despite, or perhaps because of, the controversy surrounding Fechner's logarithmic hypothesis, one prominent domain of classical psychophysics became epitomized by the search for the *psychophysical law*.

Integration psychophysics, in contrast, is epitomized by search for *psychocognitive* laws. Of foremost interest are laws that govern the integration of separate sensations into a unitary perception. Such laws typically lie at a stage beyond sensory processing, within the mental realm.

Psychocognitive laws and psychophysical laws thus address different classes of questions. In principle, there should be no conflict between them. They should work hand in hand, as they do in the **V** and **I** operations discussed later in the integration diagram of Figure 2.1. In practice, there has been conflict, reflecting a fundamental limitation of classical psychophysics, a limitation built into the very concept of psychophysical law.

The typical psychocognitive law is a function of more than one variable. This reflects the focus on stimulus integration, that is, on the joint action of multiple determinants of perception and action. This many-variable form, as it will be called, turns out to have fundamental significance.

The ideal psychophysical law, in contrast, is a function of a single variable: Sensation is a function of physical stimulus intensity. Other factors that affect sensation are mostly considered nuisance, context variables that should be eliminated to isolate the true psychophysical law.

Perceived heaviness of an object, for example, should depend only on gram weight. Context factors, especially size, also affect perceived heaviness, but these have no place in the psychophysical law. The usual practice, accordingly, has been to eliminate such context factors by presenting the weights unseen. This practice seems sensible, for these context factors have no direct relation with the sense receptors for heaviness. The focus on the psychophysical law thus mirrored J. Müller's doctrine of specific nerve energies in the sensory realm.

Three unfortunate, far-reaching consequences flowed from this conceptualization in terms of single-variable functions (Anderson, 1975). These are taken up in the next three sections (see also concluding sections).

Many-Variable Phenomena

The first consequence of the focus on psychophysical law was the relative neglect of important psychophysical phenomena that cannot be adequately represented as single-variable functions. One class of such phenomena concerns cross-modal integration, in which different sense modalities contribute jointly to a sensation. "Taste," for example, depends on several seemingly distinct senses of the tongue as well as on smell. The taste of mixtures cannot be understood in terms of the single-variable psychophysical laws for the components of the mixture (McBride & Anderson, 1991). Mixture psychophysics requires many-variable laws.

Another class of many-variable phenomena is that of context effects. This is a diverse class that includes both sensory and cognitive phenomena of great importance for behavior. There have, of course, been innumerable studies of context effects, including some by nearly every contributor to this volume. Concepts of assimilation and contrast, in particular, go back to the early years of scientific psychology. Moreover, context was a main theme of the gestalt psychologists, in particular in their concern with perceptual constancies. But general theory has been lacking. The conceptual framework of psychophysical law has been inhospitable to context effects, for they are many-variable phenomena, not amenable to one-variable, psychophysical analysis.

Nonconscious Sensation

A second limitation of classical psychophysics is its treatment of sensation as conscious. This treatment appears in the standard instructions to judge "heaviness," "grayness," or "sweetness" of a single stimulus, or to choose the "heavier," etc. of two stimuli. Although some workers might demur at the term conscious, they still consider these instructions to elicit unitary sensations, which subjects can judge with respect to the indicated dimension. This view underlies the concept of psychophysical law: The single variable of sensation is a function of the single variable of physical energy.

Nonconscious sensation is one casualty of the concept of psychophysical law. It is hardly an exception to note that Fechner, as well as modern signal detection theorists, allow that very weak sensations may not exceed "threshold" to become conscious. Indeed, it is not uncommon to read that consciousness is a defining property of sensation. The present view, in contrast, is that even strong sensations may not become conscious. What does become visible through the window of consciousness is often the integrated resultant of nonconscious sensation.

Nonconscious sensation can be meaningfully defined. In the size-weight illusion, for example, the proper effect of gram weight, processed through the kinesthetic receptors, is preconscious. What reaches consciousness is the integrated resultant of this preconscious sensation and the no less preconscious effect of the visual appearance. Within the traditional framework of psychophysical law, such preconscious sensations are more or less nonthinkable. With integration psychophysics, nonconscious sensations have a natural role and indeed become measurable.

Psychological Measurement

The third limitation is structural, and relates to psychological measurement. The approach of classical psychophysics cannot solve its own central problem of determining the form of the psychophysical law (Anderson, 1970). This limitation is logical, inherent in the single-variable conceptualization.

To see this limitation, denote the psychophysical law as:

$$\psi = \mathbf{V}(S), \tag{1}$$

where ψ and S represent psychological sensation and physical stimulus, respectively, and **V** denotes the psychophysical law. Since S may be measured with physical scales, **V** would be determinate if ψ were known. Determination of the psychophysical law is thus equivalent to measuring sensation -- and conversely.

The longstanding crux concerns the measurement of sensation. Monotone (ordinal) scales of sensation are readily available, but a true linear (equal interval) scale is necessary. Fechner's claim that **V** has a logarithmic form rested on the plausible but arbitrary assumption of equality of *jnds* (just noticeable differences). Stevens' claim that **V** has a power form rested on the no less arbitrary assumption that the method of magnitude estimation provided a true linear, even ratio, scale of sensation. The long controversy over Fechner's claim and the controversy between Fechner's and Stevens' claims continued because both were arbitrary (Anderson, 1970, 1974a; Krueger, 1989, 1991).

This crux is unresolvable within the conceptual framework of psychophysical law. The logarithmic function and the power function are monotonically equivalent. Because it is a single-variable function, the psychophysical law is mathematically insufficient to provide the constraints necessary to obtain the true scale of sensation.

Measurement of sensation becomes possible within the conceptual framework of psychocognitive law because it is a many-variable function. Even two variables can provide a validational base for measurement (*see Parallelism Theorem* and *Linear Fan Theorem* below). There is thus a qualitative, logical difference between the single-variable form of the prototypical psychophysical law and the many-variable form of the prototypical psychocognitive law. Mathematically, the psychocognitive law provides sufficient constraint to obtain the true scale of sensation (see also comparative discussion of measurement theories in Anderson, 1981, Chapter 5).

Cognitive Algebra

This many-variable approach was blessed by Nature. Numerous tasks of psychophysical integration have been shown to obey algebraic laws of addition, multiplication, averaging, and so on. These algebraic laws extend outside the domain of psychophysics to constitute a general *cognitive algebra* (Anderson, 1974a,c, 1979, 1981, 1982, 1991b,c,d). This cognitive algebra has made it possible to resolve the crux of classical psychophysics and obtain true measures of sensation.

Cognitive algebra has also helped go beyond the other two limitations of the classical conception of psychophysical law. First, it can define and measure nonconscious sensation. Second, it provides a general attack on mixture psychophysics, context effects, and other many-variable phenomena. These advantages rest on functional measurement theory, discussed in the following sections.

III. Functional Measurement Theory

Putting cognitive algebra on firm ground involved two kinds of problems: mathematical and substantive. The substantive problems, which are the more important, are taken up later. The following sections give a brief overview of the mathematical problems of the theory of functional measurement (see further Anderson, 1974a,c, 1982; McBride & Anderson, 1991).

Integration Diagram

A conceptual overview of integration psychophysics appears in the simplified integration diagram of Figure 2.1. The organism is considered to reside in a field of observable stimuli, denoted by S_1, S_2,..., at the left of the diagram. These multiple stimuli are determinants of the observable response, *R*, at the right of the diagram. Between the observable stimuli and the observable response intervene three processing operators: *valuation, integration*, and *action*, denoted by **V, I,** and **A**, respectively.

Also represented in the integration diagram is the operative goal. The goal controls all three processing operations. The purposiveness of thought and action is thus explicitly represented.

The valuation operator, **V**, extracts meaning and value from stimuli. In the diagram, it refers to processing chains that lead from the observable stimuli, S_i, to their psychological value representations, denoted by ψ_i. Valuation may be mainly

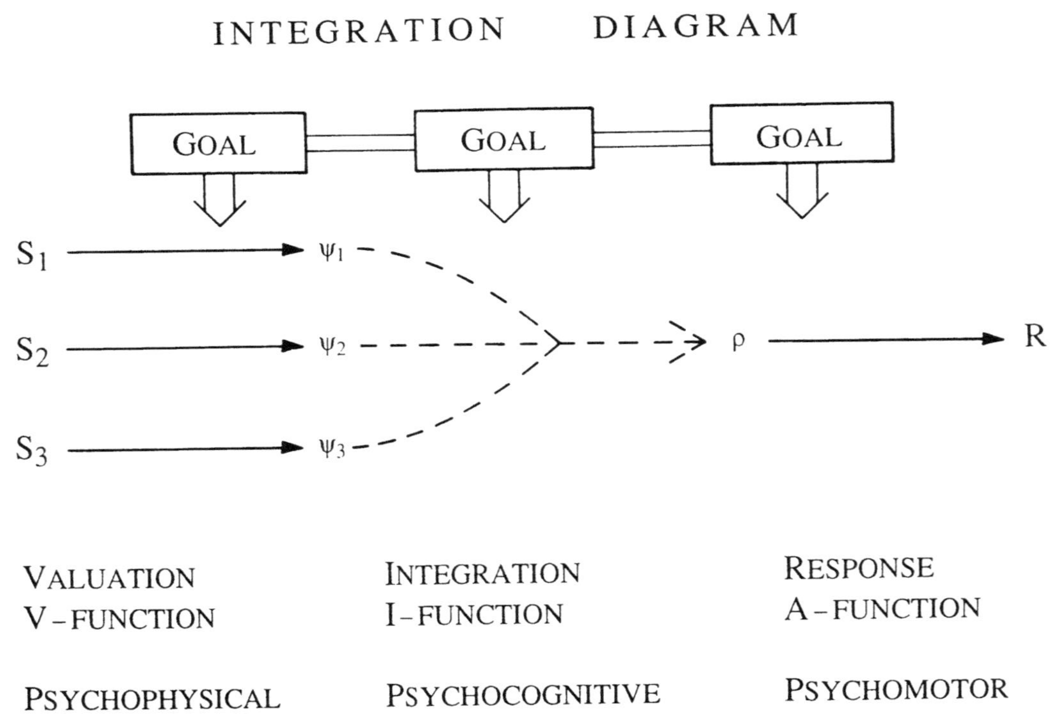

Figure 2.1: Information integration diagram. Chain of three linked operators, **V-I-A**, leads from observable stimulus field, $\{S_i\}$, to observable response, *R*. Valuation operator **V**, transforms observable stimuli, S_i, into subjective representation, ψ_i. Integration operator, **I**, transforms subjective stimulus field, $\{\psi_i\}$, into implicit response, ρ. Action operator, **A**, transforms implicit response, ρ, into observable response, *R*. (After N.H. Anderson, Foundations of Information Integration Theory, 1981).

sensory, as with the temperature of coffee; hedonic, as in judging its goodness of taste; or cognitive, as in deciding not to have another cup.

The integration operator, **I**, combines the several separate psychological stimuli, ψ_i, into a unitary response, denoted by ρ. Most psychophysical reactions of everyday life result from integration, as with taste of food and drink, feelings of comfort or pain, and motor responses.

The action operator, **A**, transforms the implicit response, ρ, into the observable response, R. This $\rho \rightarrow R$ distinction is clearest with simple sensations: ρ could be your feeling of pain, for example, and R your rating of painfulness on a 1-20 scale.

Problems of multiple determination can be extremely difficult. When even two factors are at work, pushing in different directions, their combined effect is not generally predictable without quantitative analysis. It is a blessing of nature, therefore, that some integration operators have simple algebraic forms. And this, as will be seen, carries the associated blessing of a capability for measurement of personal values.

The Three Unobservables

The most important entities in the integration diagram are all unobservable. The integration operator is clearly unobservable, usually beyond the reach of introspection. The physical stimuli, S_i, are observable, but the corresponding psychological stimuli, ψ_i, are inside the head, often nonconscious. The implicit response, ρ, may be conscious, but it also is a feeling inside the head; the observable R may be severely biased as a measure of ρ (see Figure 2.2). These three unobservables are the focus of cognitive theory.

The problem of the three unobservables seems formidable. To illustrate, suppose you are shown two gray chips and asked to select a third chip that lies midway between them in grayness. This instruction prescribes an addition rule:

$$\psi_1 - \rho = \rho - \psi_2;$$
$$\rho = \tfrac{1}{2}(\psi_1 + \psi_2).$$

Here ψ_1 and ψ_2 are the grayness sensations induced by the two given stimulus chips, and ρ is the grayness of the response chip.

These grayness values, however, are unobservable. What can be observed are the reflectance values of the chips, but these have an unknown, highly nonlinear relation to grayness sensation. To test the bisection rule depends on measurement of these three grayness sensations (see Figure 2.3 below).

This measurement problem is fundamental. It is not peculiar to grayness bisection, but applies generally to all rules of sensory summation or perceptual addition. Unless this measurement problem can be solved, even the simple addition rule - right or wrong - will remain untestable.

Parallelism Theorem

The diagnostic sign of an addition rule is a pattern of parallelism in the factorial graph. This *parallelism theorem* employs the following notation. Let *A* and *B* be two variables manipulated in a Row x Column factorial design, with stimulus levels S_{Ai}, for row i and S_{Bj} for column j. Let R_{ij} denote the observable response to stimulus combination (S_{Ai}, S_{Bj}) in cell *ij* of the design.

The hypothesis that the two stimulus variables are integrated by an addition rule may then be written:

$$\rho_{ij} = \psi_{Ai} + \psi_{Bj} \quad .$$

Here ρ_{ij} is the implicit response in cell *ij*, and ψ_{Ai} and ψ_{Bj} are the subjective values of the row and column stimuli, S_{Ai} and S_{Bj}, respectively.

This addition rule embodies the problem of the three unobservables. We do have leverage on two of them. We can manipulate the physical stimuli, S_{Ai} and S_{Bj}, thereby manipulating the unobservables, ψ_{Ai} and ψ_{Bj}; also, we can measure R_{ij}, which is a direct link to ρ_{ij}. This leverage is just enough to solve the problem of the three unobservables.

PARALLELISM THEOREM. Two assumptions are required in this simple form of the parallelism theorem:

$$\rho_{ij} = \psi_{Ai} + \psi_{Bj}; \qquad \text{(addition)} \qquad (2a)$$

$$R_{ij} = c_o + c_1 \rho_{ij}. \qquad \text{(linearity)} \qquad (2b)$$

The linearity condition says that the observable response, R_{ij}, is a linear function of the implicit response, ρ_{ij} (c_o and c_1 are zero and unit parameters whose values need not be known). If linearity holds, then the factorial pattern in the observable data will mirror that in the underlying cognition. From these two assumptions follow two conclusions (see Anderson, 1981, Section 1.2).

Conclusion 1: The factorial graph will be parallel.

Conclusion 2: The psychophysical law is determinable from the marginal means of the factorial data table. Specifically, the row means are a linear scale of $\mathbf{V}_A(S_{Ai})$, where $\mathbf{V}_A$ is the psychophysical function for the row variable. Similarly, the column means are a linear scale of the psychophysical function for the column variable, $\mathbf{V}_B(S_{Bj})$.

Functional Measurement Principle

Algebraic structure is the key to functional measurement. This structure provides the base and frame for measurement. This has just been shown in Conclusion 2 for the stimulus variables. The same holds for the response scale (see also *Monotone Analysis* below). Indeed, observed parallelism is evidence for the linearity of whatever response measure is used.

Success of this approach depended entirely on the empirical reality of algebraic laws. Without this, the parallelism theorem would be barren mathematics. The real problem was to demonstrate the theorem empirically. The heart of functional measurement lies in the empirical studies of cognitive algebra. Integration psychophysics thus makes psychological measurement an organic component of substantive theory.

This view sees measurement as functional in psychological theory. "A guiding idea of functional measurement is that measurement scales are derivative from substantive theory." (Anderson, 1970, p. 153). "The functional view is that measurement is woven into the fabric of empirical knowledge ... Measurement exists only within the framework of substantive empirical laws. The measurement of any quantity is organically related to the empirical-theoretical network into which that quantity enters; that is the true foundation of measurement theory" (Anderson, 1974a, p. 288). The work on algebraic integration models is an attempt to develop such an empirical-theoretical network.

Implications of Parallelism

The parallelism theorem provides a remarkably simple and precise test of the addition rule. Observed parallelism constitutes strong support for both premises of the theorem taken together. Hence, it supports each of them separately.

Of special importance, parallelism supports the linearity of the response measure. Response linearity is invaluable. It means that the pattern in the observable data gives a veridical picture of the pattern in the unobservable cognition; this pattern is a key to cognitive analysis.

Response linearity has been the critical issue in psychological measurement theory. Everyone has desired linear response measures, but the validity question has seemed insurmountable: How can we tell whether R is a linear function of ρ when the latter is unobservable? The perplexity of this question is highlighted by the sharp disagreement between two common methods of obtaining numerical response (see Figure 2.2). This question has been answered by the parallelism theorem.

An interesting aspect of the parallelism theorem is that nothing need be known about the stimulus values. The test of parallelism is made directly on the raw response. This may seem indirect, but it is actually more powerful than the traditional approach of reliance on separate estimates of stimulus value (see *Difference Rule* below).

The subjective stimulus values, however, can readily be obtained. By the second conclusion of the parallelism theorem, the row (column) means provide a linear scale of the row (column) stimuli of the design. Observed parallelism thus validates this functional measurement on the stimulus side.

The parallelism theory thus allows an empirical determination of the psychophysical law: Graph the functional stimulus values as a function of the physical stimulus values. This graph represents the psychophysical law, **V**(*S*).

There is thus a three-fold benefit to be gained from observed parallelism:

1. support for the addition rule;
2. support for the linearity of the response measure;
3. linear scales of each stimulus variable.

Each benefit corresponds to one of the three unobservables. In this way, the parallelism theorem solves the problem of the three unobservables.

Observed parallelism is not mathematical proof of additivity, of course, but it is strong evidence. This is shown in Table 2.1, which relates the two premises

Table 2.1: Parallelism and Nonparallelism

Case	Additivity	Linearity	Response Pattern
1	Yes	Yes	Parallelism
2	Yes	No	Non Parallelism
3	No	Yes	Non Parallelism
4	No	No	?

of the theorem to the pattern in the factorial graph. In case 1, both premises are true, so parallelism is guaranteed by the theorem. In cases 2 and 3, one premise is true, the other false; in both cases, it is straightforward to show that the data will generally be nonparallel. In case 4, both premises are false, so it is tempting to conclude that the data will be nonparallel. It is possible, however, that nonlinearity in the response just cancels nonadditivity in the integration to yield net parallelism. This may not seem likely, but it is logically possible. Subject to this qualification, however, observed parallelism supports both premises of the theorem taken together, and hence each premise taken separately.

Parallelism and Nonparallelism

It may seem odd that so simple a technique as parallelism analysis was not exploited sooner. Sensory summation and other kinds of addition models have been suggested in many domains of psychophysics. Two causes, however, conjoined to hold back the development and use of parallelism analysis. One concerned response linearity, which is discussed later.

The other cause was the empirical prevalence of nonadditive integration, especially averaging processes (see Anderson, 1981, Chapters 2-4). An averaging process yields parallelism only under the special condition of equal weighting, that is, when all levels of a given stimulus variable have equal weight. The general averaging model is nonadditive and yields nonparallelism, a consequence of differential weighting of different levels of a given variable.

To establish the parallelism theorem as a working tool was thus by no means straightforward. The difficulty concerned the interpretation of observed nonparallelism. This could reflect nonadditive integration, or nonlinear response bias, or some combination of the two. Furthermore, the nonparallelism undercut the interpretation of the parallelism, suggesting that it was not real, merely response bias or statistical accident. This perplexity was accentuated by the known fact of biases in numerical response measures. All this meant that nothing could be trusted.

It took some time, therefore, to develop experimental procedures to obtain response linearity and to establish an interlocking body of evidence associated with functional measurement. This was possible only because nature had endowed the mind with a general algebra of cognition. Of special importance was the development of averaging theory, which provided a unified account of much of the parallelism and the nonparallelism that have been observed.

Linear Fan Theorem

The linear fan theorem for multiplication rules requires two assumptions:

$$\rho_{ij} = \psi_{Ai} \times \psi_{Bj}; \qquad \text{(multiplication)} \qquad (3a)$$

$$R_{ij} = c_0 + c_1\rho_{ij}. \qquad \text{(linearity)} \qquad (3b)$$

The linearity assumption is the same as for the parallelism theorem, and it serves the same purpose. From these two assumptions follow two conclusions:

Conclusion 1: The appropriate factorial graph will be a linear fan.

Conclusion 2: The psychophysical law is determinable from the marginal means of the factorial data table. Specifically, the row means are a linear scale of $\mathbf{V}_A(S_{Ai})$, where $\mathbf{V}_A$ is the psychophysical function for the row variable. Similarly, the column means are a linear scale of the psychophysical function for the column variable, $\mathbf{V}_B(S_{Bj})$.

The second conclusion is the same as in the parallelism theorem. The linear fan pattern, however, will only be obtained if the factorial graph is constructed "appropriately." This requires that the column stimuli be spaced on the horizontal axis in proportion to their subjective values. These subjective values can be determined by virtue of the second conclusion (see Anderson, 1981, Section 1.4).

The linear fan theorem thus provides a simple, precise test of the multiplication rule. An observed linear fan pattern constitutes strong support for both premises of the theorem taken jointly. Hence it supports each of them separately. Just as with the parallelism property, accordingly, an observed linear fan provides a three-fold benefit, corresponding to the three unobservables:

1. support for the multiplication rule;
2. support for the linearity of the response measure;
3. linear scales of each stimulus variable.

Averaging

Cognitive algebra is not complete without the averaging rule, which is empirically ubiquitous. For the case of two variables, this rule may be written:

$$\rho_{ij} = \frac{w_{Ai}\psi_{Ai} + w_{Bj}\psi_{Bj} + w_0\psi_0}{w_{Ai} + w_{Bj} + w_0} \tag{4}$$

This equation differs from the addition rule by the inclusion of the w s, which are weight or importance parameters. The $w_0\psi_0$ term represents prior or background information, but will be ignored here. The numerator of Equation 4 represents an addition rule; dividing by the sum of the weights yields an averaging rule.

Parallelism analysis applies to the averaging rule in the special case of equal weighting, that is, when all levels of variable A have equal weight, $w_{Ai} = w_A$, and similarly, $w_{Bj} = w_B$. In this equal weight case, the denominator of Equation 4 is constant, and it cannot be distinguished from the adding rule.

The general averaging rule allows unequal weighting for different levels of each stimulus variable. The denominator of Equation 4 is then nonconstant, and the factorial graph will be nonparallel. This has the unique advantage that the importance weights become identifiable psychological parameters. The nonlinearity, however, requires iterative analysis that faced statistical difficulties, now mainly resolved in the publicly available AVERAGE program (Zalinski & Anderson, 1991).

The averaging model has some interesting properties. One is that it contradicts the sure-thing principle in judgment-decision theory, for addition of a good may actually average down the response. A second is that it can be disordinal, thereby demonstrating the inadequacy of ordinal theories of measurement. A third is that it can provide estimates of weight and of scale value that have common zero and common unit for different variables, thereby permitting comparisons across qualitatively different variables.

Monotone Analysis: The General Parallelism Theorem

Response linearity is not essential for functional measurement. At bottom, only a monotone (ordinal) response measure is required. As stated originally, the basic logic "consists in using the postulated behavior laws to induce a scaling on the dependent variable" (Anderson, 1962, p. 410). The idea is simple. Suppose ρ is additive and $R = \mathbf{A}(\rho)$, where **A** is some strictly monotone transformation. Then the inverse transformation, $\mathbf{A}^{-1}(\mathbf{A}(\rho)) = \rho$ is additive. $\mathbf{A}^{-1}$ is determinate, for it is the one that transforms the observed data to parallelism.

The general parallelism theorem thus requires nothing more than the one assumption of additivity. All that is at issue is the algebraic structure of the integration rule -- and that is tested in the analysis. The measurement scales, of both stimuli and response, are derivative from the algebraic structure. Because it requires no prior scaling, functional measurement is a new type of fundamental measurement.

Three problems arise in using monotone analysis. The first is to determine the best monotone transformation; this is practicable with modern computer programs (see Anderson, 1982, Chapter 5). The second is to test whether the deviations from parallelism in the transformed data are statistically reliable; this is practicable with a general method for analysis of nonlinear models developed in integration theory (Anderson, 1982, Section 4.4). An example appears in the later study of grayness bisection.

The third problem is that monotone transformation is so flexible that it may make data from a truly nonadditive process appear additive (Anderson, 1962). This is a serious problem, extensively studied in Anderson (1982, Chapter 5). This work shows that two-factor design usually lacks adequate power for monotone or ordinal analysis. Two-operation models, however, with three stimulus variables, such as $A \times (B + C)$, can provide sufficient constraint for practical use.

Statistical Analysis

Functional measurement provides an error theory, which is essential for model analysis, that is both valid and practicable. For many applications, ordinary analysis of variance is ideal. The metric test for an addition rule is the well-known interaction term of analysis of variance. The corresponding test for a multiplication rule is the residual from the bilinear component of the interaction. Monotone tests are feasible with the general method for analysis of nonlinear models cited in the previous section. Double cancellation and other ordinal tests can be handled with multiple comparison procedures (Anderson, 1982, Section 5.4), although in typical applications these tests have so little power to detect real nonadditivity that they are rather useless.

On the whole, statistical theory and practice for functional measurement is in a satisfactory state. Statistical problems are not of main concern here, however, and the reader is referred to previous discussions (Anderson, 1982). Nearly all other approaches, however, suffer serious, often-fatal shortcomings. This matter requires brief comment, which is given in the following section.

How Not to Test Algebraic Models

The key question for algebraic models of perception is whether the model fits the data. Unfortunately, many current methods used to answer this question are seriously prone to false successes. They claim support for the model without serious evidence.

One such method uses the correlation between the predictions of the model and the observed data. This method is unsatisfactory because extremely high correlations, from .96 to .99 and even higher, can be obtained from models that are seriously incorrect. Two related statistics, percentage of variance accounted for by the model and relative mean square error, suffer the same problem. It may seem odd that a model that accounts for a large percentage of variance can be invalid, but this is typically built into the main effects of the experimental design. These methods are called *weak inference* because they seem to test the model but do not really do so (see Anderson, 1982, Section 4.1).

A similar problem faces the ordinal tests of axiomatic measurement theory. An error theory is necessary to handle real data, but this has not been provided (Suppes, Krantz, Luce, & Tversky, 1989, p. *xiii*). Real data will ordinarily contain some violation of the ordinal predictions, but without an error theory there is no way to decide whether they are statistically reliable (see Anderson, 1982, Sections 5.4 and 5.5). The practice of selecting an arbitrary criterion for number of violations has little merit. The fact is that two-variable designs are generally inadequate to prevent invalid transformation to additivity of data generated by an inherently nonadditive process (Anderson, 1982, Sections 5.6 and 5.10). As a consequence, little faith can be placed in most of the experimental studies that have attempted to rely on ordinal tests.

Continuous Response Measures

Most applications of functional measurement have used continuous response measures. They have three strong advantages over choice data. First, they contain more information. Indeed, with a linear response scale, the analysis of stimulus integration can be remarkably simple, as illustrated in the parallelism theorem. Second, they allow use of well-developed statistical theory for testing goodness of fit and for estimating parameters. Third, they are almost essential for analysis of configural processing.

The well-known objection is that continuous response measures may be nonlinear. This problem is highlighted by the contrast between the rating method and Stevens' (1974) method of magnitude estimation, illustrated in Figure 2.2. Magnitude estimations of grayness (lightness) of Munsell chips are plotted on the vertical axis as a function of the grayness ratings of these same chips on the horizontal axis. If the two methods were equivalent, the curve would be a straight diagonal. Since the curve is far from a straight diagonal, at least one of the methods must be highly nonlinear.

Which, if either, method gives a true linear scale? Some writers have seen no way to answer this question. Neither method can be trusted, they argue. Instead, psychological measurement theory should be built on some other foundation.

But there is a way to answer this question. Success of the parallelism theorem, in particular, provides validational support for whatever response measure was used. Rating and magnitude estimation have equal opportunity to meet this validational criterion. The parallelism theorem is a neutral judge. As noted in a previous comment on the work of Marks (1974): "From this position, the difference between ratings and magnitude estimation becomes open to empirical investigation. Both response methods suffer various biases, and the main goal is to improve the methods. Proponents of the two methods thus become protagonists engaged with common problems" (Anderson, 1981, p. 358).

The primary issue, accordingly, is to develop experimental procedures that can eliminate the nonlinear biases in whatever method is used. An addition rule

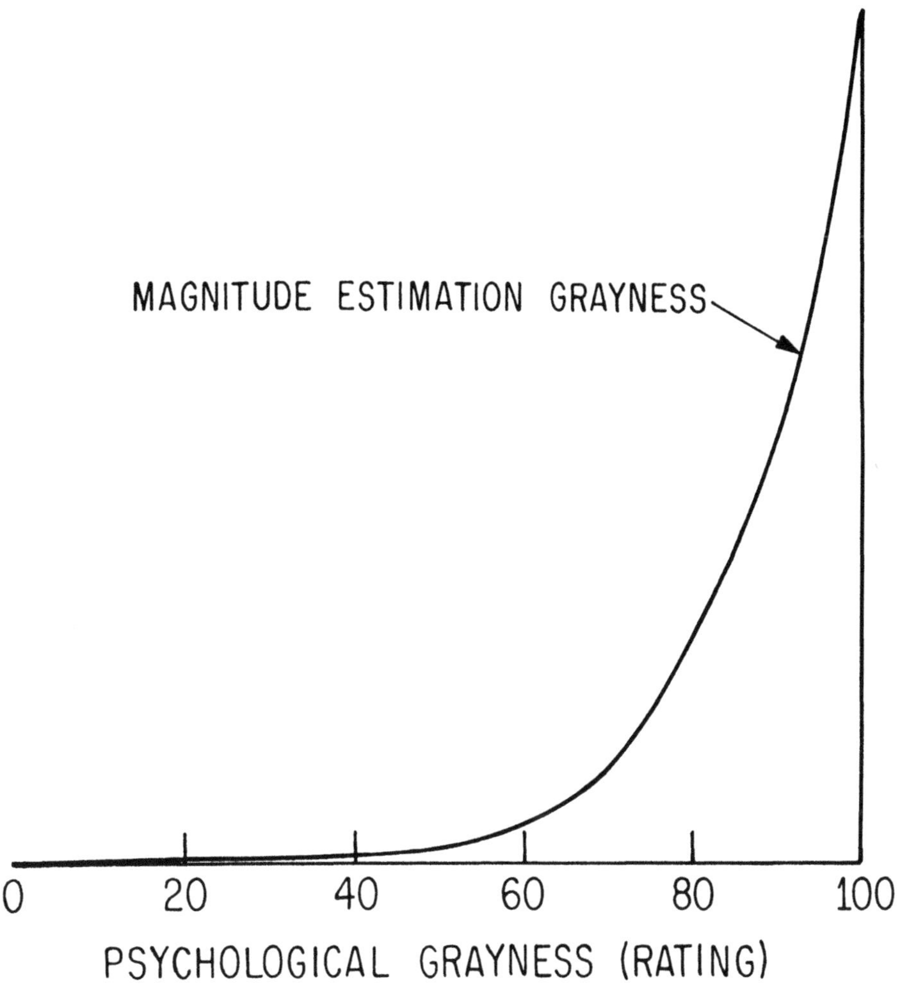

Figure 2.2: Magnitude estimation differs radically from rating. The curve represents magnitude estimations of grayness of Munsell color chips, plotted on the vertical, as a function of ratings of the same chips, plotted on the horizontal. Equivalence of the two response measures would appear as a straight diagonal curve. The curve is far from the diagonal, which means that the two response measures are far from equivalent. Since the ratings satisfy validational criteria for a true linear scale, the deviation of the curve from the straight diagonal reflects bias in magnitude estimation (see discussion of Figure 2.4 below). (After N.H. Anderson, Methods of Information Integration Theory, 1982).

provides a structural framework that makes it possible to assay and refine the response scale. The procedures developed for the rating method are noted below.

In the present view, continuous response measures are a near-necessity for psychophysical theory. They are almost essential to the study of configural and interactive processes, which will not generally obey simple algebraic rules. They are also essential when a single variable induces two processes, as illustrated later with geometric illusions in Figure 2.8.

Attempts to construct measurement theory based on choice data can hardly progress beyond simple algebraic rules. In the functional approach, the algebraic rule is used as base and frame for developing continuous response methodology. Once developed, this provides an invaluable tool for studying the more difficult problems of configural processing as well as nonsimple integration rules.

IV. Theory and Practice of Rating

The use of the rating method depends both on the theory of the rating process and on certain associated experimental procedures. These are the concern of the following two sections. For simplicity, only the standard situation will be considered, in which the ends of the response scale are explicitly defined in terms of end anchor stimuli.

Theory of Rating

Beneath the simplicity and immediacy of rating lie cognitive abilities that have been little studied. To begin, ratings are comparative and constructive. A rating of heaviness, for example, is not a direct report of the sensory experience of lifting an object. The rating involves reference to a dimension and to comparison within that dimension to other experiences stored in memory. Heaviness, moreover, is not the sensory experience itself, but only a partial, one-dimensional representation. This constructive nature of sensory judgments is also illustrated with colors, which may be judged along the distinct dimensions of brightness, hue, or saturation.

The comparative nature of rating is explicitly embodied in the end anchor procedure. The rating of any given stimulus is considered to depend on similarity comparisons between it and each of the end anchors. Specifically, let S_L and S_U be the lower and upper end anchor stimuli, corresponding to responses R_L and R_U, respectively, usually the two ends of the rating scale. Let S be a given stimulus, and denote its similarity to the lower and upper end anchors Sim_L and Sim_U. The rating of S is assumed to be located between R_L and R_U in proportion to its similarities:

$$(R-R_L)Sim_L = (R_U-R)Sim_U \quad . \tag{5}$$

Hence

$$R = \frac{Sim_L R_L + Sim_U R_U}{Sim_L + Sim_U} \quad . \tag{6}$$

The rating is thus a weighted average of the two end responses, with weights determined by the similarities. This averaging formulation can be extended to include comparisons with other stimuli, such as stimuli on preceding trials or other reference or anchor stimuli (Anderson, 1982).

Properly speaking, Equation 6 should refer to the implicit judgment, ρ, not to the observable rating, R. It is a further question whether R is a linear scale of ρ, that is, whether the observable rating is a veridical measure of the unobservable sensation. This question has been answered affirmatively for the rating method by its success in cognitive algebra.

The applicability of the rating method across diverse dimensions of judgment is thought to depend on a general metric sense. This same metric sense may underlie ratings of heaviness, expectancy, hedonic value, and other qualities of everyday life.

The linearity of the rating method, and indeed the metric sense itself, may derive from motor skills in local space. From infancy onwards, accurate movement is important for survival. The graphical form of the rating scale, which is the usual form with children, may thus embody perceptual-motor skills. The numerical rating scales used with adults may be derivative from this perceptual-motor representation.

Experimental Procedure

Two experimental procedures are important for ensuring linear rating measures. Both are intended to familiarize subjects with the range of stimuli and to set up a correspondence between it and the response scale.

The first procedure concerns *end anchors*. These are stimuli a little more extreme than the regular experimental stimuli, and are given initially to define the ends of the rating scale. If the regular experimental stimuli ranged from 200 to 600 grams in a lifted weight experiment, for example, weights of 100 and 800 grams might be used as end anchors. The 100-gram weight could be given at the very beginning with the instruction: "This is the lightest weight you will ever lift; call it 1." Next, the 800-gram weight could be given with the instruction: "This is the heaviest weight you will ever lift; call it 20."

These two end anchors thus define the range of stimuli and also the range of response. They begin the process of setting up the correspondence between the subject's feelings of heaviness and the external response scale. This process is continued with the second procedure, which involves practice stimuli. A representative set of stimuli that cover the range is presented, the subjected being instructed to "Use numbers between 1 and 20 to signify heaviness of intermediate stimuli in the natural way; just say how heavy it feels to you; it is your own personal feeling that counts." Not much practice is ordinarily needed to establish stable usage of the scale. In some cases, however, repeating the end anchors during the experiment may be desirable to refirm scale usage.

It is remarkable that subjects can use ratings in a linear way. This depends in part on the indicated procedures, which proved effective in eliminating various rating biases. More important, rating linearity depends on cognitive abilities already discussed under *Theory of Rating*. The net result, however, is that a few simple experimental procedures can yield linear response scales, even with little children (see Anderson, 1991d).

Rating Validity

An extensive, interlocking network of evidence shows that the rating method can, with suitable procedure, provide valid linear measures of psychological quantities. The main evidence is the wide empirical success of cognitive algebra. Averaging theory had special significance, as already noted. Evidence from scale invariance is illustrated in the later grayness studies. Other evidence is summarized in Anderson (1982, Sections 1.1, 1.2, 3.1, 3.2, 5.9, and 5.10).

Rating methodology is still in process of development. In at least one task, judgment of loudness, it has run into difficulty (see Anderson, 1981, Note 5.6.2a; 1982, Note 1.1.7c; Marks, 1979). Applications to new tasks, accordingly, must be approached with care. At best, some residual biases, including number and position preferences, must be expected. Further refinement and extension are thus of continuing concern.

V. Comparison Processes

Comparison processes are ubiquitous in the psychophysics of everyday life. Categorization is one example, as in recognition of a word or face, or in the various classification tasks invented by psychologists. Categorization depends on *similarity* comparison: between the stimulus object and a mental prototype in one case, and among the several stimuli of the classification task in the other case. *Difference* judgments are also common comparisons: bigger, faster, older, prettier, smarter, and richer are but a few of the comparative judgments in the daily life of child and adult. Such difference judgments seem to presuppose some factor or dimension of similarity to define the difference. They might thus be reducible to dis-similarity judgments, conditionalized on a given dimension. *Relational* judgments also need consideration. Among the many perceptual examples is the geometric illusion of Figure 2.8, in which the same center circle looks larger by comparison with the small context circles, smaller by comparison with the large context circles. Relational judgments include difference judgments, but many are more complex. Some seem to involve ratio comparison processes different from difference judgments. Others involve multiple features.

Comparison processes have been used in psychological measurement. Difference and bisection judgments are illustrated in the grayness study of Figure 2.3 below. Ratio and fractionation judgments have been used similarly. Similarity forms the foundation of multidimensional scaling.

Cognitive theory of comparison processes, however, has not progressed very far. The measurement models have usually been treated as a means to an end. When they did poorly, interest turned elsewhere. Some work has been done on particular issues, by Garner (1974) on classification analysis of dimensional stimuli, by Krantz (1972) on relation theory, by Luce (e.g., 1991) on ratio judgment, and by Parducci (e.g., 1974) on range-frequency theory. Aside from functional measurement, however, the only attempt at a general approach is that of Helson (1964), discussed later.

The functional measurement approach to comparison processes is illustrated with difference judgments in the next section, and this is followed by a brief discussion of similarity and ratio judgments. Of special interest are the little-studied problems of multiple comparison stimuli. Applications are given in later discussions of adaptation-level theory and of geometric illusions.

Difference Rule

Measurement is central to analysis of comparison processes. An instructive contrast between the functional and traditional approaches to measurement appears in the difference rule. To illustrate, let *S* and *C* denote focal and content stimuli, respectively, with perceptual values denoted by *f(S)* and *g(C)*, where *f* and *g* are arbitrary functions. The difference rule may then be written

$$\rho = f(S) - w\,g(C). \tag{7}$$

The weight parameter, *w*, is included to allow for possible asymmetry between focal and context stimuli.

The traditional approach begins by attempting to measure the three terms in this equation, planning a direct check by substitution. This substitution test has generally done poorly (Anderson, 1974a, p. 237*f*; 1981, Section 5.4; Marks, 1974, p. 257). Failure is ambiguous, however, because the substitution test is very demanding. All three terms in the equation must be measured on linear scales. The two stimulus scales, moreover, must have common zero and common unit.

The weight parameter may also need to be determined. Shortcomings in the stimulus measurement alone could cause a true difference rule to fail.

Functional measurement is at once simpler and more powerful. No prior stimulus measurement is needed; the functions *f* and *g* may be entirely arbitrary, and the weight *w* need not be known. The simple form of the parallelism theorem assumes only that the response scale is linear. If parallelism fails, that cannot be due to shortcomings in the stimulus scales. If parallelism succeeds, then stimulus values may be derived from the data, as in the later study of grayness. Instructive applications in taste psychophysics have been made by Klitzner (1975) and by De Graaf, Frijters, and van Trijp (1987), discussed further in McBride and Anderson (1991).

Functional measurement thus inverts the traditional approach. Measurement is not prerequisite to, but derivative from substantive theory (see, e.g., *Scale Invariance* below).

Similarity Rules

Similarity has been most studied in psychophysics in connection with multidimensional scaling. This area is outside the scope of this chapter, but one issue deserves comment. This concerns the integration model for similarity. Multidimensional scaling is founded on a model of addition of dissimilarities; integration psychophysics suggests an alternative model of averaging of similarities.

Multidimensional scaling assumes that complex stimuli, faces and odors, for example, can be represented in a space of a few dimensions that have psychological meaning. Similarity between two stimuli is equated with distance between two corresponding points in this space. Judgments of similarity have the potential for revealing the number and nature of the dimensions. Formally, however, the multidimensional scaling models are nearly always formulated as addition of dissimilarities along the several dimensions. Dissimilarity provides a rational zero point, namely, when the two stimuli are the same. Unfortunately, this model seems incorrect.

An alternative model was suggested in a thought experiment by Anderson (1974a, p.256), who pointed out that addition of a common element increased the similarity between two stimuli. This infirms the multidimensional scaling model, in which addition of a zero dissimilarity has no effect. Accordingly, Anderson suggested that subjects average similarities. A similar view, based on similar arguments, has been given by Tversky (1977). Critical experimental support for averaging theory has been presented by Lopes and Oden (1980).

The foregoing thought experiment brings out the more general criticism, made by several writers, that multidimensional scaling has largely ignored cognitive processing. The model of addition of dissimilarities was evidently selected for its mathematical convenience, without much concern for cognitive validity. Even the underlying idea of spatial representation comes under question when it is realized that similarity depends on context and goal. As Lopes and Oden (1980) point out, previous approaches to similarity have been dominated by the idea that the judgment process is determined by the hypothesized representation of the stimulus information in semantic memory. In the functional perspective of integration theory, judgment is constructive and depends on the operative goal, as indicated in the integration diagram of Figure 2.1. The similarity between two given stimuli may thus vary with task and context. Hence the study of similarity needs to be embedded in a functional framework.

Ratio Rule

Ratio comparisons provide an alternative to difference comparisons. With the same notation as in Equation 7, but omitting the *w*-parameter for simplicity, the ratio rule may be written:

$$\rho = f(S) \,/\, g(C) \tag{8}$$

Here again, functional measurement provides a simple test: The ratio rule implies a linear fan pattern in the factorial graph.

This form of ratio rule has been employed by a number of investigators. In Stevens' method of magnitude estimation, for example, the comparison stimulus is the standard against which the regular stimuli are to be judged in ratio terms. Different *C* standards should yield a linear fan, an implication not well supported by results in the literature.

Other psychophysical studies have also attempted to use a ratio rule, for example, in fractionation judgments. A ratio rule is also the basis for Helson's adaptation-level model, discussed later. On the whole, the ratio rule seems to have fared poorly in psychophysics (see Anderson, 1974a, Section III.B).

Herrnstein's "matching law" has a ratio form: Pigeons distribute their responses between two concurrent schedules in proportion to relative reinforcement. Studies of this ratio rule have been restricted to physical measures of reinforcement. Functional measurement can allow for subjective reinforcement values (Anderson, 1974c, p. 294; 1978, pp. 371-373, 375). This seems necessary to handle quality of reinforcement, as with size of grain or texture of wet food. The matching relation itself may be viewed as a special case of averaging theory.

Relative Ratio Rule

Also of interest is the relative ratio rule, symbolized as:

$$\rho = \frac{f(S)}{f(S) + g(C)} \quad . \qquad (9)$$

In psychophysics, this relative ratio rule has appeared as the constant-sum model, in which subjects apportion 100 points between two stimuli to represent the ratio of their magnitudes (see Anderson, 1974a, pp. 266-271). Luce's (1959) choice rule has a similar form, although it is limited to probabilistic, threshold choices. A more general relative ratio rule, which also allows for suprathreshold preferences, has been derived from averaging theory. It has done quite well in judgment-decision theory (see, e.g., Anderson, 1981, Section 1.7.4; 1991a), and a model of similar form has been applied in speech perception by Oden and Massaro (1978) and Massaro (1991).

Processing Modes with Multiple Comparison Stimuli

The context in many tasks will be compound, having multiple components. Although a compound context can sometimes be treated as a molar unit, more detailed analysis may be desirable or even necessary. The main points can be illustrated with two comparison stimuli, C_1 and C_2, varied together with the focal stimulus, S, in a three-factor design.

Under the difference rule:

$$\rho = f(S) - g(C_1, C_2) \quad , \qquad (10)$$

where $g(C_1,C_2)$ is the perceptual value of the compound comparison stimulus. This rule can be tested with the parallelism theorem, treating (C_1,C_2) as a single compound variable in a two-factor, Focal x Comparison design.

A further question concerns the integration of the two comparison stimuli. If the difference rule succeeds, the observed response measure, *R*, is presumably a true linear scale. Hence the pattern in the $C_1 \times C_2$ factorial graph will mirror the pattern in the unobservable perception. A pattern of parallelism, of course, would imply that the effect of the comparison compound an additive function of its components: $g(C_1,C_2) = g_1(C_1) + g_2(C_2)$. Nonparallelism could be more interesting, for its pattern would provide information about interaction or configurality in the comparison processing.

Focal-context comparison may also involve a ratio rule, which brings a possibility of distinguishing two processing modes. In the **C-I** mode, separate comparisons are first made between the focal stimulus and each comparison stimulus; these two separate comparisons are then integrated. In the alternative **I-C** mode, the two comparison stimuli are first integrated to form a single effective stimulus; the focal stimulus is then compared to it.

A useful test is available for the **I-C** mode, which may be symbolized:

$$\rho = f(S) \, / \, g(C_1, C_2) \qquad (I\text{-}C \ mode) \qquad (11)$$

This model makes two predictions. First, linear fans should be obtained for the Focal x Comparison design. This holds for each separate comparison stimulus and for the two considered as a compound variable. Second, the C_1 x C_2 design may be expected to exhibit nonparallelism. Even if $g(C_1,C_2)$ is additive, it appears in the denominator, and so produces nonadditivity.

Analysis of the **C-I** mode is simplest in the case of comparison additivity:

$$\rho = f(S)/g_1(C_1) + f(S)/g_2(C_2). \qquad (C\text{-}I\ mode) \qquad (12)$$

The foregoing linear fan predictions still hold for each separate comparison stimulus, but the C_1 x C_2 design will yield parallelism. The two modes of processing may thus be distinguished by this test. Such a test was found to infirm adaptation-level theory, which predicts the **I-C** mode for the line-box illusion of Figure 2.7.

The **I-C** and **C-I** modes may both be expected under certain conditions. The **C-I** mode would be facilitated by perceptual separation of the two comparison stimuli, and this might be reinforced by successive presentation. Analogously, the **I-C** mode would be facilitated by perceptual integration of the two comparison stimuli. This kind of analysis may be expected to yield useful results on the important but little-studied problem of multiple comparison or context stimuli.

VI. Comparison of Two Theories: Adaptation Level Theory and Information Integration Theory

Information integration theory (IIT) and adaptation-level theory (ALT) have a number of similarities. Both are concerned with effects of context stimuli and with stimulus integration. Indeed, Helson conceptualized adaptation level as a weighted average of relevant stimuli. Both theories are accordingly concerned with quantitative analysis and with measurement. Both are also concerned with cognitive processes in psychophysics, as with expectancy and comparative judgment. And both have been extensively applied outside the psychophysical domain.

The following sections present a critique of the theoretical structure of ALT, contrasting it with IIT. Although the concept of adaptation has the wide importance that Helson claims for it, his theoretical structure is weak, even in its primary area of application. Outside of that area, it suffers serious objections that have been brushed aside. It will be indicated, however, that IIT can make an effective contribution to pursuing the goals of ALT.

Adaptation-Level Theory

Helson stressed the importance of context effects in psychophysics and perception. The response to a focal stimulus, he argued, could not be understood without reference to context and background stimuli. In this, he sided with the gestalt psychologists and sharply criticized classical psychophysics for passing over or ignoring the importance the total stimulus field. Helson went on to criticize the gestalt psychologists in turn, arguing that they took the idea of organization of the stimulus field as a primitive, whereas Helson sought to analyze it.

This was the theme of Helson's theory: To find a quantitative analysis of the integrated action of the entire stimulus field on the response to a focal stimulus. This is an enormous task, but Helson claimed to have found a general solution with the concept of adaptation. The entire stimulus field was reduced to a single value, the adaptation level (*AL*), and the focal stimulus was judged relative to this *AL*. Helson developed a quantitative formulation in studies of vision, especially his well-known demonstrations of hue adaptation and contrast as well as in studies of grayness (lightness). He later extended this formulation beyond psychophysics to include all psychology: learning, motivation, cognition, social psychology, and personality (see Helson, 1964; Appley, 1971).

Concept of adaptation level. Sensory adaptation may be illustrated with temperature. If you put a finger into a glass of warm water, the feeling of warmth quickly fades away. If you then put this finger into a glass of lukewarm water, it feels cool. On the other hand, a finger adapted to cool water will feel warm when placed in the same luke-warm water. The same physical stimulus may thus feel warm or cold. Temperature perception is not absolute, therefore, but relative to the prevailing level of adaptation. Analogous adaptation occurs to some degree in every sense modality.

This concept of adaptation-relative perception appears also in psychophysics of everyday life. Drivers on the two-lane roads of the American West adapt to high speeds and find it painfully slow to obey the 35 miles per hour speed limit in the small villages. Even horses may be trained with heavier shoes so their feet will feel fleeter in the big race.

Such adaptation effects are widely known. Helson, however, sought to extract a single general principle: Perception was always relative to the prevailing level of adaptation, which represented the "zero of function." The effect of any given stimulus was determined by its relation to the adaptation level, as in the temperature example. This principle was elaborated as a unifying, general framework for diverse domains of psychophysics and general behavior. Two quantitative models were presented, taken up in the next two subsections.

AL model. The adaptation level (*AL*) was taken to be a pooled average of all relevant stimuli. The basic equation of the theory defines *AL* as a weighted geometric mean (Helson, 1964, pp. 129ff; see similarly Guilford, 1954, p. 329; Restle, 1971, p. 56). In mnemonic notation, this may be written:

$$AL = \bar{S}^{w} B^{b} R^{r}. \tag{13}$$

Here $\bar{S}$ is the geometric mean of the focal stimuli, *B* represents the background or context stimuli, and *R* represents the residual from past experience. The three exponents are required to sum to unity, making the expression a geometric mean.

The *AL*, it should be noted, is defined entirely in physical terms. For grayness judgments, to which Helson devoted much experimental attention, all terms would be measured in percentage reflectance. The *AL* could thus be measured by the method of constant stimuli, say, as the reflectance of that comparison patch that matched the grayness of a test patch within a given field. This AL model is notable, for it bypasses any problem of measuring psychological scale value, although it does leave the problem of measuring the psychological weight parameters. The functional measurement analysis is discussed below.

Perception model. The *AL* is only one step towards perceptual value. The perceptual value of any stimulus is determined by a ratio comparison to the *AL*. Helson attempted to use a Fechnerian assumption, namely, that the perceptual value is determined by the number of *jnd*s between the *AL* and the focal stimulus *S*.

This Fechnerian approach was pursued one step further by assuming the validity of Fechner's logarithmic formula. Thus, the perceptual value, ρ, of the stimulus *S* would be:

$$\rho = \log(S/AL) = \log S - \log AL. \tag{14}$$

This is the basic perception model of ALT. To test this, Helson would require, first, that the observed response is a veridical measure of ρ, and second, that the *AL* has been calculated from Equation 13. A much simpler analysis is possible as noted next.

Functional Measurement Analysis of Adaptation-Level Theory

The two basic ALT models of the previous section can readily be analyzed using the parallelism and linear fan theorems (Anderson, 1974a, pp. 274-279). These functional measurement analyses are at once more powerful and more general than had previously been available.

AL model. The AL model of Equation 13 is a multiplication rule, and so may be tested by varying two (or more) variables in a factorial-type design. To illustrate, suppose that the subject is presented a gray patch centered on a variable gray background, and selects a gray to match the apparent grayness of the center patch. The reflectance of this matching gray is the *AL* (ignoring possible adaptation effects on the matching patch itself). The AL model requires this matching reflectance to exhibit a linear fan in a factorial design. For a more specific case, suppose that the background is constituted of two parts, 1 and 2, each independently variable in grayness. Then $B^w = B_1^{w_1} B_2^{w_2}$, and the factorial graph of reflectance for the $B_1 \times B_2$ design should exhibit the linear fan.

No measurement of the background stimuli is needed, either of their reflectance values or of their weights. The linear fan test is made on the *AL* response, which is measured in the physical metric. If the AL model passes the test, of course, the stimulus values may be derived by virtue of the second conclusion of the linear fan theorem. Thus, if B_1 corresponds to the row factor, the slopes of the row curves would be a linear scale of the effective variable, namely, B_1^{w1}.

A remarkable advantage of this functional measurement analysis is that it can allow for complex or heterogenous stimuli. Thus, B_1 may be completely arbitrary in shape and variegated in grayness. The analysis reveals the functional values of B_1 treated as a perceptual unit.

One qualification is needed. The linear fan theorem actually tests a more general model than the AL model (see also Anderson, 1981, Section 1.4.4). This more general model may be written for the present example as:

$$AL = f(S)\, g_1(B_1)\, g_2(B_2)\, h(R),$$

where f, g_1, g_2, and h are arbitrary functions. In the IIT framework, therefore, it is not appropriate to assume that $g_1(B_1) = B_1^{w1}$ without additional evidence.

This functional measurement analysis contrasts with the traditional measurement approaches adopted in all other analyses of ALT. Thus, Helson (1971, p. 10) asserts that the basic AL model of Equation 13 is neither true nor false; "It does not become a true or false proposition until specific values are given the weighting coefficients." This assertion is incorrect. If the linear fan test fails, no set whatever of weighting coefficients can make the AL model agree with the data. If the linear fan test fails, the AL model is simply false.

The traditional conception of measurement reappears in the reiterated statements by Flock (1971, e.g., p. 141) to the effect that ALT "requires that everything within the visible scene be measured, weighted, and pooled." In Flock's view, each homogeneous part of the visual scene must first be measured for its reflectance value. Weights must then be determined, with the weight of each part depending on its size, frontal and lateral separations from the focal stimulus, and perhaps on attentional factors as well. Such analyses would certainly be complex, generally impracticable. All this is unnecessary with functional measurement methodology. It is much simpler, more flexible -- and more powerful.

Perception model. The functional measurement analysis of the perception model of Equation 14 rests on the parallelism theorem. If the observed R is a linear function of the unobservable perception ρ, then Equation 14 becomes:

$$R = c_0 + c_1 [\log S - \log AL]. \quad (15)$$

This equation is additive in $\log S$ and $\log AL$. No more is needed, therefore, than to manipulate S and AL independently in a factorial design. If ALT is correct, the factorial graph will exhibit parallelism.

A notable advantage of this test is that the problematic task of measuring *AL* is finessed. In Helson's approach, the analysis of the perception model of Equation 14 depends squarely on the validity of the AL model of Equation 13 -- and on its laborious use to measure *AL*. In IIT, the perception model is testable quite independently of the AL model. Indeed, it provides the possibility of an independent assessment of the *AL*, obtainable much more simply from the judgmental data.

One set of data is available to test the ALT prediction of parallelism. Helson and Kozaki (1968) asked subjects to give numerosity judgments of plates of dots, each preceded by an unjudged anchor plate. The anchor plate was taken to be the major determinant of *AL*. Hence the parallelism analysis should apply. In fact, the data showed a strong linear fan pattern, in agreement with a model of comparative judgment from IIT (Anderson, 1974a, Figure 10).

Two Problems of Field Organization

IIT and ALT have common concern with the operation of complex stimulus fields. ALT represents an attempt to come to grips with one problem of field organization, namely, that encapsulated in the concept of adaptation level. There are, however, two associated problems of organization that lie outside the domain of ALT.

Stimulus integration. Stimulus integration is not generally recognized in ALT. The *AL* itself, to be sure, is an integrated resultant of context and other stimuli. In contrast, analogous integration for the focal stimulus lies outside the AL domain. Instead, the focal stimulus is treated as unitary, and its perceptual value is determined by its relation to the *AL*.

One illustration of this issue appears in the later discussion of the assimilation process in the line-box illusion of Figure 2.7. A second illustration is the "taste" of coffee, which is an integrated resultant of a multitude of stimulus cues, including odor as well as the taste senses of the tongue (McBride, 1990a; McBride & Anderson, 1991). This kind of integration lies outside the adaptation-level framework. It is quite general in perception, however, and represents a different kind of organization of the stimulus field.

Multiple comparison stimuli. IIT allows a focal stimulus to be compared separately with more than one referent stimulus. The focal stimulus could be seen as large relative to one context stimulus, small relative to another. These two relative evaluations would then be integrated to form the overall judgment. This is the **C-I** mode of processing, discussed previously.

Multiple comparison stimuli are not admissible in ALT. Multiple context stimuli may be operative, to be sure, but their effects must be mediated by the *AL*. This adaptation level is unitary, and it is the sole referent for comparison. ALT thus assumes the **I-C** mode of processing. This assumption is fundamental, for it is inherent in the concept of adaptation level used by Helson.

Not much is known about multiple comparison stimuli or about the **C-I** mode of processing. The theoretical model for rating of Equation 6 is one instance of the **C-I** mode, and others have appeared in social judgment (see Anderson, 1991e). A related case arose with the line-box illusion discussed later. The diagnostic tests discussed in connection with the **C-I** mode may prove useful in pursuing this question.

Relativity of Judgment

To say that something is better than average does not imply it is positive; it might be the best of a bad lot. Such comparative terms as *better* are relative, not absolute. The same applies to rating scales in general, whether they range from 1 to 20, say, or from *very much below average* to *very much above average*. For most purposes, this relativity of judgment language causes no problem. For ALT, however, it is extremely serious, as pointed out most tellingly by Stevens (1958) and studied experimentally by Campbell (e.g., Campbell, Lewis, & Hunt, 1958; see also Anderson, 1982, Section 1.1.5).

Relativity of judgment is a problem for ALT because the *AL* is considered the neutral point, or "zero of function." This makes sense in some sensory adaptation, as in the foregoing example of temperature adaptation. However, it seems questionable that similar adaptation applies to line length or numerosity, for example, or to social phenomena.

To illustrate the problem, suppose that subjects are asked to rate length of lines ranging continuously from 6 to 20 inches. Group P gets a positively skewed distribution, with a predominance of short lines; Group N gets a negatively skewed distribution, with a predominance of long lines. The question concerns the judgment of the medium, 13-inch line common to both distributions.

ALT implies a perceptual contrast. Each group will develop an *AL* towards the mean of its distribution, so the *AL* will be less than 13 inches for Group P, greater than 13 inches for Group N. Hence the 13-inch line will be rated "above average" in Group P, "below average" in Group N. At face value, this reflects perceptual contrast, the mainstay phenomenon of ALT.

But this apparent perceptual contrast may be merely an artifact of the rating language. Subjects have a tendency to spread their ratings evenly across the scale, and this alone would produce the observed effect. No claim about perceptual contrast is warranted. The true perceptual value of the 13-inch line might be identical in both groups.

Hoping to avoid this problem, Krantz and Campbell (1961) also asked subjects to judge in inches. This appeared to reduce the apparent contrast -- thereby demonstrating the reality of the artifact obtained in their rating condition. The same artifact, however, may still operate with reduced strength with the inch response. Although the physical inch is absolute, its psychological length is vague, and this allows the artifact to intrude. Indeed, Anderson (1982, Note 1.1.5a) pointed out that the observed effect was 30% of the line length, much too large to be perceptually real. Whatever genuine contrast may appear in this task is obscured by the confounding.

Much the same difficulty besets the *experimentum crucis* of Helson and Kozaki (1968). They presented plates of 10 to 18 dots for .3 seconds, and asked subjects to judge numerosity. Each plate was preceded by an unjudged anchor plate, of 4, 13, or 32 dots for different groups, and a control, no-anchor group was also run. These numerosity judgments showed strong anchor effects. The 18-dot plate, for example, was judged about 15, 20, and 25 dots for the 32-, 13-, and 4-dot anchor plates, respectively.

What does this result mean? Does the anchor effect lie at the level of perception or merely at the level of judgment? The judgment interpretation is entirely plausible. It claims that the 32-dot plate evokes an implicit numerosity judgment that depresses the overt response to the following plate -- with no effect on the perception itself. Analogous judgment biases are well-known in judgment research.

Helson asserted that the anchor plate changed the actual perception of numerosity. Calling this an *experimentum crucis*, he then dismissed the problem completely, even for verbal category ratings. But no actual evidence was presented to demonstrate a change in perception. Helson merely assumed that the difference in response reflected a difference in perception, apparently on the ground that the physical number of dots is absolute. But this does not speak to the relative component in the number language. Moreover, even if some genuine perceptual effect were present in this study, generalization to verbal category ratings is not justified.

Evaluation of AL Theory

The ubiquity of adaptation phenomena is apparent throughout psychology. Light and dark adaptation, for example, enable organisms to function under a wide range of illumination. Outside the perceptual domain, analogous adaptation occurs to pleasant or unpleasant conditions of food, work, exercise, and so on. Such expectancies, as they might perhaps preferably be called, are important in the goal directed behavior of everyday life.

Helson seems the first to envisage the possibility of a unified theory for the whole class of adaptation phenomena. His 1964 book does signal service by collecting from the literature many instances of such effects across the entire domain of psychology. This book is an invaluable compendium.

Helson's attempt at theory construction, however, has foundered on severe conceptual and methodological problems. There are real differences between the sensory adaptation to temperature or brightness, on one hand, and to length or numerosity, on the other. There are also real differences between all these psychophysical dimensions and the social-personality dimensions considered by

Helson. But these differences are never addressed. The foregoing relativity in the judgment language is recognized as real by all who have worked on the problem -- except Helson. Helson dismissed the problem completely, recognizing no exception to his claim of "profound change in sensory character" (1964, p.136). As a consequence, Helson's analyses are often uninterpretable.

Nevertheless, Helson did call attention to an important problem, and he recognized a similarity of adaptation concepts across many situations that had previously been treated in isolation. In this way, Helson's work has made a positive contribution to the development of psychological science.

VII. Experimental Studies in Cognitive Psychophysics

Applications of integration psychophysics in five illustrative areas are presented in the following sections. The first considers the classical problem of determining the psychophysical law. Functional measurement provides a general analysis of the bisection task for grayness -- buttressed by scale invariance across two other integration tasks. Fechner's problem thus becomes resolvable.

The second section discusses mixture psychophysics. This involves functions of two or more variables, which are not generally amenable to analysis in terms of the one-variable psychophysical functions of their components. Mixture psychophysics thus highlights the need to study the integration function, or psychocognitive law.

The next two sections take up two well-known problems in perception. The first, geometric illusions, is used to compare adaptation-level theory and the theory of information integration. Among other results, contrast and assimilation, which cannot coexist in adaptation-level theory, become amenable to joint analysis in integration theory. The study of the second problem, phenomenal causality, illustrates conjoint analysis of nature and nurture.

The final section takes up intuitive, commonsense physics, that is, our naive conceptions of time, speed, force, momentum, etc. Intuitive physics involves a cognitive analog of the psychophysical task. In place of stimulus energy is the physical law; in place of sensation is the psychocognitive law, that is, the cognitive representation of the physical law. The concepts and methods of integration psychophysics can assess how this cognitive structure agrees or disagrees with the corresponding structure of the physical law.

Scale Invariance

A psychophysical scale should have some generality, being invariant across different tasks (e.g., Anderson, 1962; Garner, Hake, & Eriksen, 1956). Conversely, finding the same scale operative across different tasks confers some confidence in its validity. The empirical example of scale invariance in the next subsection is followed by some comments on scale invariance as a general heuristic.

Scale invariance for grayness. This experiment demonstrated invariance of grayness (lightness) sensation across three different tasks. The stimulus display consisted of a pair of gray chips, each varied in grayness from black to white. Three judgment tasks were used. One task was to rate the difference in grayness between the two chips. The second task was to rate the average grayness of the two chips. The last task was bisection, a nonverbal task: To choose a third (response) chip midway in grayness between the two stimulus chips.

All three tasks yielded equivalent scales of grayness. The lower half of Figure 2.3 shows near-parallelism for the average and difference tasks. This parallelism supports the prescribed integration rule, and, by virtue of the second conclusion of the parallelism theorem, determines the psychophysical law.

The bisection data, in the upper left panel, show small, systematic deviations from parallelism, noticeable for the two top curves. In this graph, the response measure is the Munsell value of the response chip. The nonparallelism is considered to reflect a mild nonlinearity in the Munsell scale; its steps are too

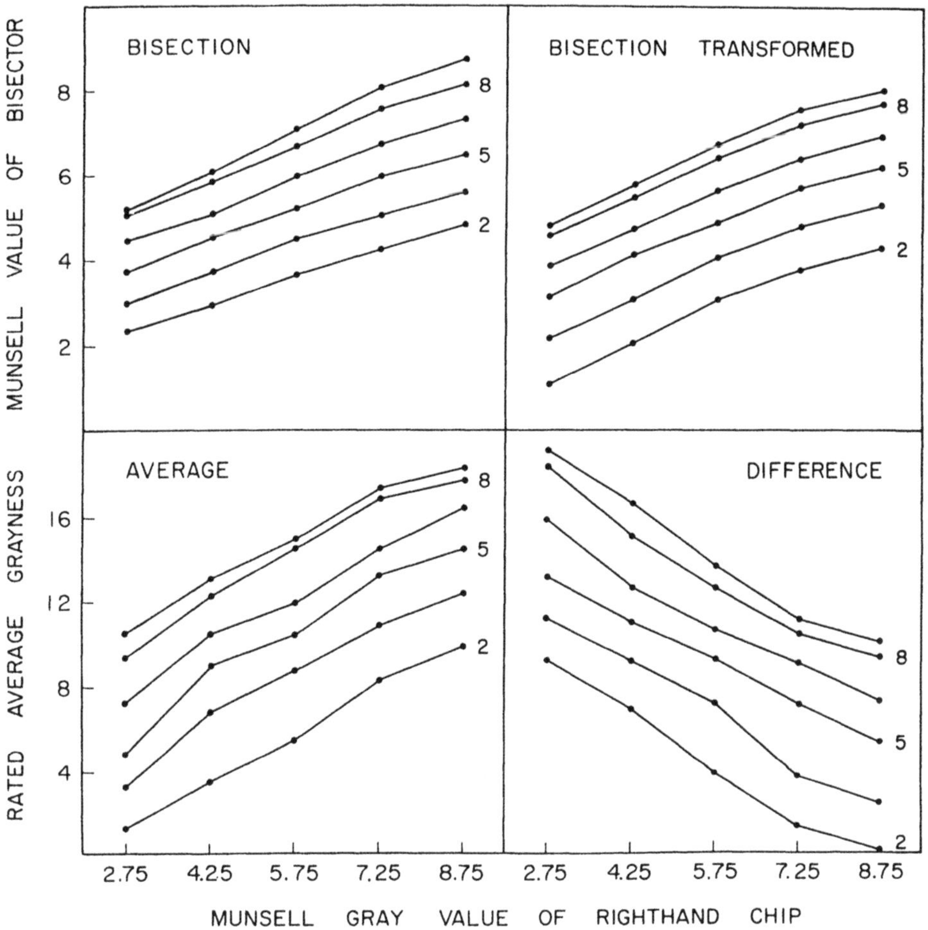

Figure 2.3: Grayness judgments for three tasks: averaging, differencing, and bisection. Stimulus display was a pair of gray chips in a 6 x 5, row x column design. Munsell values ranged from 2 (black) to 9.5 (white) for the row chip, as listed by the curves, and from 2.75 to 8.75 for the column chip, as listed on the horizontal axis. In each panel, the curves are closer together near the top, which indicates that the Munsell values deviate from equal intervals at the high reflectance end. (From Anderson, 1976).

close together towards the white end of the scale. (This nonlinearity is apparent to visual inspection of the Munsell chips). Application of monotone transformation made the curves virtually parallel, as shown in the top right panel.

Scale invariance is shown in Figure 2.4. The six row means from the averaging task are plotted as a function of the corresponding means from the bisection task. The curve is essentially linear, showing that the two scales are equivalent. Similar scale invariance was obtained for the difference task, as is also visible in the figure.

The format of Figure 2.4 shows that the two rating tasks, which use a verbal response, yield the same grayness scale as the nonverbal bisection response. Hence the scale invariance also provides support for the rating method. This conclusion needs to be qualified, however, by the fact that some individual subjects showed substantial nonparallelism in the difference task.

The psychophysical law for grayness (lightness) is shown in Figure 2.5. The row and column means from the bisection task were interlaced to yield 11 points on the curve. A power function fit yielded an exponent of .14, nine times less than the exponent of 1.2 obtained with magnitude estimation (Stevens, 1974). Stevens' exponents, however, have not satisfied proper validity criteria. In contrast, the validity of the exponent determined with functional measurement has three-fold support in this experiment: first, by the success of the integration models for each separate task; second, by the invariance of the stimulus scales across the three tasks; and third, by the agreement of the response scales between the verbal and nonverbal tasks.

Scale invariance as a heuristic. Scale invariance, in the present view, is a heuristic, suggestive of a common sensory store across different tasks and contexts (Anderson, 1981, Section 5.6.2; 1982, pp. 109-112, 147-149). Many

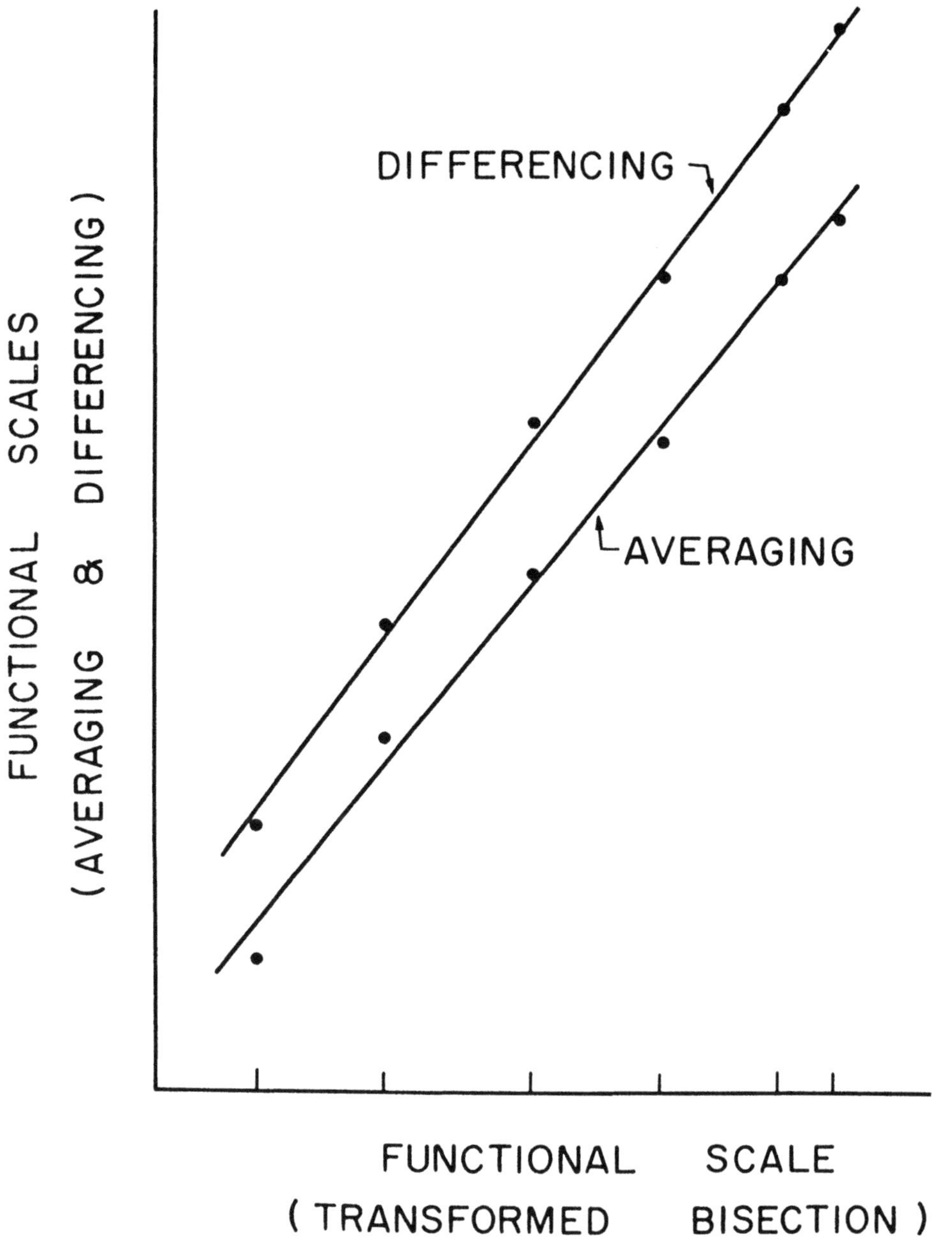

Figure 2.4: Scale invariance for grayness. Functional scales for average and difference judgments are plotted as a function of the functional scale from the bisection task; data from Figure 2.3. The linearity demonstrates scale invariance. (From Anderson, 1976).

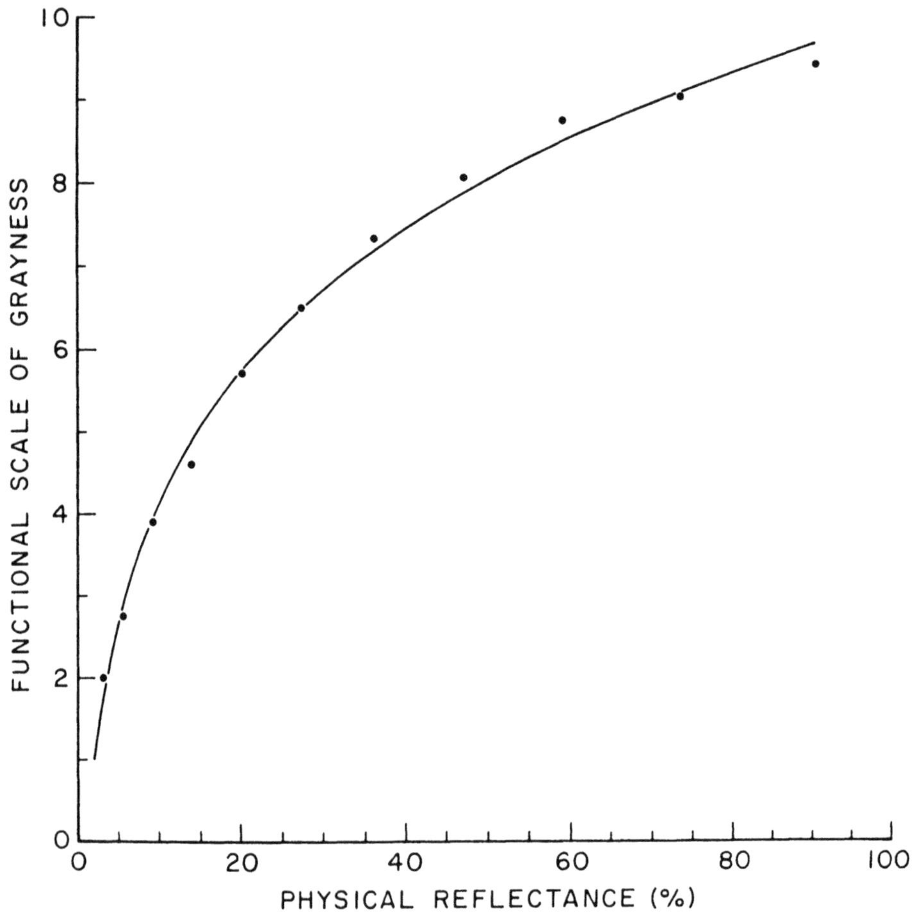

Figure 2.5: Psychophysical law for grayness (lightness). (From N.H. Anderson, Foundations of Information Integration Theory, Figure 1.12, 1981).

writers take a stronger view, treating scale invariance as an axiom, a self-evident principle that can provide powerful constraints on theory construction. In the integration diagram of Figure 2.1, however, the valuation operation depends on the goal, so the same stimulus may have different values in different tasks and contexts. Indeed, the three foregoing grayness tasks impose somewhat different perceptual-cognitive requirements, so scale invariance should not be postulated but taken only in a heuristic role. The obtained scale invariance is not unexpected, of course, but it is a useful result on sensory-cognitive processing. And it helps solidify the empirical-theoretical network of the theory of information integration.

The present results argue against Marks' (1974; see similarly Algom & Katzir, 1990) view that ratings and magnitude estimation elicit different sensory scales, the former referring to discriminability relationships, the latter to sensory magnitudes. The averaging task clearly involves judgments of sensory magnitude, yet it yielded the same grayness scale as the bisection task and the difference task.

Furthermore, magnitude estimation could still satisfy the parallelism theorem for the averaging task - even if it did yield different scale values. Valuation does not constrain integration, as indicated in Figure 2.1. But in fact, magnitude estimation of average grayness yields marked nonparallelism (see Anderson, 1982, Figure 1.3). In the present Figure 2.2, it thus appears that ratings yield a valid measure of sensation, whereas magnitude estimation is biased and invalid. In a related vein, Birnbaum (e.g., Birnbaum & Elmasian, 1977) has argued that the ratio instructions used in magnitude estimation may actually elicit difference judgments.

Context can have real effects on phenomenal stimulus value, as with the adaptation effects studied by Helson and others. Suggestions that such effects can be produced merely by differences in stimulus range for loudness have been given by Algom and Marks (1990; see also Marks, 1988). Such studies of stimulus interaction constitute an important domain for analysis of sensory-cognitive processing. Still, it should be kept in mind that scale invariance may hold at the preconscious level even with genuine contextual effects on conscious sensation.

Mixture Psychophysics

The concept of psychophysical law has limited relevance for mixture psychophysics. With taste and smell, especially, the operative stimulus is usually heterogeneous, a mixture or blend of two or more components. The psychophysical functions for the separate components are not too useful for analysis of their mixtures.

Two-variable functions. To see the limitation of traditional one-variable psychophysical functions, denote the response to a single stimulus by $R(S)$ and the response to a two-stimulus mixture by $R(S_1,S_2)$. Whereas it is meaningful to ask if $R(S)$ is a power function, it is not meaningful to ask if $R(S_1,S_2)$ is a power function. One could hypothesize that $R(S_1,S_2) = S_1^{n_1} \times S_2^{n_2}$ or $S_1^{n_1} + S_2^{n_2}$, for example, but this involves some assumption about the integration of S_1 and S_2.

The basic issue thus concerns the integration function, not the psychophysical function. The two cited hypotheses can be tested using the linear fan and parallelism theorems. Actually, these functional measurement analyses test more general hypotheses, $R(S_1,S_2) = \mathbf{V}_1(S_1) \times \mathbf{V}_2(S_2)$ or $\mathbf{V}_1(S_1)+\mathbf{V}_2(S_2)$, in the two respective cases. Here $\mathbf{V}_1$ and $\mathbf{V}_2$ are arbitrary psychophysical functions; no assumption about power functions is needed. However, some assumption about the integration function is essential.

Chemical senses as mixture psychophysics. Eating is a basic biosocial activity, heavily involved with the chemical senses, taste and smell. Taste and smell are thus prime domains of mixture psychophysics. A functional measurement approach has been applied in a number of studies (Algom & Cain, 1991b; De Graaf, Frijters, & van Trijp, 1987; Frank & Archambo, 1986; Hornung & Enns, 1984; Klitzner, 1975; see review in McBride & Anderson, 1991).

Special mention should be made of the cogent, dedicated research of McBride (see McBride, 1989, 1990a,b, in press; McBride & Anderson, 1991). Besides various findings of additivity and subadditivity, McBride has also obtained a tantalizing nonadditive result on mixture suppression interpreted as the *dominant component model*. In this model, the intensity of sensation is determined by the stronger component alone; the weaker component has no effect.

The response pattern implied by a dominant component model is shown in the factorial graph of Figure 2.6. Subjects tasted sweet-sour solutions and judged overall intensity. The top curve shows the mean judgment for the highest acid concentration. This curve is essentially flat; total intensity is the same for the acid alone (leftmost point) as for acid combined with the very sweet (.80M) sucrose concentration (rightmost point). A similar pattern appears in the second curve from the top. The judgment appears to be determined solely by the acid component.

The two bottom curves show the complementary pattern. The lowest curve is for sucrose alone, so the upward trend shows the intensity of the sucrose component per se. The next lowest curve is essentially identical over the three largest sucrose concentrations; the level of acid has no effect. The judgment appears to be determined solely by the dominant sucrose component. Thus, it seems that the sweet and sour components of a mixture are not integrated into the perception of total intensity.

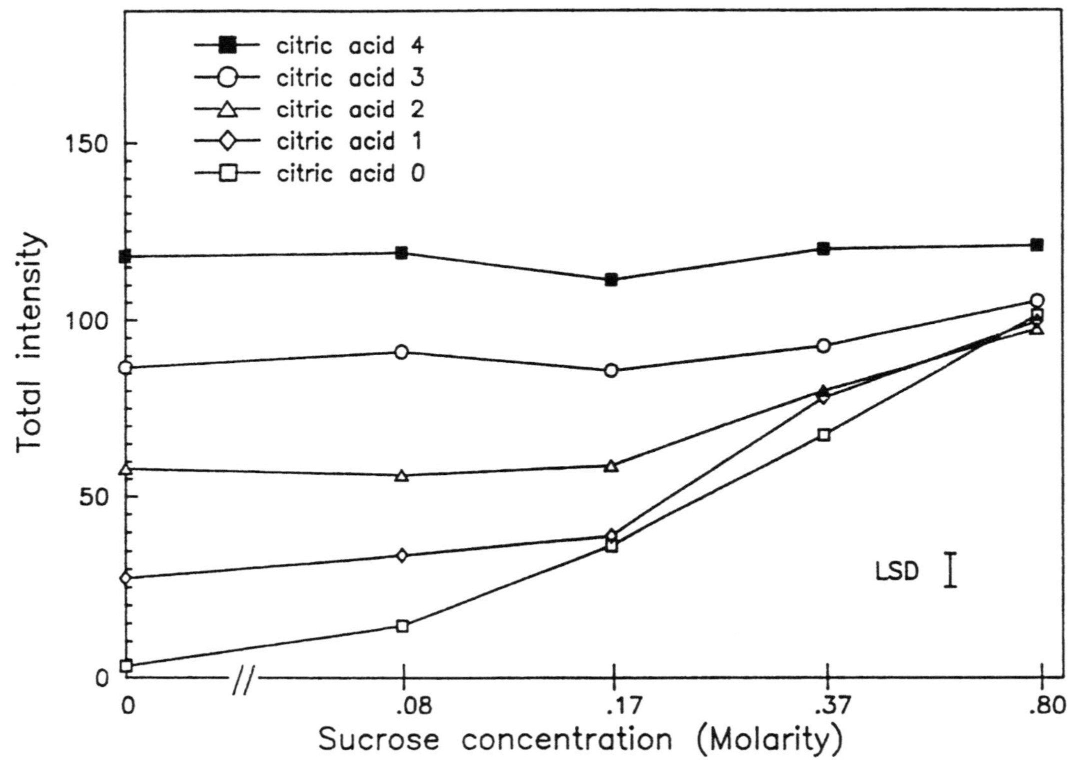

Figure 2.6: Dominant component response pattern for judgments of total intensity of sucrose-acid mixtures. (After McBride, 1989).

An interesting complication is that judgments of sweetness or sourness of the mixture, as distinct from its overall intensity, do obey an integration rule. In fact, the rule is subtraction: Each level of acidity causes a fixed decrease in perceived sweetness (above threshold); similarly, each level of sugar causes a fixed decrease in perceived sourness. This mixture suppression rule for these two quality judgments contrasts sharply with the non-integration rule for overall intensity. Although these results are still tentative, they may provide penetrating information on information processing in the chemical senses.

Also, these results are important in everyday psychophysics. As McBride (1990a) points out, the universal appeal of soft drinks depends on the joint action of sugar and acid. Sweet drinks alone are no more than mildly pleasant. The acid component provides high intensity, the "hit" of the drink. But acid at the needed concentration is distinctly unpalatable. The sugar has a strong suppressant effect on the perceived acidity, whereas the acid has substantially less suppressant effect on perceived sweetness. Hence the sweet and sour qualities of the drink are both desirable and so is the "hit." McBride's analysis thus explains the international prosperity of the cola companies.

Synergism and physiology. McBride (1989) has presented a cogent integration explanation of the previous puzzling "synergism" effect, that sugar mixtures seem sweeter than the sum of the separate sweetnesses. A 5%:5% fructose:sucrose solution, for example, tastes sweeter than either a 10% fructose or a 10% sucrose solution. Various writers have attempted to explain this seeming supra-additivity, or synergism, as it has been called.

McBride argued that there is no real synergism. Instead, fructose and sucrose activate separate receptor sites. Adding 5% fructose to 5% fructose to get 10% fructose will not double sweetness because the first 5% uses up receptor sites, leaving fewer or less reactive sites available for the second 5%. But adding

5% sucrose activates fresh receptor sites, thereby causing a greater increase in sweetness. Instead of being a puzzle, the effect provides evidence on receptor physiology.

Geometric Illusions

The two basic processes of contrast and assimilation were used as explanations in the very first studies of illusions over a century ago. Contrast was commonly taken to result from comparative judgment, assimilation from figural confusion or amalgamation. Analysis of contrast and assimilation, however, did not make much progress.

The difficulty is that contrast and assimilation often act in opposing directions. Hence virtually any result can be explained -- but almost nothing can be predicted. Illusion theorists, accordingly, have sought pure cases, in which only one or the other process would operate. Each theory seemed to explain most available data, yet contrary cases were soon found. In despair, some writers concluded that many processes were involved, virtually abandoning the possibility of general theory.

Integration psychophysics has provided a new approach. Two illustrative studies are noted here.

Baldwin line-box illusion. When a line is flanked by boxes, as in Figure 2.7, its apparent length changes. It seems as though the large boxes make the line look shorter, and the small boxes make it look longer. This has long been considered a contrast illusion.

Two theories have attempted to provide quantitative accounts of this line-box illusion: adaptation-level theory and information integration theory. An experimental test was obtained by manipulating the sizes of the left and right boxes in factorial design (Clavadetscher & Anderson, 1977). Only one line-box figure was presented at a time, and subjects made a graphic judgment of the length of the center line.

The critical result was the finding of box-box additivity. This infirms adaptation-level theory, which predicts nonadditivity, and supports integration theory (see earlier discussion of **I-C** and **C-I** modes of comparison).

An unexpected result was also obtained that threw a very different light on the illusion process. The process is not contrast, as everyone had thought, but assimilation. The right panel of Figure 2.7 shows apparent length of a 4-cm centerline as a function of box size. All but the last point lie above the control value (open circle at left). Even the 10-cm box makes the 4-cm line look longer. The apparent contrast in the left panel is really the difference between two assimilation effects, one large and one small.

This example of the importance of control conditions is doubly instructive. The standard form of the illusion, given in Figure 2.7, seems so clearly a contrast effect that no one had previously thought to include the control. Restle (1971) included a related condition, but misinterpreted the result because of theoretical precommitment to adaptation-level theory, which, in his application, required a contrast effect.

For present purposes, however, the main point is that this study signalled the demise of the standard approach of attempting to develop quantitative illusion theories based on just a single process. Both assimilation and contrast processes must be allowed. Restle (1978) attempted to revise his contrast model from adaptation-level theory to explain the assimilation effect, but this revision still failed to account for the box-box additivity (see Clavadetscher, 1991, pp. 253-254).

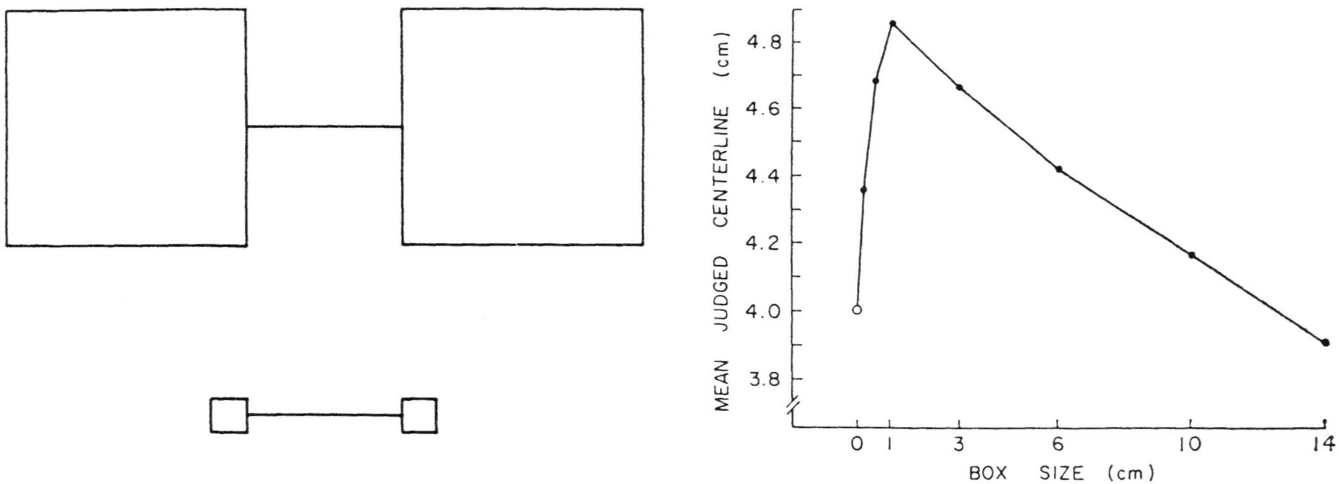

Figure 2.7: Line-box illusion. Left panel illustrates the illusion figure. Right panel shows magnitude of illusion as a function of box size. (After J.E. Clavadetscher & N.H. Anderson, "Comparative judgment: Tests of two theories of comparative judgment," *Journal of Experimental Psychology: Human Perception and Performance*, 1977, **3**, 119-135. Copyright 1977 by American Psychological Association, reprinted by permission).

Pressey (Pressey & Wilson, 1980) similarly attempted to extend his assimilation theory to include contrast, but this was merely an ad hoc assumption of a "field of contrast" at greater distances to account for observed contrast. The results of Clavadetscher and Anderson (1977), however, indicate that contrast is strongest at closer distances. Conceptually, Pressey's revised theory is inappropriate because it assumes that only one of the two processes can operate at any point. The same difficulty appears in the treatment of the parallel lines illusion by Jordan and Schiano (1986). Instead, both processes should be allowed to act jointly, as in Clavadetscher's two process integration theory discussed next.

Two process theory of illusions. Joint operation of contrast and assimilation was demonstrated by Clavadetscher (1977/1978, 1991) with the Ebbinghaus-Titchener circles illusion of Figure 2.8. Consider only the figure on the upper right, with the large context circles. Assimilation will make the center circle look larger, but contrast will make the center circle look smaller. Clavadetscher reasoned that assimilation, being presumably a figural amalgamation, would decrease rapidly with distance between center and context circles. Contrast, on the other hand, being a matter of comparative judgment, would decrease slowly. Hence large context circles could produce a U-shaped curve.

Clavadetscher's ingenious U-shape prediction is verified for the 18- and 23-cm curves in Figure 2.8. At the nearest distance of 1 mm, assimilation and contrast are equally strong, but cancel to leave a net judgment approximately the same as the no-context control. As distance increases, assimilation decreases rapidly, contrast decreases slowly, so the curves slope down. At the middle distance, assimilation is near zero, but contrast is still substantial, so the curves reach a minimum. As distance increases still further, contrast continues to decrease, and the curves rise towards the control. This appears to be the first study in which joint operation of both processes in geometric illusions has been

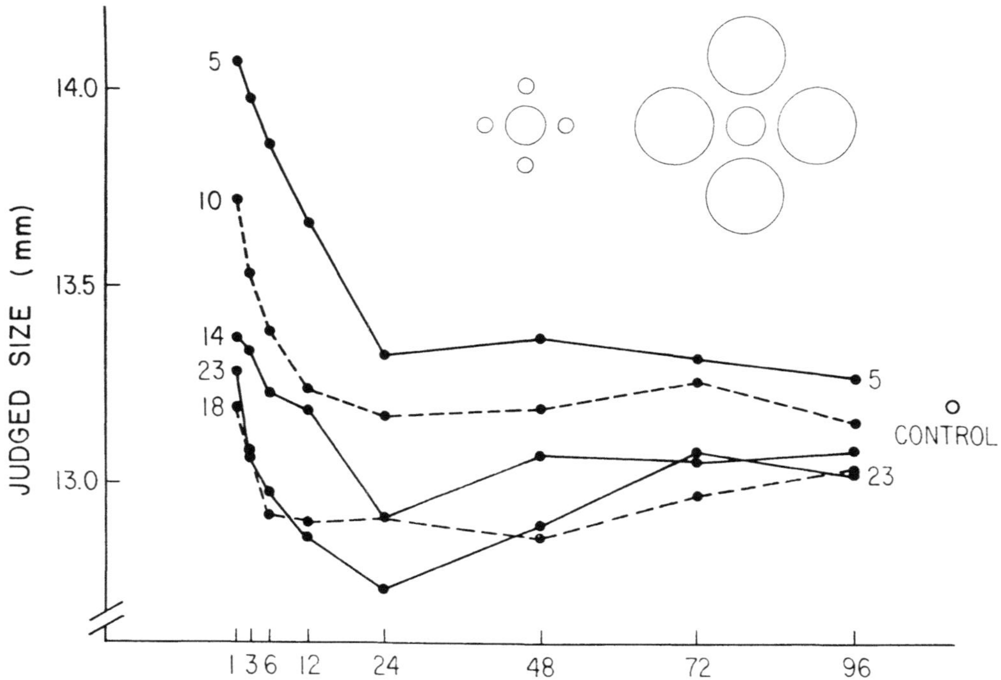

Figure 2.8: U-shaped curves demonstrate joint action of contrast and assimilation. Upper figure shows the circles illusion. Curves show apparent diameter of center circle as a function of size of surrounding context circles (horizontal axis). Control point represents apparent size of center circle with no context circles (From Clavadetscher, 1977, 1991).

definitely established. Comparisons with other illusion theories are given in Clavadetscher (1991).

Fitting the integration model to the data, assuming exponential decay, yielded decay rates of .10 for assimilation and .01 for contrast. Integration psychophysics thus provides a potential for quantitative analysis of contrast-assimilation processes that may extend to other areas such as color vision (e.g., Boynton, 1979, Figures 2.4 and 2.5).

Michotte's Phenomenal Causality

The nature-nurture issue has long been prominent in psychology, but most discussion has been strongly polarized, a characteristic that tends to perpetuate itself. In less adversarial moments, however, almost everyone recognizes that both genetic and environmental determinants are important. What is in short supply are concepts and methods that can deal with nature and nurture together. The following study illustrates the potential of integration psychophysics for conjoint analysis of nature and nurture.

In Michotte's (1946/1963) well-known studies, subjects report immediate perception of causality in artificial "launch events." In the case studied here, which embodies a typical Michotte condition, Square A moves up to stationary Square B, stops, and, after a very short delay, Square B moves off in the same direction. Most subjects perceive a causal relation, even though the two squares are only images on a computer screen. In Michotte's view, perception of causality is innate, a gestalt tendency to see the two motions as a unified whole.

Michotte's views have been controversial. Critics have demonstrated substantial individual differences and effects of prior experience, which they have claimed are inconsistent with Michotte's thesis of immediate, innate causal perception. Other investigators, however, have emphasized that most subjects do experience some sense of phenomenal causality (see Schlottmann, 1987; Schlottmann & Anderson, 1990).

The present integration approach differs from previous studies in important ways that deserve notice. First, the focus shifts to stimulus integration. Previous investigators have studied how one or another variable affects the goodness of the causal perception, but little evidence is available on joint effects of two or more variables. Second, each subject made judgments for a battery of visual scenes. This provided a data *pattern* for each individual that allowed individual analysis. Third, two different instruction conditions were used: To judge causality and to judge naturalness. This instruction interacted with individual differences to allow more informative analysis. Fourth, subjects made graded judgments of goodness of the perception. This avoids difficulties that trouble the categorical response measures used in virtually all previous work.

The visual scenes were presented on a computer screen with 17 msec update time, sufficiently rapid to provide smooth visual motion. A gray square (A) began moving from the left at a constant velocity of 49 cm/sec, stopping close to a black square (B), which, after a short delay, moved off to the right at a constant velocity of 49, 24.5, 12.2, or 6.1 cm/sec. A three-factor design was used: The *gap* between A's stopping place and B was 2.1, 1.4, 0.7, or 0 mm. The *delay* between A's stopping and B's starting was 170, 119, 68, or 17 msec, the last of which is not considered here. B's speed was varied as indicted to yield A:B *speed ratios* of 1:1, 2:1, 4:1, and 8:1.

An important technical issue concerns the selection of the levels of each stimulus variable. These were carefully chosen on the basis of Michotte's specifications and extensive preliminary work to cover a transition range between a clear causal and a clear noncausal relation. Hence the visual scenes had graded levels of causality or naturalness, which justified the use of a continuous response measure. Graded levels of causality could result, for example, from graded confidence that A caused B. This approach is consistent with Michotte's report of graded differences in "goodness" of the causal perception.

The *causality group* judged degree of confidence that A's motion had caused B's motion. The *naturalness group* judged how natural the collision looked. Judgments were made on an 11-cm graphic rating scale on the computer screen, which had a resolution of 300 points. There were 30 subjects in each group, and each subject judged the entire set of scenes in six successive replications. Six replications were used in order to have enough data for reliable analyses at the individual level.

The overall results can be summarized simply. The *integration* of the three cues followed an invariant averaging rule, the same across all individual difference subgroups. The *valuation* of each cue, however, exhibited large individual differences.

A key to the analysis lay in the interaction between the two instruction conditions and individual differences, which revealed meaningful subgroupings of individual response patterns. Under the causality instructions, spatial contiguity had large effects, whereas speed ratio had small effects. Under the naturalness instructions, speed ratio had large effects, whereas spatial contiguity had small effects. In the ordinary way, each instruction condition would have been analyzed in terms of group means. Because each subject had served in six replications, however, individual analysis was possible. Inspection of these individual analyses indicated a spectrum of behavior patterns between the modal patterns elicited by the two instructions. Serendipitously, it was found that meaningful subgroupings appeared when subjects were classified according to which speed ratio they found most causal or natural (see arrows in Figure 2.9). It would seem that subjects have a pre-experimental predisposition for one or the other of the two kinds of judgments. This individual predisposition interacted with the experimental instructions to produce five distinctive patterns of response -- patterns that correspond to the valuation processes for the three separate cues.

An overview of the results is given in Figure 2.9, in which each layer of the graph corresponds to one of the five subgroupings. Each separate panel shows the integration pattern for the listed pair of variables. Group I, in the upper layer, shows large effects of gap and delay (upper left panel) but near-zero effect of speed ratio (center and right panels). This pattern is the modal causality pattern; all but 1 of 13 subjects in Group I were from the causality instruction condition.

Group V, in the bottom layer, shows large effects of delay and speed ratio (bottom right panel), but small effects of the gap variable (left and center panels). This pattern of behavior is the modal naturalness pattern; all but 3 of the 14 subjects in this subgroup are from the naturalness instruction condition.

A theoretical account of the data can be given in terms of the **V** and **I** operations of Figure 2.1. The **I** operation is one of averaging, invariant across all groups. The curves in Figure 2.9 are theoretical, obtained by fitting the averaging model of Equation 4 for three variables. A distinctive feature of the data patterns is the taper shape. This corresponds to differential weighting within the averaging process, and is reproduced in the theoretical curves. Even the crossover in the bottom right panel is accounted for by the model. Quantitatively also, the fit seems good, for the mean magnitude deviation is only 5.1 on the 300-point scale.

The diverse response patterns in Figure 2.9 represent different valuation strategies induced by the instruction condition and by individual differences. These **V** strategies were found to emphasize the more diagnostic evidence in

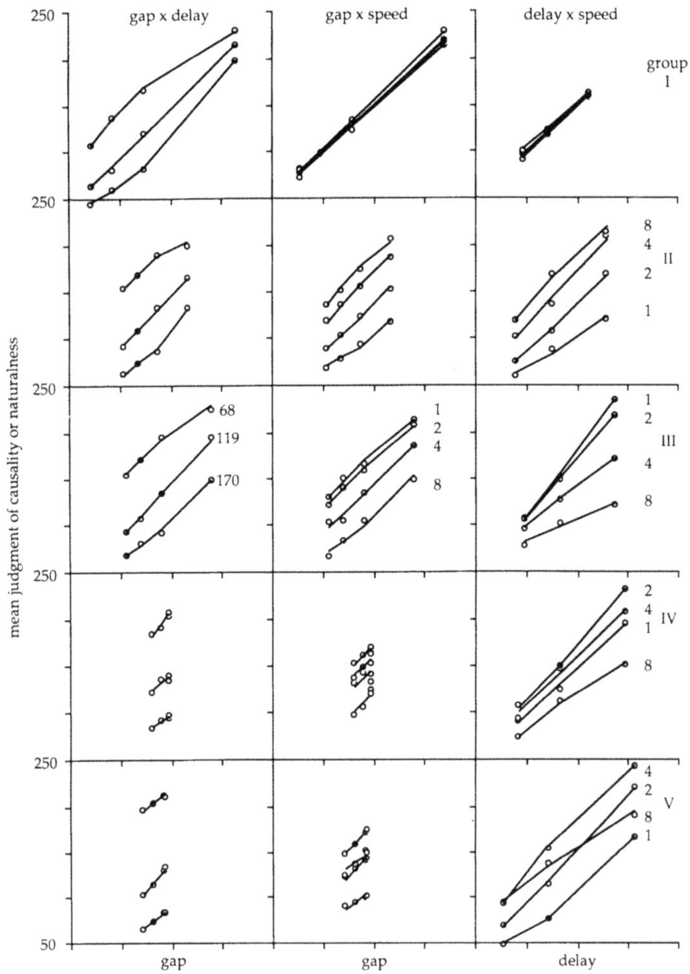

Figure 2.9: Comparison of theoretical predictions from averaging model (curves) and observed judgments of causality or naturalness (data points). Each layer of the graph represents one group of subjects, classified according to the speed ratio that yielded the highest judgment. The left, center, and right columns show the two-factor integration patterns for the variable pairs: Gap x Delay, Gap x Speed Ratio, and Delay x Speed Ratio, respectively. In left column, curves correspond to delays of 68, 119, and 170 msec, as listed in the center panel. In center column, curves correspond to speed ratios of 1, 2, 4, and 8, as listed in center panel. In right column, curves correspond to listed speed ratios, which had different order for different groups. Theoretical curves obtained from AVERAGE program (Zalinski & Anderson, 1991). (From Schlottmann & Anderson, 1990).

order to facilitate the judgment-decision process. A large gap, for example, may be taken as fairly clear evidence against a causal event, and hence would receive low scale value and high weight in the overall judgment.

Diagnosticity of the stimulus cues may appear in both the weight and value parameters. Hence the valuation strategies reveal themselves in the parameter estimates obtained from the model. The estimated parameters are shown in Table 2.2. For ψ-values, 150 is neutral, with larger (smaller) values being favorable (unfavorable) for a judgment of causality or naturalness. Values for delay, in the middle layer of Table 2.2, show a uniform trend across all groups: high values for a short delay, low values for a long delay. The bottom layer of Table 2.2 shows a similar trend for gap: high values for small gap and low values for large gap. Both trends are phenomenologically correct, since short delay and small gap characterize natural collisions.

For speed ratio, in the top layer, values are near 150 for Group I, reflecting the near-zero effect of speed in this group. For the other four groups, the highest value corresponds to the highest curve in the right panels of Figure 2.9 and the lowest value corresponds to the lowest curve. For speed ratio, in contrast to gap and delay, the subjective values show neither a uniform relation to the physical values nor a uniform trend across groups.

The weight estimates point to a "good-bad" strategy in the valuation process. Specifically, subjects seemed to use one cue to define "good" launch events, another cue to define "bad" launch events. To illustrate, consider Group I. Weights for gap range from 9.2 for the largest gap to 2.6 for zero gap. Since large gap has a low value, being noncausal, the cited pattern of weights means that the gap variable was used to define bad causal events. The delay variable, in contrast, was used to define good events in Group I: The pattern of weights is opposite to that for gap, with higher weights for small delays.

Table 2.2

Weight and Value Estimates for Three Cues from Averaging Model

Speed Ratio	Group I		Group II		Group III		Group IV		Group V	
	w	ψ	w	ψ	w	ψ	w	ψ	w	ψ
1:1	1	151	7.9	87	3.5	186	5.6	158	6.9	126
2:1	1	145	4.7	122	3.9	177	5.5	180	5.5	165
4:1	1	154	3.7	166	5.0	146	5.8	170	5.6	160
8:1	1	167	3.9	189	7.2	108	5.9	136	8.4	160
delay										
68 msec	7.4	167	2.9	240	1.6	206	2.9	180	4.1	235
119 msec	4.6	124	1.7	107	2.5	97	5.5	120	2.4	99
170 msec	3.8	100	2.2	19	5.7	66	7.1	80	4.5	48
gap										
0 mm	2.6	240	4.5	199	5.7	237	1	187	1	202
0.7 mm	4.5	151	2.7	159	2.4	178	1	192	1	192
1.4 mm	6.4	113	3.0	122	1.8	133	1	152	1	136
2.1 mm	9.2	86	3.2	97	1.6	96	1	112	1	86

Similar good-bad weighting can be seen throughout the table, especially in Group III. Different groups differ, however, in their selection of good and bad variables. These good-bad weighting strategies are evidently cognitive in nature. Short and long delay, for example, are both physically diagnostic, for and against causality, respectively, whereas medium delay is ambiguous. Weighting patterns that reflected physical diagnosticity would thus be a U-shaped function of delay. But most of the weight patterns in Table 2.2 are unidirectional, not U-shaped, which implies that the weighting operation is cognitive, not simply perceptual. More detailed discussion is given in the original paper.

To sum up, the present study may have provided some resolution of the controversy between Michotte and his critics. On one hand, the present analyses of valuation strategy clearly show the operation of cognitive process not recognized in Michotte's view. Large individual differences were demonstrated through the use of continuous response measure and individual subject design, and this confirms and solidifies previous criticisms of Michotte. But even large individual differences may be tolerated by Michotte's innatist view, as can effects of instructions and prior experience. Learning effects are important in many "automatic" perceptual events, as illustrated by various sensory adaptations, such as adaptation to inverting spectacles.

What is novel in the present approach are the model parameters. The "good-bad" strategy visible in the weight estimates demonstrates that higher-level cognitive process influence cue evaluation. An innatist position can hardly allow the spectrum of different good-bad strategies that were found here. Even for temporal delay, which showed the most uniform main effect across subjects, different groups showed very different diagnosticity patterns in their weighting strategy. To arrive at this conclusion, however, required going below the observable data to analyze the processes of valuation and integration.

On the other hand, the present finding of an invariant integration rule would seem to agree with Michotte, corresponding to his emphasis on a uniform perceptual structure. Michotte recognized that experiential factors would overlay judgments of causality, but he argued for an underlying "pure" perception of causality. The integration approach takes full cognizance of individual differences and experiential factors, which have been the concern of Michotte's critics, and unifies them into a phenomenal experience of causation.

The importance of experiential factors has been strongly emphasized in the historical development of psychology. In recent times, however, innate determinants have received increasing attention. Much of the nature-nurture argument, however, has been polarized, with attempts to demonstrate prepotency of one or the other. The present study illustrates how innate and experiential factors can both be included within a cognitive framework -- and yield a more penetrating analysis than was possible with previous theory.

The Physical Law: Intuitive Physics

Classical psychophysics has focused on the internalization of stimulus information along sensory pathways. Another kind of internalization pertains to the structure of physical laws, many of which have simple algebraic forms. One of the simplest is for area of rectangles: Area = Height x Width. Another is travel time for uniform motion: Time = Distance ÷ Speed. In both cases, interest goes beyond the psychophysical functions for the single variables to study the cognitive representation of the algebraic rule for the pair of variables. The following experimental studies indicate, moreover, that the psychophysical functions in many such tasks are cognitive in nature (Anderson, 1983a,b).

Galileo's incline. Subjects judged travel time for a ball rolling down an incline. The left panel of Figure 2.10 shows naive judgments prior to any ball rolling. Each curve corresponds to one angle of inclination; the five points on the curve refer to distance between the ball and the bottom end of the incline. The near-linear fan pattern in the left panel agrees with the multiplicative structure of

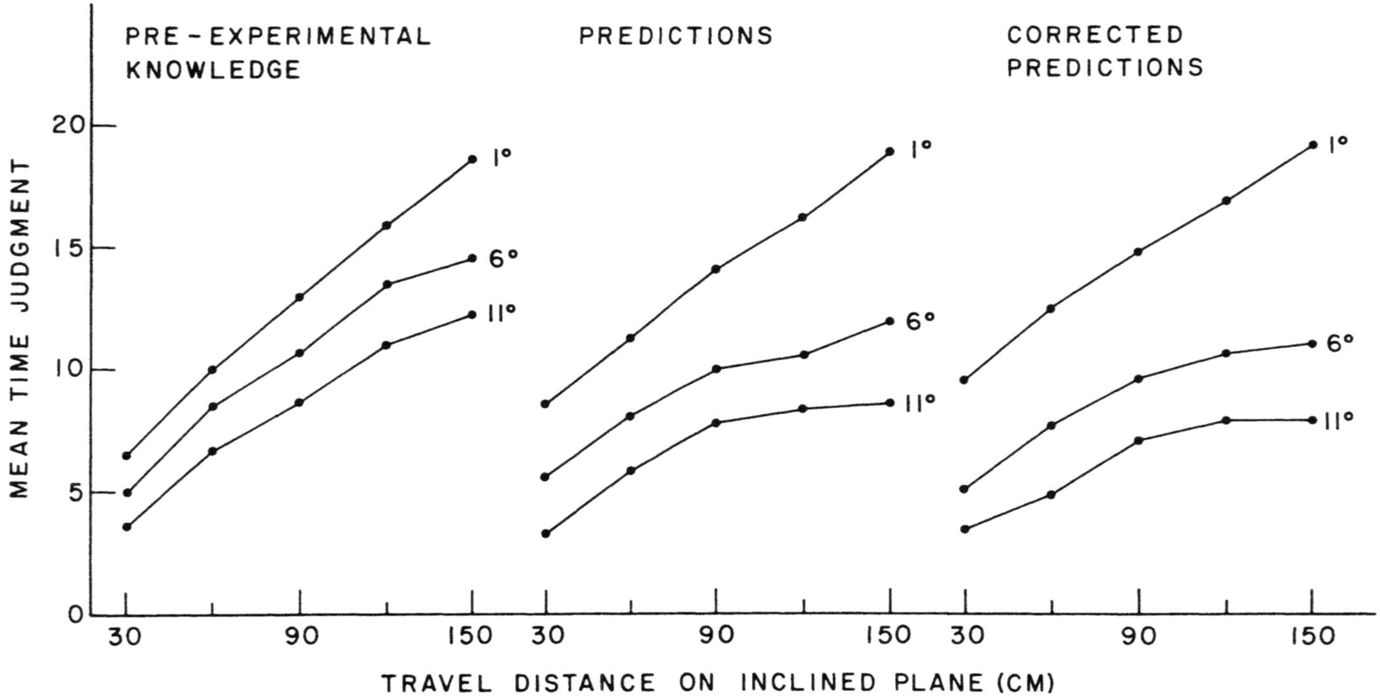

Figure 2.10: Predictions of travel time for ball on incline. Left panel shows pre-experimental knowledge: Predictions are for each of 15 distance-angle combinations prior to any observation of ball rolling. Right panel shows judgments of actual observed travel times. Center panel represents predictions followed by ball rolling; similarity between center and right panels shows that learning was rapid. (From Anderson, 1983b, p.243).

the physical law. This important feature of the physical law has thus been internalized in pre-experimental experience.

In the second part of the experiment, subjects again made a prediction for each angle-distance combination, but the ball was then released and they corrected their predictions, that is, they judged the actual travel time. These predictions and corrected predictions are plotted in the center and right panels of Figure 2.10. Comparison with the left panel shows that observations of the rolling ball had two effects. First, angle has much larger effects than in pre-experimental knowledge, which agrees with the physical facts. Second, the near-linear fan pattern has disappeared; the 1° curve remains linear, but the 6° and 11° curves show pronounced curvature, which disagrees with the physical facts.

Observation of the events thus had two learning effects: Accuracy increased, but the psychocognitive law shifted away from the physical law. Other studies in this series showed that observation of the physical event sometimes helped, sometimes hindered performance. In one case, predictions of travel *distance* up an incline remained seriously in error even after observation of the motion.

In these studies, the cognitive elements were evidently entire functions. These function shapes are represented directly in the factorial graphs, as in Figure 2.10. These functional relations are basic components of knowledge structures of intuitive physics. Efficient instruction needs to be pointed towards learning and calibration of function shape.

Nature faced a difficult problem to endow organisms with function concepts. Function shapes are not usually observable. Observation of a rolling ball gives only a single point on the function. In the natural world, information usually comes as single events, which correspond to single points on the function.

Psychological studies of learning have aped Nature by using trial-wise reinforcement and knowledge of results. Nature, however, evidently found a way to transcend individual events to confer function knowledge. This sets an ideal for the psychology of learning to understand and emulate.

General purpose addition rule. Insight into Nature's endowment of function knowledge appeared in the finding that 5-year-olds judge rectangle area by adding height and width (Anderson & Cuneo, 1978). This psychocognitive, Height + Width rule contrasts sharply with the physical Height x Width rule, but it has been amply confirmed by findings of parallelism in Height-Width factorial graphs (see especially Figure 2.11 following).

The Height + Width rule was interpreted to represent a general purpose addition rule. Young children do not possess adult concepts of multidimensional quantities. They do, however, perceive one-dimensional cues and understand their relevance, and they integrate them by applying a general purpose addition rule.

Critical tests of this interpretation come from similar findings of parallelism for other tasks in which the physical rule implies a linear fan. Thus, Cuneo (1982) found an additive Length + Density rule for judgments of number of beads in a row. Similarly, Wilkening (1982; see Anderson & Wilkening, 1991) found a subtractive Distance − Speed rule for judgments of travel time along a straightaway. Especially notable, Wilkening's work thus showed that 5-year-olds possessed true metric concepts of time and speed, thereby producing a developmental picture radically different from that in Piagetian theory.

Ecologically, an addition rule is not unreasonable. It would select the larger rectangle most of the time, for example. As a general purpose rule, applicable across many tasks, it is a useful survival skill. It exemplifies the biosocial heuristic (Anderson, 1991a) that Nature and society provide small brains with utility tools that facilitate survival by evoking reasonably good performance across a variety of situations rather than optimal behavior in a few situations.

Memory psychophysics. Memory psychophysics deals with relations between physical stimuli and their remembered properties, as well as with actions based on such memories. A pioneering approach to this little studied field has been given by Algom and his colleagues. The study by Wolf and Algom (1987) provides a striking illustration of the potential of the integration approach in memory psychophysics. In the training session, children learned to associate circles of different hue with each of eight 3-dimensional parallelopipeds. In the later test session, two conditions were used. Children in the Perception condition saw the parallelopipeds again and judged their volume. Children in the Memory condition were presented only the colored circle, asked to remember the shape and judge its volume.

Data for the memory condition are shown in Figure 2.11. The 3-dimensional parallelism in this graph is the diagnostic sign of the 3-variable addition rule:

$$\text{Volume} = \text{Height} + \text{Width} + \text{Depth}.$$

This result confirms the Height + Width rule discussed in the previous subsection, and extends it in two ways. First, it adds a third variable. Second, of central interest, the information processing was based on memorial representation of the stimulus.

The Perception condition showed the very same pattern of data. Since the information processing was necessarily cognitive in the Memory condition, the same was presumably true in the Perception condition. This conclusion was supported in collateral experiments.

This pioneering study points to a new path for psychophysical analysis, which has previously had little contact with memory theory. Data patterns from integration studies, illustrated in Figure 2.11, can shed new light on both memory and perception, when they differ no less than when they agree. In place of the traditional conception of reproductive memory, moreover, the Algom-Wolf approach emphasizes the functional conception of memory as it functions in purposive behavior (see further Algom & Cain, 1991a,b; Algom, Wolf, & Bergman, 1985).

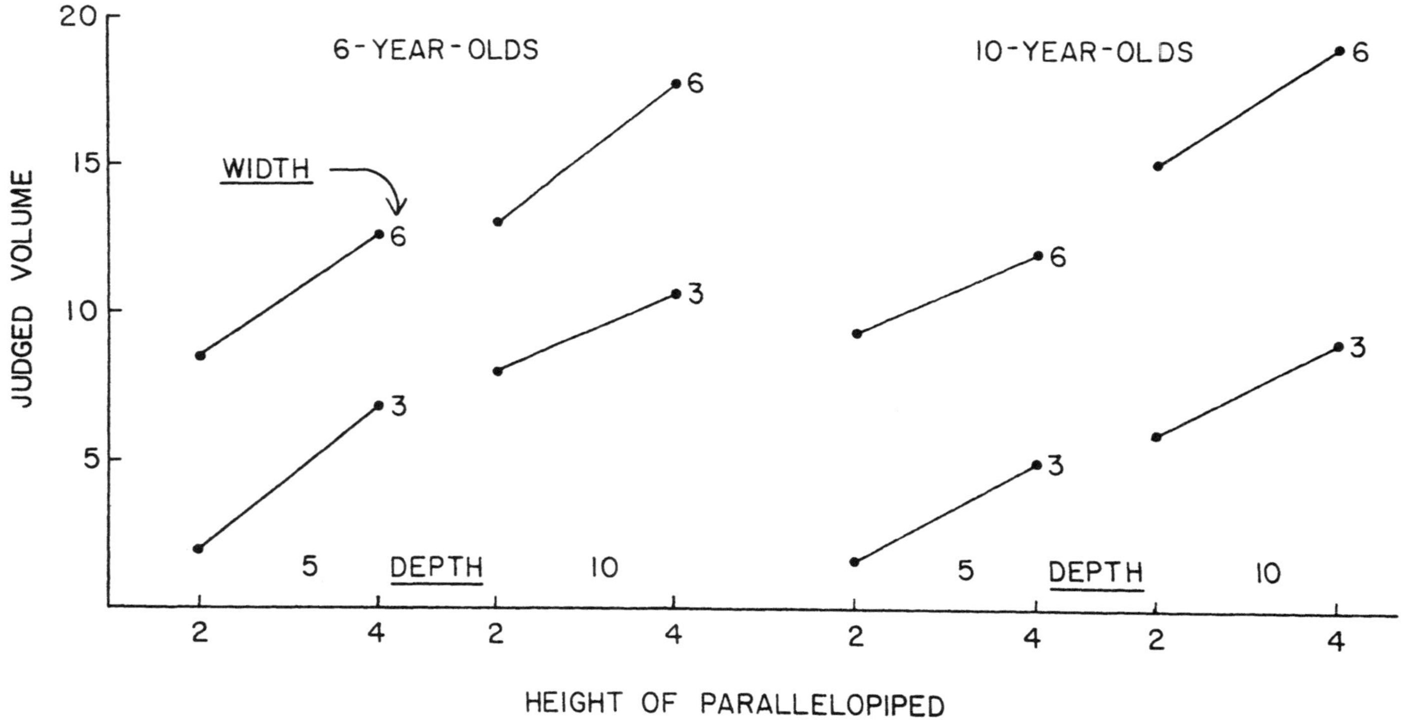

Figure 2.11: Memory psychophysics. Children judge volume of 3-dimensional parallelopipeds by addition rule: Volume = Height + Width + Depth (After Wolf & Algom, 1987).

VIII. Cognition in Psychophysics

Psychophysics has two levels of primary interest: sensory and central. Discovering the pathway between these two levels was a goal set at the earliest stages of scientific psychology, reviewed so well by Boring (1950).

Exploration of this pathway may begin at either level: from the sensory level with an inward direction, or from the central level with an outward direction. The sensory-inward direction has virtually defined classical psychophysics. The main branch is characterized by experimental analysis at the level of the sense organs, with some attention to processes farther down the neural pathway. Much has been learned, and the results cause ever increasing admiration for the engineering capabilities of Nature. The pathway to the center, however, remains shrouded in darkness.

A second branch of classical psychophysics took a more cognitive tack. It sought to traverse the pathway to the center with one bold leap. This was the hypothesis of psychophysical law promulgated by Fechner. Although primarily sensory, the concept of psychophysical law was cognitive in its focus on conscious sensation. It has not, however, been able to solve its own central problem of measuring conscious sensation.

Integration psychophysics differs from classical psychophysics by beginning at the center and working outward. It is essentially cognitive. It shifts the conceptual base from the psychophysical law to the psychocognitive law. The following sections consider some advantages of this cognitive approach.

The Psychophysical Law

The psychophysical law has largely been a conceptual misdirection (Anderson, 1975). It embodies the preconception that a simple mathematical function, the same across all sensory modalities, governs the transformation between physical stimulus and psychological sensation. This preconception became crystallized in Fechner's proposal for a general logarithmic law. Subsequent criticism, although it raised questions about the logarithmic function, only reinforced the preconception. The proposals for a power function (Guilford, 1932; Stevens, 1974) took for granted the basic idea of a simple, general psychophysical law.

This conception of psychophysical law seems inadequate on physiological grounds. "Physiologically, many successive stages lie between the physical stimulus and the conscious sensation. To treat their combined action as a lumped unit may have practical utility, but such a lump seems unlikely to have much psychological meaning" (Anderson, 1975, p.479). The importance of multiple processes or stages in sensory transduction has, of course, been emphasized by many writers (see, e.g., Boynton, 1979, p.203, on color vision and Kroeze, 1990, p. 55f, on taste).

Cognitive considerations also bring out the inadequacy of the concept of psychophysical law. Cognitive psychophysics must be able to handle context effects, nonmetric stimuli, and nonconscious sensation, as well as hedonics, which are discussed in the following sections. All four problems lie outside the conceptual framework of the psychophysical law.

Context Effects

Context effects, as indicated in the title of a previous article (Anderson, 1975), can play a basic role in psychophysical analysis. They have intrinsic importance, as shown in many studies of diverse context effects. Beyond that, they can provide a conceptual-methodological foundation for psychophysics.

The concept of psychophysical law, however, has been inhospitable to context effects. The prototypical psychophysical law is a single-variable function, intended to define "the" relation between the physical stimulus and conscious sensation. Context effects, especially from other sensory modalities, complicate this relation and tend to be avoided. Such simplification strategy is common in science. Often it pays off. Sometimes it goes astray, as did the quest for the psychophysical law.

The ecological importance of context effects needs no argument, as illustrated by the perceptual constancies. These are illusions, in a psychophysical sense, because our perception differs from what is given by the immediate sensory stimulus itself. Size constancy and hue constancy are ecologically useful, however, because they promote stability and veridicality in perception of the environment.

Context effects are a special case of multiple determination. Taste , which generally depends on multiple sensory cues, is just one domain of mixture psychophysics. Various perceptual "illusions," the size-weight illusion, for example, appear to embody ecologically useful integration of past experience in the utilization of present cues.

But although many particular context effects have been studied, general theory is lacking. The conceptual framework of psychophysical law has been an obstacle, partly because it is a single-variable concept, partly because it adopts the sensory-inward direction of investigation.

General theory of context effects requires a fundamental shift. The search for order and law must be cognitive, within the mental realm, not at the sensory periphery. The direction of investigation must be from the center outward. Focus on psychocognitive law makes possible a direct attack on context effects. They need not be an embarrassment; instead, they can be a foundation for theory, as already illustrated in the foregoing empirical studies of context integration.

Nonmetric Stimuli

Nonmetric stimuli are important in psychophysical judgment, but they tend to be passed over in the classical approach. The psychophysical law for grayness, for example, refers to a focal stimulus of uniform reflectance under uniform illumination. This says little about the action of a nonuniform stimulus with variegated reflectance. The effective metric is not then definable in purely physical terms because, in particular, that cannot provide attentional coefficients for different parts of the visual field.

The difficulties increase when context effects are admitted. In the size-weight illusion, for example, the weight can be quantified in grams, but analogous quantification of the visual stimulus is not generally possible. A similar situation appears if the boxes in the illusion of Figure 2.7 are replaced by arbitrary geometric figures. Even with a square box, size is not the effective stimulus because its proximal and distal parts would have different effects.

Classical psychophysics has general difficulty with nonmetric stimuli. This is clearest in the branch concerned with the psychophysical law, which requires a physical metric by definition. It also applies in the sensory branch of psychophysics, which is founded on manipulation of physical parameters (e.g., Boynton, 1979, Chapter 3). This approach has produced impressive results, but it embodies a basic limitation that at some point will halt the sensory-inward direction of investigation.

Functional measurement is not tied to any physical metric. The parallelism and linear fan theorems require only nominal definition of the stimulus. They do not require a prior stimulus metric. Rather, they can measure the subjective values that were functional in the response. This allows psychological metrication of stimuli that have no physical metric. Thurstonian scaling, it may be noted, is not effective with non-metric stimuli for practical reasons stemming from its reliance on imperfect discrimination (Anderson, 1981, Section 5.3). This measurement capability of integration psychophysics is not within the purview of classical psychophysics.

Nonconscious Sensation

Cognitive psychophysics needs a concept of nonconscious sensation. Much sensation, perhaps most, is nonconscious. What reaches consciousness is often, if not typically, the integrated resultant of preconscious sensations.

Apparent length of a short stick, for example, changes noticeably with minor variation in room level illumination (Anderson, 1977). This represents a central integration, since the illumination level has little effect on the retinal image. A preconscious apparent length, independent of illumination, is one factor in this integration. The other factor is brightness, the effect of which may be mediated by learning of the environmental correlation between brightness and distance.

The conscious percept of length is thus preceded in the processing flow by a different, preconscious percept of length.

This situation seems fairly general. Other examples of nonconscious sensation arise in the size-weight illusion (Anderson, 1972, 1975), the circles illusion of Figure 2.8 (Clavadetscher, 1991; Massaro & Anderson, 1971), in taste, already discussed, and in apparent rarefaction (Bressan, Masin, Vicario, & Vidotto, 1985). Conscious sensation is only the tip of an iceberg.

Nonconscious sensation can be defined and measured with integration psychophysics. If an integration function can be established, it can be used to fractionate the conscious sensation into its determinants, which will be nonconscious in many cases. This begins the central-outward analysis: towards the stimulus in one direction -- and towards motor behavior in the other.

Hedonics

Affective reactions are involved in much of everyday behavior. Comfort and discomfort, pleasure and pain, characterize the goal directed approach and avoidance of everyday purposiveness. This functional role of the senses is prominent with taste, smell, pressure, the temperature senses, and pain itself. The importance of these affective reactions is highlighted by cases of their absence, as with hypothermia or with congenital insensitivity to pain.

Affect, however, has been rather neglected. Psychophysics has largely cast itself in the mold of vision and audition, in which affective aspects have minor importance. The study of taste, accordingly, has been much more concerned with intensity than with hedonics.

Affect has been no less neglected by modern cognitive psychologists, many of whom treat affect as outside the pale of cognition. Those who do allow affect to be a legitimate aspect of cognition rarely get farther than saying they have little to say about it.

Affect is information. This is a basic premise of the general theory of information integration (Anderson, 1989). Pleasure and pain are signal information associated with motivational knowledge systems that facilitate survival.

The classical concept of psychophysical law is ill-suited to hedonics. Affective reaction typically has a "bliss point" (McBride, 1990a), an optimum level with a fall-off on either side. Such inverted-U functions obey neither the logarithmic law nor the power law.

Integration psychophysics provides a straightforward approach to hedonics, from the chemical senses (McBride, in press; McBride & Anderson, 1991) to pain (see references in Anderson, 1989). A special advantage is that sensory and nonsensory determinants can be included in the same analysis. The influence of visual appearance on taste of a food, for example, can be assessed using functional measurement methodology.

Integration Psychophysics: The Psychocognitive Law

Integration psychophysics involves a conceptual shift: away from the concept of psychophysical law to the concept of psychocognitive law. In terms of the integration diagram of Figure 2.1, this is a shift away from the valuation function, **V**, which corresponds to the psychophysical law, to the integration function, **I**, which corresponds to the psychocognitive law. This is the foundation of integration psychophysics.

This conceptual shift entails a direct attack on the problem of multiple determination. It then becomes clear that multiple determination is central to psychophysical theory. The traditional single-variable approach of the psychophysical law is not adequate even for sensory psychophysics, much less for the multimodal effects of cognitive psychophysics.

Moreover, the psychocognitive law provides a validational base for the two measurement problems: measurement of stimulus and measurement of response. The psychophysical law, **V**(S), thus becomes determinate. The action function, **A**(ρ), also becomes determinate, an accomplishment almost beyond the horizon of the traditional conception of psychophysical law. All this rests on using the integration function as the base and frame for measurement (Anderson, 1962, 1970).

Integration psychophysics aims to complement sensory psychophysics. It aims to work from the center outward, to link up with work inward from the sensory periphery. An earnest advantage of this approach is its capability for measuring nonconscious sensation.

Integration psychophysics is not really new. "A conception of the organism as an integrator of stimulus information is time honored in perception and judgment" (Anderson, 1974c, p.236). This may be seen in the many studies by many workers on mixture psychophysics, sensory summation, cross-modal effects, adaptation, contrast-assimilation, and other context effects.

Other contributors to this volume have also done important work on integration problems in psychophysics. Foremost, of course, are Marks and

Algom, both of whom have emphasized the role of algebraic models as a foundation for psychophysical investigation. Marks has pursued with imaginative flair integration problems too numerous and diverse to catalog here. Of special interest are the studies of memory psychophysics by Algom and his collaborators (e.g., Algom & Cain, 1991b; Wolf & Algom, 1987). Algom has also contributed to integration analysis of the chemical senses (Algom & Cain, 1991a,b) and pain (Algom, Raphaeli, & Cohen-Raz, 1986) as has Rollman (1983), a topic also discussed in Anderson (1989). Feldman and Baird (1971) introduced a novel task of judging total intensity of paired stimuli of different quality, and this has been followed up by others (Anderson, 1974b; see Ward, 1991, p. 90f). Gescheider (1988) has discussed the use of algebraic rules as a foundation for measurement, and the extensive work of Verillo (1991) and Gescheider, Bolanowski, and Verillo (1989) on vibrotactile sensitivity appears to offer a prime opportunity for the study of sensory integration. Of special interest would be integration studies for cross-modal comparison with work of Algom, Marks, and many others on the other vibration sense of audition. Ward (1990) has done basic work on assimilation-contrast processes in sequential judgment. Melara and Marks (1990a,b) have introduced a new look at the fundamental problem of the psychological reality of the usually taken-for-granted common stimulus dimensions of psychophysics.

Integration psychophysics entails a new way of thinking, different from traditional psychophysics. Some old problems lose their interest; others take on new luster. The problem of context effects, in particular, is seen to provide a new foundation for psychophysical theory (Anderson, 1975), a theme that has been amplified and extended by Algom and Marks (1990) and by Ward (1990). New problems also open up, an "endless frontier" for psychophysical science.

References

Algom, D., & Cain, W.S. (1991a). Chemosensory representation in perception and memory. In S.J. Bolanowski, Jr. & G. Gescheider (Eds.), *Ratio scaling of psychological magnitude* (pp. 183-198). Hillsdale, NJ: Erlbaum.

Algom, D., & Cain, W.S. (1991b). Remembered odors and mental mixtures: Tapping reservoirs of olfactory knowledge. *Journal of Experimental Psychology: Human Perception and Performance*, **17**, 1104-1119.

Algom, D., & Katzir, B. (1990). Sweetness magnitudes and sweetness differences: multiple psychological scales for sucrose. *Chemical Senses*, **15**, 75-85.

Algom, D., & Marks, L.E. (1990). Range and regression, loudness scales, and loudness processing: Toward a context-bound psychophysics. *Journal of Experimental Psychology: Human Perception and Performance*, **16**, 706-727.

Algom, D., Raphaeli, N., & Cohen-Raz, L. (1986). Integration of noxious stimulation across separate somatosensory communications systems: A functional theory of pain. *Journal of Experimental Psychology: Human Perception and Performance*, **12**, 92-102.

Algom, D., Wolf, Y., & Bergman, B. (1985). Integration of stimulus dimensions in perception and memory: Composition rules and psychophysical relations. *Journal of Experimental Psychology: General*, **114**, 451-471.

Anderson, N.H. (1962). On the quantification of Miller's conflict theory. *Psychological Review*, **69**, 400-414.

Anderson, N.H. (1970). Functional measurement and psychophysical judgment. *Psychological Review*, **77**, 153-170.

Anderson, N.H. (1972). Cross-task validation of functional measurement. *Perception & Psychophysics*, **12**, 389-395.

Anderson, N.H. (1974a). Algebraic models in perception. In E.C. Carterette & M.P. Friedman (Eds.), *Handbook of perception* (Volume II, pp.215-298). New York: Academic Press.

Anderson, N.H. (1974b). Cross-task validation of functional measurement using judgments of total magnitude. *Journal of Experimental Psychology*, **102**, 226-233.

Anderson, N.H. (1974c). Information integration theory: A brief survey. In D.H. Krantz, R.C. Atkinson, R.D. Luce, & P. Suppes (Eds.), *Contemporary developments in mathematical psychology* (Volume 2, pp. 236-305). San Francisco: Freeman.

Anderson, N.H. (1975). On the role of context effects in psychophysical judgment. *Psychological Review*, **82**, 462-482.

Anderson, N.H. (1976). Integration theory, functional measurement, and the psychophysical law. In H.-G. Geissler & Yu.M. Zabrodin (Eds.), *Advances in psychophysics* (pp.93-129). Amsterdam: North-Holland.

Anderson, N.H. (1977). Failure of additivity in bisection of length. *Perception & Psychophysics*, **22**, 213-222.

Anderson, N.H. (1978). Measurement of motivation and incentive. *Behavior Research Methods & Instrumentation*, **10**, 360-375.

Anderson, N.H. (1979). Algebraic rules in psychological measurement. *American Scientist*, **67**, 555-563.

Anderson, N.H. (1981). *Foundations of information integration theory*. New York: Academic Press.

Anderson, N.H. (1982). *Methods of information integration theory*. New York: Academic Press.

Anderson, N.H. (1983a). Cognitive algebra in intuitive physics. In H.-G. Geissler (Ed.), *Modern issues in perception* (pp. 229-253). Berlin: VEB Deutscher Verlag.

Anderson, N.H. (1983b). Intuitive physics: Understanding and learning of physical relations. In T.J. Tighe & B.E. Shepp (Eds.), *Perception, cognition, and development* (pp. 231-265). Hillsdale, NJ: Erlbaum.

Anderson, N.H. (1989). Information integration approach to emotions and their measurement. In R. Plutchik & H. Kellerman (Eds.), *Emotion: Theory, research, and experience* (Volume 4, pp.133-186). New York: Academic Press.

Anderson, N.H. (1991a). A cognitive theory of judgment and decision. In N.H. Anderson (Ed.), *Contributions to information integration theory* (Volume I, pp.105-142): *Cognition*. Hillsdale, NJ: Erlbaum.

Anderson, N.H. (1991b). *Contributions to information integration theory*. Volume I: *Cognition*. Hillsdale, NJ: Erlbaum.

Anderson, N.H. (1991c). *Contributions to information integration theory*. Volume II: *Social*. Hillsdale, NJ: Erlbaum.

Anderson, N.H. (1991d). *Contributions to information integration theory*. Volume III: *Developmental*. Hillsdale, NJ: Erlbaum.

Anderson, N.H. (1991e). Schemas in person cognition. In N.H. Anderson (Ed.), *Contributions to information integration theory* (Volume I, pp.57-103): *Cognition*. Hillsdale, NJ: Erlbaum.

Anderson, N.H., & Cuneo, D.O. (1978). The Height + Width rule in children's judgments of quantity. *Journal of Experimental Psychology: General*, **107**, 335-378.

Anderson, N.H., & Wilkening, F. (1991). Adaptive thinking in intuitive physics. In N.H. Anderson (Ed.), *Contributions to information integration theory*. (Volume III, pp.1-42): *Developmental*. Hillsdale, NJ: Erlbaum.

Appley, M.H. (Ed.). (1971). *Adaptation-level theory*. New York: Academic Press.

Birnbaum, M.H., & Elmasian, R. (1977). Loudness "ratios" and "differences" involve the same psychophysical operation. *Perception & Psychophysics*, **22**, 383-391.

Bressan, P., Masin, S.C., Vicario, G., & Vidotto, G. (1985). A functional-measurement study of apparent rarefaction. *Perception & Psychophysics*, **23**, 415-417.

Boring, E.G. (1950). *A history of experimental psychology* (2nd ed.). New York: Appleton-Century-Crofts.

Boynton, R.M. (1979). *Human color vision*. New York: Holt, Rinehart and Winston.

Campbell, D.T., Lewis, N.A., & Hunt, W.A. (1958). Context effects with judgmental language that is absolute, extensive, and extra-experimentally anchored. *Journal of Experimental Psychology*, **55**, 220-228.

Clavadetscher, J.E. (1977). *Two context processes in the Ebbinghaus illusion* (Unpublished doctoral dissertation). La Jolla, CA: University of California, San Diego. *Dissertation Abstracts International*, 1978, 38(9), 4500B.

Clavadetscher, J.E. (1991). Studies of a two process theory for geometric illusions. In N.H. Anderson (Ed.), *Contributions to information integration theory* (Volume I, pp.217-257): *Cognition*. Hillsdale, NJ: Erlbaum.

Clavadetscher, J.E., & Anderson, N.H. (1977). Comparative judgment: Tests of two theories using the Baldwin figure. *Journal of Experimental Psychology: Human Perception and Performance*, **3**, 119-135.

Cuneo, D.O. (1982). Children's judgment of numerical quantity: A new view of early quantification. *Cognitive Psychology*, **14**, 13-44.

De Graaf, C., Frijters, J.E.R., & van Trijp, H.C.M (1987). Taste interaction between glucose and fructose assessed by functional measurement. *Perception & Psychophysics*, **41**, 383-392.

Feldman, J., & Baird, J.C. (1971). Magnitude estimation of multidimensional stimuli. *Perception & Psychophysics*, **10**, 418-422.

Flock, H.R. (1971). Toward a theory of brightness contrast. In M.H. Appley (Ed.), *Adaptation-level theory* (pp.129-146). New York: Academic Press.

Frank, R.A., & Archambo, G. (1986). Intensity and hedonic judgments of taste mixtures: An information integration analysis. *Chemical Senses*, **11**, 427-438.

Garner, W.R. (1974). Attention: The processing of multiple sources of information. In E.C. Carterette & M.P. Friedman (Eds.), *Handbook of perception* (Volume II, pp.23-59). New York: Academic Press.

Garner, W.R., Hake, H.W., & Eriksen, C.W. (1956). Operationism and the concept of perception. *Psychological Review*, **63**, 149-159.

Gescheider, G.A. (1988). Psychophysical scaling. *Annual Review of Psychology*, **39**, 169-200.

Gescheider, G.a., Bolanowski, S.J. Jr., & Verillo, R.T. (1989). Vibrotactile masking: Effects of stimulus onset asynchrony and stimulus frequency. *Journal of the Acoustical Society of America*, **85**, 2059-2064.

Guilford, J.P. (1932). A generalized psychophysical law. *Psychological Review*, **39**, 73-85.

Guilford, J.P. (1954). Psychometric methods (2nd ed.). New York: McGraw-Hill.

Helson, H. (1964). *Adaptation-level theory*. New York: Harper & Row.

Helson, H. (1971). Adaptation-level theory: 1970 - and after. In M.H. Appley (Ed.), *Adaptation-level theory* (pp. 5-17). New York: Academic Press.

Helson, H., & Kozaki, A. (1968). Anchor effects using numerical estimates of simple dot patterns. *Perception & Psychophysics*, **4**, 163-164.

Hornung, D.E., & Enns, M.P. (1984). The independence and integration of olfaction and taste. *Chemical Senses*, **9**, 97-106.

Jordan, K., & Schiano, D.J. (1986). Serial processing and the parallel lines illusion: Length contrast through relative spatial separation of contours. *Perception & Psychophysics*, **40**, 384-390.

Klitzner, M.D. (1975). Hedonic integration: Test of a linear model. *Perception & Psychophysics*, **18**, 49-54.

Krantz, D.H. (1972). A theory of magnitude estimation and cross-modality matching. *Journal of Mathematical Psychology*, **9**, 168-199.

Krantz, D.L., & Campbell, D.T. (1961). Separating perceptual and linguistic effects of context shifts upon absolute judgments. *Journal of Experimental Psychology*, **62**, 35-42.

Kroeze, J.H.A. (1990). The perception of complex taste stimuli. In R.L. McBride & H.J.H. MacFie (Eds.), *Psychological basis of sensory evaluation* (pp.41-68). New York: Elsevier Applied Science.

Krueger, L.E. (1989). Reconciling Fechner and Stevens: Toward a unified psychophysical law. *Behavioral and Brain Sciences*, **12**, 251-320. (Includes commentary and reply).

Kreuger, L.E. (1991). Toward a unified psychophysical law and beyond. In S.J. Bolanski, Jr. & G.A. Gescheider (Eds.), *Ratio scaling of psychological magnitude* (pp. 101-114). Hillsdale, NJ: Erlbaum.

Lopes, L.L., & Oden, G.C. (1980). Comparison of two models of similarity judgment. *Acta Psychologica*, **46**, 205-234.

Luce, R.D. (1959). *Individual choice behavior.* New York: Wiley.

Luce, R.D. (1991). What is a ratio in ratio scaling? In S.J. Bolanowski, Jr. & G.A. Gescheider (Eds.), *Ratio scaling of psychological magnitude* (pp.8-17). Hillsdale, NJ: Erlbaum.

Marks, L.E. (1974). *Sensory processes.* New York: Academic Press.

Marks, L.E. (1979). Sensory and cognitive factors in judgments of loudness. *Journal of Experimental Psychology: Human Perception and Performance*, **5**, 426-443.

Marks, L.E. (1988). Magnitude estimation and sensory matching. *Perception & Psychophysics*, **43**, 511-525.

Massaro, D.W. (1991). Language processing and information integration. In N.H. Anderson (Ed.), *Contributions to information integration theory* (Volume I, pp.259-292): *Cognition*. Hillsdale, NJ: Erlbaum.

Massaro, D.W., & Anderson, N.H. (1971). Judgmental model of the Ebbinghaus illusion. *Journal of Experimental Psychology*, **89**, 147-151.

McBride, R.L. (1989). Three models for taste mixtures. In D.G. Laing, W.S. Cain, R.L. McBride, & B.W. Ache (Eds.), *Perception of complex smells and tastes* (pp. 265-282). Sydney: Academic Press Australia.

McBride, R.L. (1990a). *The bliss point factor.* Melbourne: Macmillan.

McBride, R.L. (1990b). Three generations of sensory evaluation. In R.L. McBride & H.J.H. MacFie (Eds.), *Psychological basis of sensory evaluation* (pp. 195-205). New York: Elsevier Applied Science.

McBride, R.L. (in press). Integration psychophysics: The use of functional measurement in the study of mixtures. *Chemical Senses*.

McBride, R.L., & Anderson, N.H. (1991). Integration psychophysics in the chemical senses. In N.H. Anderson (Ed.), *Contributions to information integration theory* (Volume I, pp.295-319): *Cognition*. Hillsdale, NJ: Erlbaum.

Melara, R.D., & Marks, L.E. (1990a). Perceptual primacy of dimensions: Support for a model of dimensional interaction. *Journal of Experimental Psychology: Human Perception and Performance*, **16**, 398-414.

Melara, R.D., & Marks, L.E. (1990b). Processes underlying dimensional interactions: Correspondences between linguistic and nonlinguistic dimensions. *Memory & Cognition*, **18**, 477-495.

Michotte, A.E. (1963). *The perception of causality*. (T.R. Miles & E. Miles, trans.). London: Methuen. (Original work published 1946).

Oden, G.C., & Massaro, D.W. (1978). Integration of featural information in speech perception. *Psychological Review*, **85**, 172-191.

Parducci, A. (1974). Contextual effects: A range-frequency analysis. In E.C. Carterette & M.P. Friedman (Eds.), *Handbook of perception* (Volume II, pp. 127-141). New York: Academic Press.

Pressey, A.W., & Wilson, A.E. (1980). Assimilation theory and the Baldwin illusion. *Italian Journal of Psychology*, **7**, 65-73.

Restle, F. (1971). Visual illusions. In M.H. Appley (Ed.), *Adaptation-level theory* (pp.55-69). New York: Academic Press.

Restle, F. (1978). Assimilation predicted by adaptation-level theory with variable weights. In N.J. Castellan, Jr., & F. Restle (Eds.), *Cognitive theory* (Volume 3, pp.75-91). Hillsdale, NJ: Erlbaum.

Rollman, G.B. (1983). Measurement of experimental pain in chronic pain patients: Methodological and individual factors. In R. Melzack (Ed.), *Pain measurement and assessment* (pp.251-258). New York: Raven.

Schlottmann, A. (1987). *Judgments of causality in the perception of launch events*. Unpublished M.S. Thesis. La Jolla, CA: University of California, San Diego.

Schlottmann, A., & Anderson, N.H. (1990). An information integration approach to perception of causality. Unpublished paper. La Jolla, CA: University of California, San Diego.

Stevens, S.S. (1958). Adaptation-level vs. the relativity of judgment. *American Journal of Psychology*, **71**, 633-646.

Stevens, S.S. (1974). Perceptual magnitude and its measurement. In E.C. Carterette & M.P. Freidman (Eds.), *Handbook of perception* (Volume II, pp.361-689). New York: Academic Press.

Suppes, P., Krantz, D.H., Luce, R.D., & Tversky, A. (1989). *Foundations of measurement* (Volume II). New York: Academic Press.

Tversky, A. (1977). Features of similarity. *Psychological Review*, **84**, 327-352.

Verrillo, R.T. (1991). Measurement of vibrotactile sensation magnitude. In S.J. Bolanowski, Jr. & G.A. Gescheider (Eds.), *Ratio scaling of psychological magnitude* (pp. 260-275). Hillsdale, NJ: Erlbaum.

Ward, L.M. (1990). Critical bands and mixed-frequency scaling: Sequential dependencies, equal-loudness contours, and power function exponents. *Perception & Psychophysics*, **47**, 551-562.

Ward, L.M. (1991). Associative measurement of psychological magnitude. In S.J. Bolanski, Jr. & G.A. Gescheider (Eds.), *Ratio scaling of psychological magnitude* (pp.79-100). Hillsdale, NJ: Erlbaum.

Wilkening, F. (1982). Children's knowledge about time, distance, and velocity interrelations. In W.J. Friedman (Ed.), *The developmental psychology of time* (pp. 87-112). New York: Academic Press.

Wolf, Y., & Algom, D. (1987). Perceptual and memorial constraints in children's judgments of quantity: A law of across-representation invariance. *Journal of Experimental Psychology: General*, **116**, 381-397.

Zalinski, J., & Anderson, N.H. (1991). Parameter estimation for averaging theory. In N.H. Anderson (Ed.), *Contributions to information integration theory* (Volume I, pp. 353-394): *Cognition*. Hillsdale, NJ: Erlbaum.

Psychophysical Approaches to Cognition
D. Algom (Editor)

3

"WHAT THIN PARTITIONS SENSE FROM THOUGHT DIVIDE": TOWARD A NEW COGNITIVE PSYCHOPHYSICS[1]

Lawrence E. Marks

John B. Pierce Laboratory

and

Yale University

[1] Preparation of this chapter was supported in part by grant DC-00818 from the National Institutes of Health. I thank Daniel Algom and Bonnie Potts for comments on an earlier version. Please direct correspondence to Lawrence E. Marks, John B. Pierce Laboratory, 290 Congress Avenue, New Haven, CT 06519.

Table of Contents

I. Overview

O for a life of sensations rather than of thoughts.

-- John Keats

The Window Hypothesis

While reviewing research on iconic memory, Paul Kolers (1983) questioned the claim that visual icons -- the immediate, very short-term "residue" of optic stimulation -- simply reflect the output from an early precategorical stage of information processing:

> It was never exactly clear how reports of the unrecoded information could be made, however. To claim them implies an Unbiased Reporter: a reporter of mental events that can accurately reveal the contents of an operation without influencing it or being influenced by it.
>
> The assumption of the Unbiased Reporter is similar to the assumption made by the advocates of analytical introspectionism as the model technique of cognitive psychology ..., and is subject to the same complaints. The introspectionists sought the sensory elements of experience, the first stage in the mind's acquisition of information from physical objects. In doing so, they assumed that the remainder of the mind could be disconnected from its "front end" that responded to sensory stimuli, and that an Unbiased Reporter could report selectively on the features processed there .... The Introspectionists did not always appreciate that what they

> experienced as sensations were the result of extensive processing by mind, not some initial stage. Many students of cognition now seem to miss the same point -- that what can be reported as a perceptual event is the result of extensive operations carried out by the visual mechanisms, and not some selected content or stage. (pp. 134-135).

Let us not fail to include among the "many students of cognition" many psychophysicists; for I suspect, indeed I fear, that a kind of insidious neotitchenerianism continues today, largely unabated despite the widespread disavowal of Titchener's explicitly formulated research program, and relatively unfettered by the considerable body of empirical evidence -- a very small part of which I shall review later on -- suggesting that cognitive processes permeate the so-called "sensations." Perception is not merely a constellation or bundle of sensory elements, with each element reflecting some sort of underlying -- though typically unconscious and not otherwise directly accessible -- *Urprozess*.

But even though psychophysicists as well as other cognitive psychologists "know" this, there is a strong tendency nevertheless on the part of some students of the senses and the mind often to assume that, under certain well-controlled and well-constrained experimental conditions, the "back end" of the mind -- with all of its experiences and expectancies and strategies -- can be made transparent, and consequently that perceptual judgments may thereby provide a window into the transduction and subsequent sensory processing that take place at the perceptual "front end." For convenience, I shall call this assumption the Window Hypothesis.

Now, I have little doubt that the Window Hypothesis sometimes is correct. Consider, for example, absolute thresholds for detecting visual stimuli of various wavelengths falling on the retinal periphery of a dark-adapted eye. Whether the Window Hypothesis fails or succeeds will depend on our perspective -- on whether we examine the individual thresholds per se, or the relationship amongst them. On the one hand, the particular values of threshold depend not only on relatively early, peripheral processing of sensory information but also on the location of the internal criterion that the person uses to decide when to respond, "yes, I see it," and therefore also on subsequent high-level decisional processes sensitive to expectations, pay-offs, and so forth, all of which contribute to the location of the response criterion; this is to say that thresholds per se reveal how cognition can infiltrate perception.

On the other hand, it is possible to hold the decisional processes constant, thereby keeping the response criterion constant, while measuring the way that thresholds change as a function of the stimulus wavelength. The *spectral sensitivity curve* determined in this manner does very largely if not wholly represent a concatenation of early visual processes: the filtering of incident light energy by the optic media and the absorption spectrum of the photopigment rhodopsin in retinal rods. In this regard, it is also important to note that, at scotopic threshold, stimuli of different wavelengths are indistinguishable (see the later discussion of metamerism in color vision). Consequently, in this example it seems reasonable to uphold the Window Hypothesis -- reasonable to the extent that we are concerned with this high-order feature of the psychophysical data, namely a constant-response function or invariance function known as spectral sensitivity.

To repeat, then, the Window Hypothesis surely is sometimes correct. Still, it is not self-evidently correct; neither is it wholly clear under just what conditions it will be correct, nor whether there is a general set of principles that will make it possible to discern when it will be correct. And without such principles it is necessary to "bootstrap," that is, to decide on a case-by-case, ad hoc basis. Contrary to William Blake, it seems unlikely that "if the doors of perception were cleansed everything would appear as it is ...."

Recall that Kolers (1983) disputed the contention that perceptual reports based upon visual icons reflect nothing but afterimages (which is not to say that reports of afterimages reflect only early processing in the visual system; Emmert's law suggests otherwise). In a similar vein, later in this chapter I shall dispute the view that psychophysical judgments of loudness reflect nothing but some measure of excitation in the auditory system.[2] Of course there are times in which perceptual reports or psychophysical judgments *do* tell us something directly about "front-end" sensory processes; but I believe that the number of circumstances in which this is so is very limited and, therefore, rarely encountered. Consequently, we should be duly cautious whenever we may be tempted to apply the Window Hypothesis; for it is imperative to keep in mind a rather simple dictum or postulate -- that every psychophysical judgment, no matter how seemingly elementary, is fundamentally a cognitive act.[3]

Perception and Sensation

To suggest that cognitive processes infuse perception may seem hardly to say anything that is new or provocative. After all, Helmholtz (e.g., 1866/1925) made the same point more than a century ago, when he proposed that perception involves the superposition of an inferential structure, his well-known *unbewusster Schluss*, onto sensory inputs. So let me make an additional suggestion, intended to be more clearly provocative: that cognitive processes also penetrate *sensation*.

---

[2] Perhaps we should always be wary of the "nothing buts" of psychology: Animals are nothing but hydraulic machines, thought Descartes; the mind is nothing but a computer, think some contemporary cognitive scientists. (Do computers think so too?)

[3] Many years ago, while I was still in graduate school, it was the late Paul Kolers who repeatedly insisted to me that all percepts, even the perceptions of single pure tones heard in silence or lone spots of light seen in darkness, involved cognitive processing. It has taken many years for the impact of this observation fully to infiltrate my mind.

It is commonplace to contend that cognitive processes affect perception. But is it provocative to contend that they affect sensation? To answer affirmatively is, I would claim, to adhere to the neotitchenerianism I mentioned before, a position in which I identify three main components: (a) that sensory processes precede perceptual processes, (b) that the sensory processes form the "front end" of perceptual information processing, and (c) that some seemingly basic or primitive properties of perceptual experiences can provide windows into the early sensory processes. These basic or primitive properties we often call "sensations."

One of my goals in this chapter is to explain why this account of sensation and perception is inadequate, which is analogous to saying that one goal is to recount some of the ways in which cognition can infiltrate the kinds of processing that are usually considered "sensory." But there is another goal, and perhaps an even more important one: to assess the historical roots for the distinction between sensation and perception and thereby to explore certain deep implications that I believe to inhere in that distinction; for it is my position that the distinction between sensation and perception -- and its cousin, the Window Hypothesis -- entail a particular vision of sensory and perceptual science; to state it crudely, it is a vision of sensory science as a Platonistic system of universals and perceptual science as an Aristotelian system of concrete particulars.

II. Psychophysics and Cognition; Causality and Representation

Sweet exists by convention, bitter by convention, color by convention; atoms and void (alone) exist in reality.

-- Democritus

Psychophysics, even when construed in its narrowest and most esoteric form is in its methods and concepts an intimate to cognitive psychology. Although the psychophysical analysis of perception may seem, like that *rara avis*, an obedient child, quietly to inhabit one modest corner of the edifice of human information processing, nevertheless, it was the broadly-based psychophysics of the last century that gave birth to the procedures, indeed the very styles, of much (though surely not all) of contemporary cognitive research. We might even say, paraphrasing Wordsworth, that "the psychophysical child is father to the cognitive man."

Of course, to view psychophysics and cognition as in some wise cognate domains would hardly have surprised dear old Gustav Fechner (1860), whose own definition of psychophysics -- as the science that concerns itself with quantitative relations between mental phenomena and their physical correlates -- was so broad that it could encompass, or at least touch on, virtually every aspect of psychological science. It may be useful to keep in mind, as Scheerer (1987) tells us, that Fechner's "inner psychophysics is virtually extensive with his psychology" (p. 200) and that, as Boring (1957) surmised, Fechner intended his psychophysics to buttress his metaphysics. Many a psychophysics is linked to a metaphysics, but few scientists are as explicit about their philosophies as Fechner, whose speculations on mind in the universe evoked little sympathy among psychologists of the last century or the present one -- with the notable exception of William James (1909) who wrote enthusiastically about Fechner's "thick" philosophy, much richer and more dense than those "thin" philosophies of his time that so dismayed James.

In any case, to put it anachronistically, Fechner's psychophysics of sensation aimed to serve as a prototype or model system for a much more pervasive discipline -- and in particular, as a prototype for a generic psychophysics that was in principle coextensive with cognitive psychology, or at least with cognitive neuroscience. Unfortunately, through the century that followed Fechner, in a route that would take me too long to retrace, psychophysics came to wither in the imagination of many psychologists, until it found itself taking on its contemporary status, to numbers of those outside the field, of an esoteric and largely methodological discipline. This view, however, I think is mistaken, and one of my aims is to show how psychophysics falls squarely in psychology's main arena.

At the very least, it seems necessary to affirm that the borders of psychophysics -- however rigid or elastic we may view them -- are contiguous with those of cognitive psychology (see, for example, Baird, 1970a, 1970b, for a relatively early characterization of psychophysics as cognitive). Cognition deals broadly with the acquisition, characterization, and use of knowledge, and given this definition it seems clear to me that the psychophysical approach to sensory and perceptual processing falls squarely within cognition -- as a couple of thousand years of history also reminds us. For when the early Greek philosophers began to ask questions that became central to Western epistemology -- What do we know? How do we know what is real? -- and began to explore multitudinous Nature, these philosophers inquired, among other topics, into the processes of perception, in a quest to determine whether, when, or how we may trust perception to provide us with accurate and valid knowledge about the world around us.

Roots of Psychophysical Thinking

This is no place, of course, to try to recount in detail the early history of epistemological inquiry, which in many instances tended to laud Reason as the highest cognitive faculty, often if not typically at the expense of Perception. But it is useful nevertheless, I think, to sketch very briefly a couple of related but distinct theories that emerged around the fifth century BCE, for those theories will be relevant to my primary issues.

Effluence theories of perception. First of all, it was this period, nearly two and a half millennia ago, that saw the emergence of *eidola* or effluence theories of perception, that is, theories that conceived of perception as the reception of images or likenesses of objects, copies of themselves that objects emit and that subsequently impinge upon sensory systems. According to such a theory, the table in front of me, for instance, sends out its *eidolon* or image, which subsequently enters my eyes and thereby makes it possible for me to see its source, the table itself. In its earliest versions we may characterize such *eidola* theories as *realist* theories of perception, though from the vantage of our modern eye they exemplify a rather primitive sort of realism.

At first glance, the theory of *eidola* suggests an indirect sort of realism, since the perceiver does not respond directly to stimulus objects but instead responds to their effluences, which presumably resemble their sources. But for a sense modality like vision, which responds to objects located some distance away from the eyes, effluence theories are about as direct as causal realist theories get. Consequently, it may be more fruitful to think of *eidola* theories as being in some vague sense forerunners of modern theories of *direct* perception -- and thus to think of Empedocles as an intellectual forerunner to Gibson (1979) -- at least, *if* we are willing to conceive *eidola* as conveying not just some kind of stimulus energies, but high-level stimulus information.[4] In informational terms, *eidola* would presumably correspond to, contain, or simply be the internal structures of their objects, structures that in turn could, would, or should be defined through an appropriate set of quantitative functions, mathematical or geometric. I shall leave it to others, however, to explore the further implications of this last suggestion -- and in particular to examine any implications to the intriguing though perhaps irrelevant historical note that Empedocles himself supposedly was a Pythagorean.

Atomist theories of perception. Let me turn now to a second theory, which arose roughly contemporaneously with *eidola* theory. This was the theory of *atomism*. According to the early Greek atomists, notably Leucippus and his student Democritus, the universe comprises nothing but an infinitude of tiny, solid, indivisible particles -- the atoms; and betwixt and amongst these atoms resides only empty space. According to Theophrastus, a rough contemporary of Aristotle, and from whom we learn a good deal about early Greek views on perception, the atoms that constitute perceptual objects vary in three ways, to wit: "[S]ome [Democritus] distinguishes by the size [of their atoms], others by the shape, and a few by the [atomic] order and position" (De sensibus, 60, in Stratton, 1917, p. 121). Thus, in Democritus's theory all perceptible objects reduce to multidimensional variations in spatial configuration, or what, two millennia later, John Locke (1690) would include within the domain of "secondary qualities" of objects.

[4] It is not clear, however, whether the distinction between stimulus energy and stimulus information can easily be made with respect to Empedocles's theory of sensation.

A bit of thought can easily lead us to see why Democritus's atomism entailed an early kind of psychophysics. By implication, this theory demands that the plethora of perceptual qualities -- colors, sounds, tastes, smells -- depends in some fashion on the spatial dimensions of atoms, since it is only their spatial characteristics that individuate them; and unlike Empedocles, who had little to say about the psychophysical relations of percepts to their objects (though he did try to explain why the senses are specialized to perceive different objects, to wit, that each sense has a different size of pores, or apertures, that permit the *eidola* to enter), Democritus speculated systematically about what such functional relations between percepts and atoms might be:

> What is 'sour', he holds, is at once 'angular' in its [atomic figure] and is 'twisted', minute, and thin. By its keenness it swiftly slips in and penetrates everywhere, and by its roughness and 'angularity' it draws the parts together and binds them .... 'Sweet' consists of [atomic figures that are rounded and not too small; wherefore it quite softens the body by its gentle action, and unhastening makes its way throughout. (Theophrastus, De sensibus, 65, in Stratton, 1917, pp. 123-124).

Democritus's psychophysics appears to rest largely on analogy or metaphor between the qualities of sensory experience and the physical properties of atoms that he presumed to underlie these qualities (see also Hartshorne, 1934), and it has as its starting point the inference that because colors and tastes are not themselves spatial, then, consequently, colors and tastes themselves are not "real":

> Other than hardness and heaviness, none of the other sensory objects has an objective reality, but ... one and all are effects in our sensuous faculty as it undergoes alteration, -- and ...

> from this faculty arises the inner presentation .... Proof that [these sensory qualities] are not objectively real is found in the fact that they do not appear the same to all creatures; what is sweet to us is bitter to others, and to still others it is sour or pungent or astringent; and similarly of the other [sensory qualities]. (Theophrastus, De sensibus, 63, in Stratton, 1917, p. 123).

Indeed, in what is undoubtedly Democritus's best-known adage -- the epigraph to this section -- he says that sensory qualities such as sweet and salty, black and white, exist only "by convention," which is to say, only as a set of qualities in a percipient organism, as effects that depend upon but nevertheless are ontologically distinct from the atoms and empty space that alone constitute physical reality.

Atomism and causal theories of perception. It has doubtless struck the reader that Democritus's theory denies perceptual realism, for it denies that what we perceive corresponds accurately to the reality presumably lurking behind our perception. Quite to the contrary, the theory constitutes a brand of representationalism, in that it postulates the existence of an inner "presentation" or *phantasian*; furthermore, we should note that Democritean theory by its very nature entails a causal model of perception, in which atomic configurations *cause* the perceptions of variegated qualities.

Now, there is a trivial version of causal theory, by which all theories of perception are causal -- to the extent that all may be cast in the form "X causes Y," where X is an object or event (or its effluence) and Y is the perception of that object or event. But Democritus's theory implies more than this; it implies an *intermediate* causal stage, where X causes X', and where X' (somehow) causes (or constitutes) Y. The intermediary X' itself constitutes a change in the sensorium -- a change wrought by the particular configuration of the atoms that fit into sensory passages. By this interpretation of "causal," causal theories are representational, though representational theories need not be causal; similarly, atomistic theories like that of Democritus are predictably representational, though representational theories need not rely on an atomistic physical theory.

More than two thousand years later, with the emergence of modern science in the seventeenth and eighteenth centuries, Galileo, Newton, Locke, and others would speculate on the correspondences between stimulus and sensation, thereby following a line of thought analogous to that established by Democritus (though not necessarily derived from Democritus); many of these later speculations -- Isaac Newton's visual theory, for example -- would be even more explicit in postulating intermediate stages of causality. Moreover, because all of these theories rest on the assumption that the qualities of perception differ from the qualities of the physical world, such theories must entail at least implicitly a set of rules or laws that relate the former to the latter, rules or laws that tell us how percepts depend on their stimuli.

Representationalism and psychophysics. From this brief survey, I shall pick up the two main, intertwined threads that can be identified in Democritus's atomistic theory of perception: The first is the notion that perceptions exemplify, *inter alia*, mental representations; and the second is the notion that a certain class of natural laws -- a set of psychophysical rules -- regularly and systematically can serve to connect these perceptions, or perceptual representations, to the physical stimuli that cause them.

The general notion of representation, incorporating perceptual representations, lies at the heart of contemporary cognitive psychology, at least, as cognitive psychology is practiced in its majoritarian form. To many, perhaps most cognitive psychologists, knowledge consists of a set of mental representations, often though not always conceived to be "symbolic" information that is stored, retrieved, and otherwise acted upon by a set of "well-defined" processes, procedures, or computations. The use of quotations in the last sentence is meant to serve as a warning: For one, though it is often tempting to treat "symbolic" as equivalent to "propositional" or "linguistic," it is useful to recognize that perception (visual, auditory, olfactory, and so forth) can equally well be conceived as symbolic; and for another, the processes, procedures, or computations may be well-defined in principle -- if we only knew what the principles were!

Sensory psychophysics deals in large measure with the (again, in principle) equally well-defined correspondences between external stimuli and resulting perceptual representations. By linking sensory meanings to their stimulus objects, sensory psychophysics provides, in Fodor's (1981) terms, a kind of semantic theory of perception -- a limited one to be sure, a semantic minitheory -- of the sort that perhaps is needed more broadly if cognitive psychology is not only to interpret behavior in terms of the internal manipulations of abstract symbols, but to relate those hypothetical symbols-being-hypothetically-manipulated to their less hypothetical referents.

Primary and secondary qualities. Causal theories of perception may seem "natural". If so, then they may seem so "natural" in part because causal theories are ... well ... so patently *scientific*. After all, physical science has done remarkably well for centuries by relying on causal theories. Indeed, in Newton's time, the notion that physical forces had to act locally -- a familiar example is the way billiard balls impart momentum when they strike one another -- made it hard for some of his contemporaries to accept the notion that certain forces, like gravity, can act at a distance, without direct contact between objects. So perhaps it should not be surprising that as physical science met greater and greater success in the seventeenth and eighteenth centuries, notions about the processes of perception piggybacked along.

Newton himself tried to bridge the gap between the physical specification of the world and the perceptual. He expressed very nicely a causal view of visual perception when he wrote

> ... when a Man views any Object, ... the Light which comes from the several Points of the Object is so refracted ... as to converge and meet again ... in the bottom of the Eye, and there to paint a Picture of the Object upon [the retina] .... And these Pictures, propagated by Motion along the Fibers of the Optick Nerves into the Brain, are the cause of Vision. (Newton, 1730/1952, p. 15).

Like Galileo before him, Newton distinguished sharply between the domains of physics and psychology; and to each domain would be rendered its proper due. Where Newton, like Democritus, an atomist (of sorts), pointed out that light, which belongs to the physical realm, can vary in its refrangeability (refraction, which depends on wavelength), color is a whole different kettle of fish. We shouldn't confuse what is in the external object with what is in our minds, a psychophysical distinction that had not been lost on Galileo, a generation earlier:

> I do not believe that for exciting in us tastes, odors, and sounds there are required in external bodies anything but sizes, shapes, numbers, and slow or rapid movements; and I think that if ears, tongues, and noses were taken away, shapes, numbers, and motions would remain, but not odors or tastes or sounds (Galileo, 1623/1960, p. 311).

In modern parlance, we might say that the colors black and white, the musical pitches corresponding to A-flat and C-sharp, and the tastes sour and sweet are *subjective*, or perhaps that they are attributes characterizing internal representations of external events. They constitute the "perceptions of secondary qualities," to use the terminology of John Locke (1690) -- himself in several respects a Newtonian: not only because he accepted Newton's views on physics, but perhaps even more importantly because he latched onto Newton's scheme in the realm of physics and extended it into the realm of ideas, into the realm of mental representations, which is to say, into the realm of psychology.

Two main distinctions emerge in Locke's theory, the one distinguishing physical qualities from the perception of them, and the second distinguishing primary qualities from secondary qualities (and from tertiary ones, which I shall not consider here). To start, note that Locke follows the tradition of referring to qualities per se as properties of objects (or events) in the physical world. Qualities belong to the domain of physics. Two main subdivisions of qualities are primary and secondary -- or, roughly speaking, macroscopic and microscopic. Primary qualities characterize the relatively large-scale spatial and temporal properties of objects, and, according to Locke, we do perceive these qualities much "as they are." So it is that the texture of the keys on my computer's keyboard, the shape of its monitor, and the number of lines of text on the screen, all of these primary qualities are discernible by vision (and the first two also by touch; primary qualities include what Aristotle called the "common sensibles").

Secondary qualities, by way of contrast, exist on a much smaller scale; they are like Democritus's atoms, *individually* invisible or inaudible or intangible -- and consequently too small, too finely grained to be perceived "as they are." Instead, secondary qualities produce within us perceptions that are intrinsically dissimilar to their causes. So it is that my computer's keyboard is mauve, and the border around the screen and the text itself are colored black.

Where Democritus, Galileo, and Locke had speculated upon the possibilities of a perceptual psychophysics, Newton and others would begin to construct an empirical psychophysics of perceptual systems -- so that it's fair to say that by the time psychology emerged in the mid-nineteenth century as an independent and identifiable experimental discipline, new generations would seek to catch up to the experimental psychophysics of Newton and Young, of Helmholtz and Johannes Müller, of Weber and Fechner, a psychophysics that was already grounded epistemologically in notions of causality and representation.

Let me say something here about what a causal/representational theory is or can be, and what it is not or need not be. In particular, such a theory need not displace the object of perception from outside to inside the organism, though some versions of the theory mistakenly do so. So, for example, when Johannes Müller (1838/1842) translated Locke's theory of the perception of secondary qualities into the realm of sensory physiology, Müller suggested just such an incoherent interpretation: that the object of sensation resides in the sensorium:

> That which through the medium of our senses is actually perceived by the sensorium, is indeed merely a property or change of conditions of our nerves; but the imagination and reason are ready to interpret the modifications in the state of the nerves produced by external influences as properties of the external bodies themselves. This mode of regarding sensations has become so habitual in the case of the senses which are more rarely affected by internal causes, that it is only on reflection that we perceive it to be erroneous .... (p. 1061).

> VIII. *The immediate objects of the perception of our senses are merely particular states induced in the nerves, and felt as sensations either by the nerves themselves or by the sensorium; but inasmuch as the nerves of the senses are material bodies, and therefore participate in the properties of matter generally occupying space, being susceptible of vibratory motion, and capable of being*

> *changed chemically as well as by the action of heat and electricity, they make known to the sensorium, by virtue of the changes thus produced in them by external causes, not merely their own condition, but also properties and changes of condition of external nature, varies in each sense, having a relation to the qualities or energies of the nerve*. (p. 1073).

To talk about perceptions of secondary (or even of primary) qualities risks the danger of talking, as Müller does, of "the immediate objects of the perception of our senses" being "the particular states induced in the nerves," and consequently of perception as the act of observing an internal representation -- as if what I now "see" is the mental representation in my mind, or the neural representation in my brain, of the computer resting on my desk. But of course what I *see* is the computer itself. To be sure, the activity in my brain is somehow related to my seeing the computer, and perhaps this neural activity bears some type-type relation to the mental representation of the computer. But I don't *see* that representation; presumably, my seeing is that representation.

III. Psychophysics, Information Processing, and Perception: The Search for Invariances

He is a barbarian, and thinks that
the customs of his tribe and island
are the laws of nature.
-- George Bernard Shaw

Endemic to many theories of human information processing in general, and to psychophysical theories in particular, is the notion of sequential processing. Indeed, it seems hard to imagine how to conceptualize the processing of information in any terms that fail to incorporate logically distinct mechanisms, if not at least partially temporally distinct ones -- however interactive these mechanisms may be. Moreover, the view that information is processed in such a fashion that outputs from one stage form inputs to the next stage has seen at least a few notable successes.

The Perception of Color

Consider, to take a prominent example, the matter of human color vision, for which we have a well-developed, "normative," contemporary theory, grounded in reliable, coherent, and often quite precise psychophysical, anatomical, and physiological evidence. The theory incorporates the following sequence of stages or zones, which, for present purposes, I shall simplify as follows: (a) passive optical filtering of light by the ocular media; (b) spectrally selective absorption of light quanta by distinctive classes of receptors (most importantly, by the three types of cone; I ignore for this purpose any residual role that retinal rods may play types of cone; I ignore for this purpose any residual role that retinal rods may play in color perception); and (c) transformation of trireceptor responses to a set of color-opponent processes (for reviews, see Boynton, 1979; Hurvich, 1981).

This generic color theory, with its crucial distinction between an early receptor stage and a later opponent-process stage, has several virtues: For one, the theory explains different sorts of phenomenological and psychophysical results (for instance, it explains color blindness and color matching in terms of processes that are inherent in the sensitivities of individual receptor-types; and it explains color contrast and color interactions in terms of the characteristics of opponent processes). For another, as already indicated, the theory squares rather well with known anatomical and physiological structures in the visual system.

Color as a model system. In many respects, color vision might seem to provide an ideal system for characterizing perceptual information processing more generally. For instance, the information processed at each stage in the system can be considered to provide a kind of local representation, with one stage linked causally to another stage or set of stages. The underlying principle of sequential processing need not exclude all sorts of parallel processes, including interactions between different subsystems, feedback and feedforward within systems, and so forth. That is, spatial or temporal sequencing need not be complete or exclusive. What the presence of such interactions means, however, is that it will be so much more difficult to isolate the events that arise at a given stage. And more importantly, such interactions, especially feedback and what are often called "top-down" interactions, make more problematic than many of us would like the discovery of basic invariances.

Metamerism and the limitations of color as a model. Having just made the case that color vision provides a good model system, I would now like to argue that color may in fact provide a dangerously misleading *generic* model for perceptual information processing. Color is misleading, I think, because a primary dichotomy between color stages -- the split between receptor-based processing and later opponent processing -- derives from what is largely a peculiarity of the color system that may have few significant parallels elsewhere. I refer here to the property of *metamerism*.

Color vision is said to be metameric because, or to the extent that, it is possible to identify physically different optical stimuli -- lights that differ in their spectral composition -- that nevertheless are perceptually indistinguishable. For instance, it is possible to mix long wavelength (red) light, say of 700 nm, and middle wavelength (yellow) light, say of 560 nm, to produce an orange that looks just like an intermediate wavelength, say of 600 nm -- to which perhaps a dram of white light needs be added so as to compensate for the desaturation that invariably arises from mixing pure colors.

Now, the crucial point is that metamerism in color vision finds its physiological basis in what has been termed the "principle of univariance" (e.g., Rushton, 1972), according to which the outputs of visual receptors depend solely on the number of quanta of light that the receptors absorb, and not at all on the wavelength of the light. Though Nature may have tried to make visual receptors work like coarse light meters, it did not, or could not, get them to work like even crude spectrometers.

<u>Individual visual receptors are color blind</u>. Given the principle of univariance, we may draw the following inference: From the output from any one receptor alone it is impossible to determine anything at all about the wavelength of light. This is to say, as long as a receptor catches a constant number of light quanta, the receptor's output will be fixed. Consequently, there is a potential infinitude (or at least, a very great number) of possible ways to make a given receptor cell produce a given level of output; for regardless of the wavelength of

light, it is always possible to adjust the physical intensity of light impinging on the receptor in order to produce a given output. In this sense, therefore, any single receptor is "color blind", and its response to any and all wavelengths can be metameric.

With three different kinds of receptor, to be sure, the system as a whole is more constrained -- but the general principle remains as true for the triumvirate as it does for any member: Whenever the quantum catches of all three receptors are identical, their outputs will be identical, and thus the lights are metameric, which is to say, they will appear identical perceptually. For if the outputs from the receptors are identical under two different stimulus conditions, it is safe to presume that all subsequent processes imposed on those outputs will also yield identical outcomes.

By definition, the metamerism of color vision means that a wide range of different stimuli can give rise to a constant perceptual effect. There are lots of ways to make orange or turquoise or white. Another way to think about this is as follows: When two lights are metameric, from which we infer that the outputs at the trireceptor level are identical, either light could be substituted for the other without any consequence for subsequent processing. So, for example, regardless of the language that I use to describe or carve up the domain of colors, regardless of my prior experience with colored objects and chromatic illuminations, either recent or remote in time, or regardless of any other factor that may influence just how I encode, judge, compare, or remember colors, all of these behaviors will be subject to the constraints imposed by metameric properties of color vision. No matter what happens at the mind's "back end," the way I perceive, describe, categorize, or remember a monochromatic orange, produced by a single wavelength of light at 600 nm, will be identical to the way I perceive, describe, categorize, or remember a metamerically equivalent orange compounded of lights of 560 and 700 nm.

Metamerism and Cognitive Impenetrability

Perhaps it is useful to cast metamerism within the framework of Pylyshyn's (1984) dichotomy between phenomena that are cognitively penetrable and those that are impenetrable. According to Pylyshyn, certain phenomena or processes are not "hard-wired", but can depend on what takes place at the mind's "back end"; these processes are not immune to a person's experiences, beliefs, desires, and so forth, but depend in a coherent and rationally explicable way on some inferential, cognitive structures; such phenomena are said to be cognitively penetrable. Other phenomena or processes are not readily affected in these ways by cognition, and consequently are called cognitively impenetrable. With regard to perception, Pylyshyn (1984) wrote

> Without doubt, the perceptual process is cognitively penetrable in the sense required by our criterion. What one sees -- or more accurately, what one sees something to be -- depends on one's beliefs in a rationally explicable way. In particular, it depends in a quite rational way on what one knows about the object one is viewing and on what one expects .... Nonetheless, as Fodor and I have argued ..., a clearly noninferential component is required as well, one that is part of the functional architecture. This component, called a transducer, may well be extremely complex by biological criteria, yet it counts as a cognitive primitive.... Furthermore, the transducer is cognitively impenetrable. (134-135).

The processes giving rise to metamerism in color vision are cognitively impenetrable, for different objects that take on the same color will do so quite independently of any rationally explicable scheme of belief or knowledge, even if that belief or knowledge should change the particular hue or saturation ascribed to a given object. For even if, say, I infer that the yellowish-looking book on my shelf is really gray -- and that it only seems vaguely yellow because of the peculiar tint of the illumination that is cast right now in my office -- still, the laws of metamerism entail that I would make exactly the same perceptual judgment about any other object whose color in the identical environment is similarly yellowish. In brief, metameric lights are substitutable -- the overarching principle of Grassman's laws of color vision. Hence by Pylyshyn's criterion some properties of color perception are clearly impenetrable.

To repeat, then, metamerism entails cognitive impenetrability. But even though the converse is not necessarily true -- a failure of metamerism does not preclude cognitive impenetrability -- still, a lack of metamerism does set the stage for penetrability, does make it possible for later cognitive processes to modulate perceptual outcomes. For once it happens that two stimuli produce nonidentical responses in the "front end," these responses may subsequently be modified in different ways in the "back end."

It is unfortunately the case that the metamerism so prominent in color vision has few relatives to be found in other perceptual realms -- where, therefore, cognitive impenetrability is probably the vast exception rather than the rule. For it is unusual to be able to manipulate two or more dimensions of physical stimuli in order to keep perceptions identical.

Let me give a concrete example. There are no metameric musical notes -- except perhaps with the trivial exception of tones differing infinitesimally in some relevant physical property. Thus, if I strike two piano keys, and thereby produce notes having different fundamental frequencies, say C and F#, perhaps these notes will be identical in timbre; and certainly by changing the impulsive force I exert on the keys I can make the notes equal in loudness. But to most people with normal hearing, F# will be clearly distinguishable in pitch from C; and there is no way to make these notes indistinguishable in all respects, including pitch, without making them physically identical, that is, without changing either C to F# or F# to C. Alternatively, I can play C on the piano and C on a violin, so that the pitches will be the same. And again, I can adjust the relative intensities of the two notes to make them equally loud. But in this case the timbres will differ. Tones can be made partially equivalent, but not perceptually identical. Most importantly, given that notes are distinguishable in pitch, or a piano note and violin note distinguishable in timbre, they are at least potentially cognitively penetrable.

Invariance in Psychophysics

From the perspective of psychophysics, we can divide the world into two greatly unequal parts: a rather small body -- the mass of land -- where perceptual experiences produced by stimuli that vary multidimensionally can be metameric, or identical to perception; and a considerably greater body -- the vast sea -- where perceptual experiences produced by multidimensionally-varying stimuli can be made equivalent with respect to one attribute or sometimes more, but not with respect to all attributes, and thus not identical. Correspondingly, that primary operation of psychophysical measurement -- the operation of matching -- divides into two classes, essentially into what Brindley (1960) distinguished as Class A or Class B operations. The one treats perceptual relations of identity, the other perceptual relations of equivalence.

Where appropriate Class A operations exist -- which is to say, when the physiological substrate and the corresponding perceptual events permit metamerism -- it *may be* a relatively straightforward matter to use the invariance characteristics to draw inferences about the processing that takes place at early stages, despite all of the sundry complexities that can be superimposed by subsequent, later processing mechanisms. For example, the coefficients of trichromatic color matching -- the proportions of three primary lights used to match every possible color -- are linearly related to the spectral absorption coefficients of the three cone pigments; nevertheless, color matches do not by themselves specify the three absorption spectra.

Moreover, when only Class B operations exist -- which is to say, when perceptual experiences can vary in several dimensions, as they do most of the time, and where percepts can be made partly equivalent but not wholly identical -- inferences about so-called early perceptual processes, and about invariance properties of these processes, are especially risky. For example, there is now considerable evidence, some of which will be recounted in the next section, showing that when tones of different sound frequencies are made partially equivalent with respect to loudness (but not wholly identical because they differ in pitch), the invariance characteristics, or spectral sensitivity function, is cognitively malleable.

In particular, I believe that it is all too easy to misapply the metameric model -- the model of color vision -- to inappropriate conditions. Where metamerism suggests that *different stimuli that produce* identical percepts (metamers) *have identical underlying representations at some stage in processing*, it is tempting to generalize to the claim that *different stimuli that produce* partially-identical (equivalent) percepts *have identical underlying representations for that particular perceptual dimension at some stage in processing.* But as I have already argued, only the former -- only metamers -- must *necessarily* be cognitively impenetrable.

There is, I believe, a strong but dangerous temptation, emanating from the causal theory of perception, to identify several properties of perceptual experience, properties such as color and brightness of objects seen, or pitch or loudness of events heard, as psychologically primitive, and therefore as cognitively impenetrable -- at least under the kinds of reductive stimulus situations that psychophysicists often employ. When subjects in a psychophysical experiment listen to pure tones, heard otherwise in silence, or view patches of color against a black backdrop, it is tempting to consider the resulting perceptions as largely based on fixed, impenetrable, front-end processes of transduction and sensory excitation, as if their lack of strong semantic content and context eliminates the need to consider any possible effects of inferential or other so-called "higher" cognitive processes. But even in such reduced and simplified situations, all stimuli are multidimensional. So too are virtually all representations of stimuli, especially perceptions.

Perceptual systems in particular -- and cognitive systems more generally -- strive to order and organize their representations within the constraints, or limitations, that the finiteness and neural instantiation of these systems necessitate. In the forthcoming section, I shall try to give some indication of the substantial role that higher-level, back-end, cognitive processes play in determining invariance properties of perception when perceptions, as well as stimuli, vary multidimensionally.

IV. Contextuality in Perceptual Representation

Probable impossibilities are to be preferred to improbable possibilities.

-- *Aristotle*

The squirming facts exceed the squamous mind.

-- *Wallace Stevens*

The present section picks up a promissory note: I shall take the opportunity here to review results of several lines of recent empirical research, mostly my own and that of colleagues, that bears directly on the issue of prime concern -- the deep contextuality displayed by what seem to be primitive and simple properties of perception, such as the loudness of sounds. Although I focus here on loudness, the underlying principles are clearly general ones, and pertain to perception much more generally.

Processing of Auditory Intensity

There is a pervasive view among students of sensory functioning, to wit, that the perception of loudness, or the intensity of sound, depends on an internal process of excitation, that the processing of auditory intensity consists of the transduction of acoustical energy into a set of neural responses, propagated through several anatomical stages; at some point, the level of excitation -- the magnitude of the nerve responses -- constitutes the code for loudness. Given the possibility that transmission and transduction alike may involve nonlinear as well as linear processes -- that sensory processing may invoke, for instance, nonlinear transduction by hair cells, binaural interactions in the central nervous system, and so forth -- we might wish to consider the excitation found at any given stage in auditory processing as corresponding intimately to the "representation" of auditory intensity at that stage; phenomenal access to these processes -- the perception of loudness proper -- presumably takes place at some relatively late stage, perhaps, for instance, where the pertinent neural events arise at the level of auditory cortex.

Stages in processing intensity. What affects loudness? Clearly, changes in sound intensity can affect loudness, presumably because these changes can modify the levels of excitation. So too can changes in the sound's frequency, in its spatial location, or in its duration. And so can the introduction of noisy backgrounds, or preadaptation of the ear to very loud sounds. But it is just as important to ask the complementary question: What does *not* affect loudness? That is, what kinds of changes or trade-offs in the world have no effect on the loudnesses of sounds, and thus, by implication, have no effect on the levels of excitation at the various stages of processing sound intensity, or at least at the final stage?

Once we find ourselves in the cognitive-psychophysical mode of thinking -- in thinking of processing intensity through a series of linear and nonlinear transformations of sensory excitation -- we have at least part of the answer to the question, What leaves loudness unchanged? The answer is, those manipulations of the stimulus world that have no effect on excitation -- including those manipulations that exert their psychological effects *after* the sensory transformations are completed, that is, after the "representation of loudness" is determined.

A simple diagram can show what I mean. Figure 3.1 shows a hypothetical series of stages in the processing of sound intensity. Both peripheral and central mechanisms can come into play by the time we reach the stage where "loudness" (L, for short) is represented, and, consequently, we can characterize the variables that impinge on this system as being of two types: One type includes those variables that directly or indirectly affect loudness, by inducing changes at one level or another before we reach stage L. As a matter of convenience, consider all levels up to and including L part of the "front end" of processing. The other category includes those variables that induce changes later on in the sequence -- at the back end rather than the front end -- perhaps by affecting the person's decision rule, choice of response, or interpretation of loudness, but presumably not by affecting the "experience of loudness" itself.

Let me give a couple of concrete examples. Say that person is exposed to a series of tones whose loudnesses she is supposed to rate on some sort of qualitative or quantitative scale. We might take a baker's dozen tones at 100 Hz, with SPLs ranging between 30 and 90 dB in steps of 5 dB, and present these 13 tones one at a time, each for 1 second, to the person's right ear. If we ask her to rate these tones on a scale that ranges from "1" (corresponding to the 30 dB tone) to "10" (for the 90 dB tone), her judgments will enable us to derive a psychophysical function relating the ratings of loudness to the SPL. Now, let us repeat the experiment, but ask the same person to rate the very same set of tones on a new scale, one that now goes to "100" at the top end rather than "10." In this case, we would obtain some other function relating the ratings of loudness to the sound intensities. Clearly the relation between stimulus intensity and numerical response will depend on the response scale, perhaps as shown in Figure 3.2.

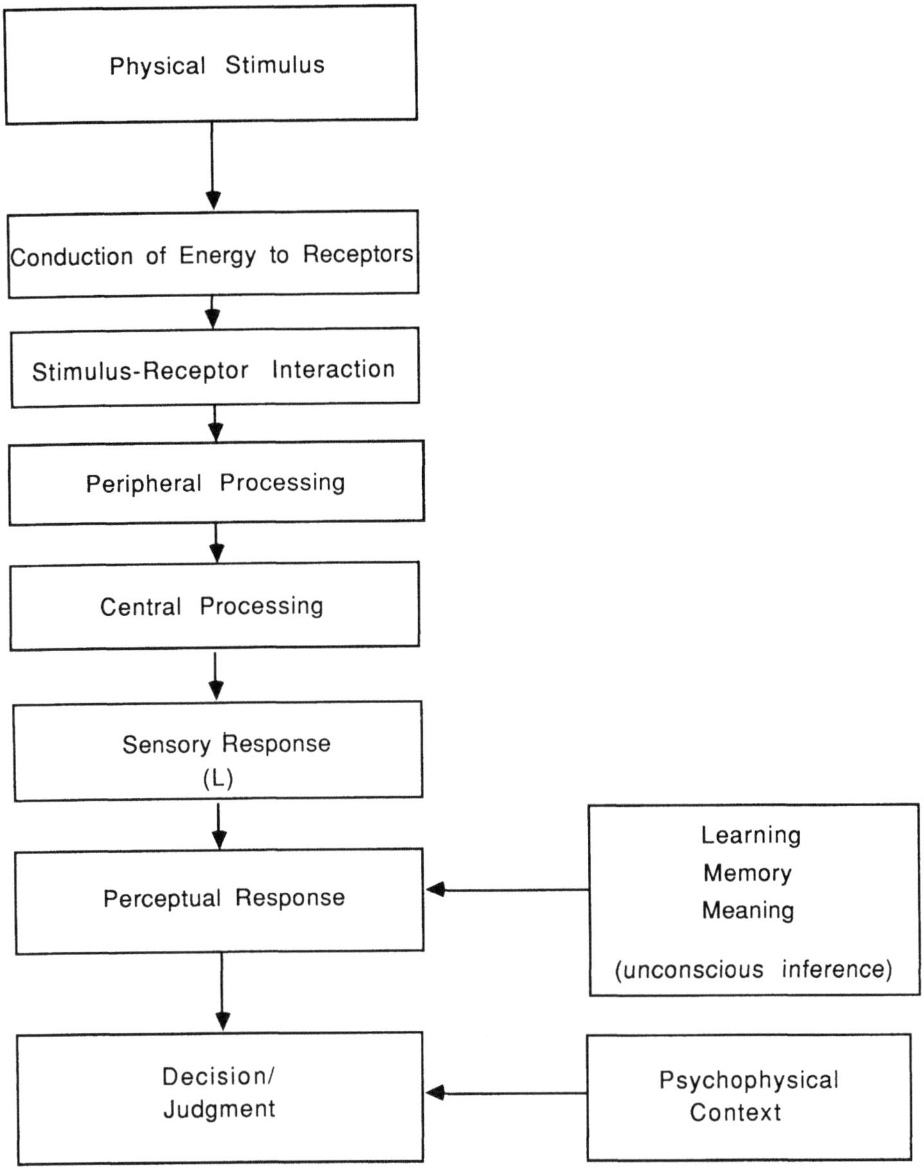

Figure 3.1: Hypothetical sequence of stages in perceptual processing of sound intensity, under the assumption that certain contextual factors affect only overt perceptual decisions, but not the underlying perceptions themselves.

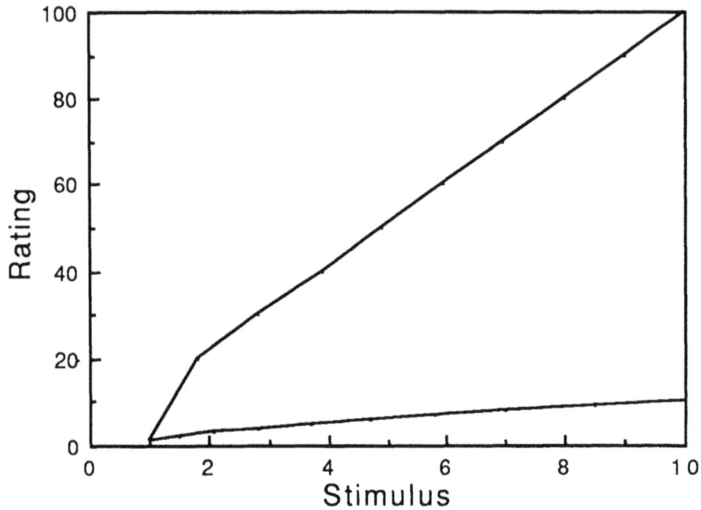

Figure 3.2: Judgments of intensity on rating scales whose end points are 1 and 10 in one instance and 1 and 100 in another.

There is nothing remarkable about all of this. With appropriate instruction, and sometimes without instruction, people are able to modify the decision rules by which they choose the response to give to any particular stimulus. Accordingly, the fact that a person may assign the response "9" to an 85 dB tone under one instruction, but assign the response "88" to the same tone under another instruction, could simply mean that the change in instruction affected the person's set of decisional rules. Presumably, the underlying experience of loudness itself -- the internal representation of sound intensity -- is the same under both circumstances.

By this view, loudness per se is invariant -- invariant, at least, as long as the sensory-perceptual system, and hence the level of neural excitation, is not perturbed (as it might be altered by the introduction of a masking noise; by prior selective adaptation of the ear to a loud tone or narrow band of noise: Young people do this all the time at rock concerts). On the other hand, there are lots of ways we might get folks to change their overt responses -- for instance, by changing instructions or by changing the contextual set of stimulus levels that are presented -- without effecting any change in the underlying process of neural excitation in the auditory system, and thus, we would like to believe, without effecting any change in the underlying perception of loudness.

Effects of sound frequency and intensity. The only problem with this scenario is that it is wrong. That it is wrong becomes evident when we consider how people actually perceive and judge sounds, with respect to loudness, under conditions in which the sounds vary multidimensionally, which is to say, under virtually all mundane conditions, where we hear voices, music, and a plethora of other constantly changing environmental signals and noises.

In many situations where stimuli vary in many dimensions -- as they generally do in the "real world" -- there is increasingly abundant evidence that the model just described is inadequate. This evidence comes largely from experiments in which subjects are asked to judge the loudness of sounds that vary not only in their intensity but also in their frequency. Perceptually, then, the subjects perceive the various stimuli to take on different pitches as well as different loudnesses. The crucial feature to these studies is the way the set of stimuli varies from one experimental condition to another; in different conditions the subjects are given different contextual sets of stimuli.

A basic measure of the way that frequency and intensity jointly determine loudness appears in the measurement of equal-loudness curves, the earliest of which date back to the first few decades of this century (e.g., Fletcher & Munson, 1933; see also Robinson & Dadson, 1954). Figure 3.3 characterizes these curves. Each contour shows the sound pressure levels (SPLs) needed at various frequencies to produce a constant loudness. Note that there is an important difference between loudness matches at different sound frequencies and metameric color matches. Unlike metameric color matching, equal-loudness curves represent a set of *equivalences*, not *identities*; as one moves along a given contour, loudness does remain constant (by definition), but pitch changes continuously. Consequently, the various stimuli whose joint values of frequency and SPL fall along a given equal loudness curve can be distinguished by the typical perceiver quite easily.

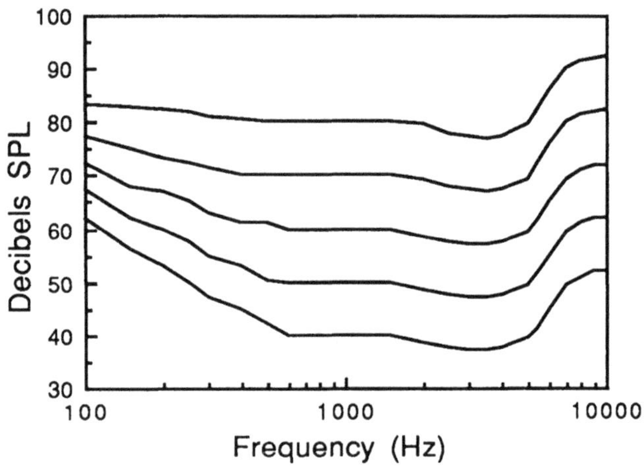

Figure 3.3: Equal-loudness curves, showing how sound pressure level (SPL) must vary with sound frequency to maintain constant levels of loudness. Based on data of Fletcher and Munson (1933).

The particular shapes of equal-loudness curves are usually conceived to represent the sum of two main factors. The first factor comprises the several mechanical filtering properties of the external auditory system: the shape of the pinna, the resonance of the ear canal, the impedances and resonances of the eardrum, middle ear cavity, and ossicles, and so forth; the second comprises those subsequent neural processes (perhaps temporal integration) that may differentially affect the relation of loudness to stimulus intensity at different frequencies (see, for example, Zwislocki, 1965).

Are equal-loudness curves "hard wired"? The notion that equal-loudness curves reflect a "hard-wired" property of intensity processing rests on two implicit premises that I have just enumerated: The first premise is that equally loud sounds remain equally loud (are judged to be equal) even when such "higher-order" factors as instructions or contextual set change, as long as the underlying level of neural excitation does not change, that is, as long as there is reason to believe that the level of excitation within the sensory system remains constant. This is the neotitchenerian premise of "front-end" constancy, to which sensations (unlike monads) presumably do provide a window.

A second premise is that equal loudness can be defined through a set of fundamental, psychophysically determined relations amenable to mathematical formulation. These relations include equal-loudness curves characterizing the interplay of sound frequency and intensity, like those of Figure 3.3 (with whatever proviso is needed to allow for the idiosyncracies of individual subjects). Analogous quantitative rules can characterize temporal integration (the way that loudness depends jointly on intensity and duration of a pulse of sound), the summation of loudness when multiple sound frequencies combine, the summation of loudness by the two ears, and so forth.

Equal-loudness curves do not define equal loudness. Let me proffer a seeming paradox: Equal-loudness curves fail to define equal loudness. What I intend by this apparent contradiction is to indicate that *neither the equal-loudness curves of Figure 3.3 nor any other such set of equal-loudness curves can serve as a universal indicant of equal loudness relations among sounds that vary in frequency and intensity*. Instead, I shall argue that *the perceptual representation of loudness is quintessentially contextual*. This is to say either that loudness is not just the end-product of excitation -- or that, if it is, then excitation is itself not based solely in the absolute characteristics of the stimulus and the local sensitivity of the auditory system, but instead is itself contextually relative.

The basic paradigm of the experiments involves shifting the stimulus context from one experimental condition to another -- where stimulus context is defined as the set or ensemble of possible stimuli that might appear over the course of testing; speaking operationally, stimulus context, or contextual set, is defined in terms of the distribution across all possible levels of the stimulus intensities that might appear at any given time, on any given stimulus trial. Moreover, it is important that the perceptions as well as the stimuli vary multidimensionally, so that there are both a perceptual dimension being judged -- the criterial dimension -- and a perceptual dimension over which the contexts vary -- the vehicle. In many of the experiments I shall describe, the criterion was loudness, and the vehicle over which contexts varied was pitch.

Because the stimulus ensembles are multidimensional, the critical variation in context involves changes in multiple subcontexts. The question is, then: How does the context -- the available set of stimuli -- affect encoding, perception, and judgment?

Of course, stimulus context has for a long time been known to affect judgments per se. A six-story building may be small in midtown Manhattan, but large on the wheatfields of Kansas. It is relativism of this sort that many theories have sought to explain -- notable in this regard is Helson's (1964) adaptation-level theory, which states that responses tend to gravitate toward the adaptation level, or AL, where the AL depends on some measure of the stimulus context, amongst other factors.

As already indicated, my experiments deal specifically with multiple (multidimensionally changing) contexts, a situation that, compared to single contexts, is much more in keeping with contextual variations in the real world -- and that, I think, is theoretically much more interesting and provocative. Imagine listening to a fife and a drum, one of which is relatively much louder than the other, or hearing different voices, maybe a soprano and a bass, whose sources are located at different distances, and consequently that have different overall or average loudnesses. If the fife and drum players are part of a band that walks past you, or if the soprano and bass are stationary but you walk past them, the relative intensities of these sounds at your ears will change. When the soprano is distant and the bass close by, the low-pitched voice will generally be the louder; but as you approach the soprano and distance yourself from the bass, the relative intensities switch, so that now the high-pitched voice is louder. Although most of the experiments I'll describe were concerned with loudness, the results are not limited to loudness but apply just as well to visual, tactile, and taste perception.

As Figure 3.4 shows, the main paradigm involves a double-contextual shift. That is, the paradigm presents the subjects with two possible experimental conditions, which I'll call A and B. In each condition, the stimulus context -- the overall set of stimuli -- contains two subsets consisting of different levels of sound intensities at two different frequencies.

	Condition A	Condition B
low frequency	low intensity	high intensity
	+	+
high frequency	high intensity	low intensity

<u>Figure 3.4</u>: The double shifting-context paradigm: In one contextual condition the set of stimuli comprises low-frequency tones at low SPLs and high-frequency tones at high SPLs; in the other condition the assignment of SPLs to frequencies is reversed.

In a typical experiment, the subjects might judge the loudnesses of low-frequency and high-frequency tones; on different days, the subjects receive the two different stimulus ensembles or contexts. Stimuli are presented one at a time, chosen randomly from the entire set, and therefore randomly with regard both to sound frequency and to the sound intensity within each subset. The task is to rate the loudness of each tone quantitatively, by assigning numbers in proportion to perceived intensities -- the method of magnitude estimation. If one prefers, one may think of the paradigm as a kind of identification procedure, in which the mapping of responses to stimuli is defined individually by each subject, not predefined by the experimenter. In any case, I am not greatly interested here in the numbers themselves -- in their quantitative properties -- except to the extent that these properties bear on the ways that the mappings of stimuli to responses at the two frequencies change with context.

In these experiments, the subjects are told to ignore the pitch of each sound, which may vary from trial to trial, and just to attend and judge loudness. Now, to repeat, it is possible to think of this task as one of identifying levels of loudness, where a particular numerical response should indicate a particular level of loudness, regardless of sound frequency. Recall the notion that loudness depends on excitation and is characterized through equal-loudness curves like those of Figure 3.3. If this is so, then, as Figure 3.5 implies, every possible sound in the stimulus ensemble -- every sound intensity at each frequency -- should have associated with it a given internal representation of loudness; every sound should produce a level of loudness as represented abstractly. The subject's task, then, is to map each of these abstract representations in some systematic and presumably monotonic way onto a response scale of her or his choosing. Thus in each contextual condition, we obtain from the subjects two identification functions, one function for each sound frequency, on the basis of which we may ask: How do these identification functions change, if at all, with stimulus context?

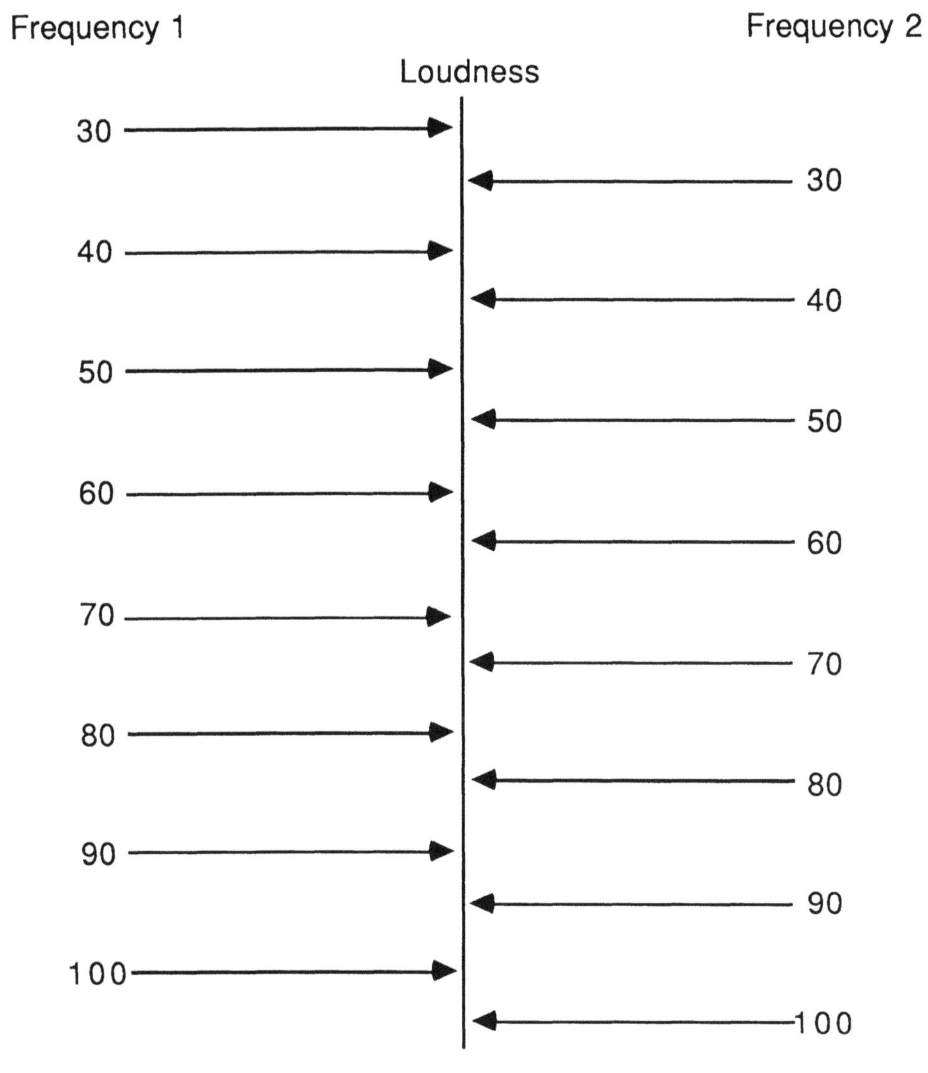

Figure 3.5: The internal representation of loudness at two sound frequencies, under the assumption that every SPL at each frequency is associated with a fixed level of loudness, as long as the sensitivity of the system is held constant.

Figure 3.6 shows the results obtained in an early experiment (Marks, 1988). In Condition A, where the low sound frequency (500 Hz) always took on relatively low intensities and the high frequency (2500 Hz) took on high intensities, I obtained one pair of identification functions, as indicated by the circles on the left. To a rough first approximation, the functions relating the loudness judgments to SPL are much the same at both frequencies; that is, equal SPLs gave roughly equal response. But in Condition B, where the low-frequency tones took on high intensities (the SPLs were shifted up 20 dB compared to those of Context A) and the high-frequency tones took on low intensities (the SPLs were shifted down by 20 dB relative to those of Context A), the two identification functions now differ, as indicated by the filled symbols. Their relation changed markedly with the shift in stimulus context: Instead of the two functions overlapping, they are now displaced laterally by about 17 dB.

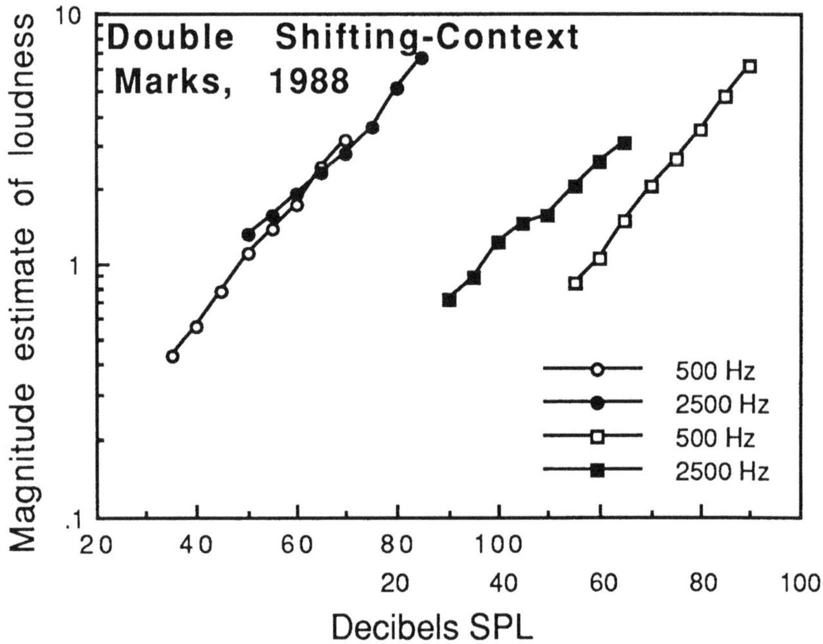

Figure 3.6: Magnitude estimates of loudness as a function of SPL at 500 and 2500 Hz, under two contextual conditions, defined as in 4. Data of Marks (1988).

A shift in loudness matches of 17 dB is a big displacement! Note that this differential effect -- this effect on the relationship between responses to two sound frequencies -- is not simply an extension of the relativity of judgment often observed when there is only a single kind of stimulus whose levels change across conditions; for in that case there is no way to decide whether the changes in response reflect changes in perception, taking place at the front end, or merely, as we may reasonably infer, changes in the way responses map onto stimuli, as a result of decision processes made relatively late, in the back end. That is, if I listen to 500 Hz sounds that vary from 40 to 70 dB, and call the lowest, 40 dB tone "soft" and the loudest, 70 dB tone "loud," then subsequently listen to tones ranging from 70 to 100 dB and now call the 70 dB signal "soft," there is little reason to believe that the underlying representations of loudness changed. It is perfectly possible that all that changed was the rule by which I apply labels to these representations.

With contextual shifts in the levels of unidimensionally-varying stimuli, there is generally no change in the rank ordering of the stimuli: biggest is still biggest and smallest smallest. But with multidimensionally varying stimuli -- and, consequently, with multiple contexts -- the very rank orders of the subjects' responses can change. For instance, Figure 3.6 reveals that a 60 dB tone at 2500 Hz was judged softer than a 65 dB tone at 500 Hz in Condition A, but louder than the same 500 Hz tone in Condition B.

Just as importantly, this effect of shifting multiple contexts is not trivial in size. One of the important implications of these findings is that equal-loudness curves are far from being universal characteristics of auditory processing. In Figure 3.7 I have redrawn one of Fletcher and Munson's (1933) equal-loudness curves (for tones equal in loudness to a 1000 Hz signal at 70 dB), together with two pairs of equal-loudness points for 500 Hz and 2500 Hz tones, as derived from my results shown in Figure 3.6. The circles correspond to loudness matches derived from Condition A (left side of Figure 3.6), and the triangles correspond to matches derived from Condition B (right side of 3.6). Whatever Fletcher and Munson's prototype may represent, it surely does not very accurately represent equal loudness when the contextual set of possible stimulus values can vary widely. Or put another way, the local form of the equal-loudness function varies enormously with changes in context.

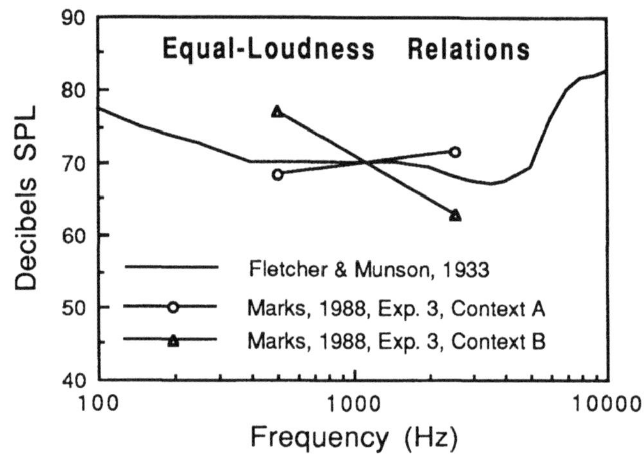

<u>Figure 3.7</u>: An equal-loudness curve from 3 (data of Fletcher and Munson, 1933), and equal-loudness curves based on data derived from the double shifting-context paradigm (6).

<u>Do changes in context really affect loudness</u>? Of course, these initial results leave lots of questions unanswered. We might ask, for example, Does this differential context effect depend on procedure? In particular might it depend on the use of a numerical rating procedure? I'll defer until later a full answer to this question, but simply to anticipate briefly, the evidence strongly supports the view that differential context effects emerge with a wide variety of tools for measurement, and consequently that the effects do indeed reflect changes in perception itself, not just changes in overt responding.

One piece of evidence comes from a study by Schneider and Parker (1990), who asked their subjects to make paired-comparisons of loudness differences. On each trial the subject heard two pairs of tones, which could take on frequencies of 500 or 2500 Hz at various SPLs. The subjects' task was to decide which pair differed more in loudness. Moreover, in different test sessions, the experimenters varied the contextual sets of tones. The results showed that changing context in this paradigm too exerted differential effects at the two frequencies, just like those obtained when subjects gave magnitude estimates of the loudness of individual tones (magnitude estimates were obtained from the same subjects as a control). Schneider and Parker concluded that changes in context affect loudness, not just overt responding.

More recently, I reported preliminary results of two experiments in which I had subjects make direct comparisons between the loudness of 500 Hz and 2500 Hz tones; these direct-comparison trials were embedded within test sessions in which the subjects were also judging the loudness of individual tones, different contexts of such tones presented in different sessions (Marks, 1991). That is, within experimental sessions identical to those used to generate the results shown in Figure 3.6 (different contextual sets of SPLs at the two frequencies in different sessions), subjects were also asked on some trials to compare directly the loudnesses of 500 Hz and 2500 Hz tones. Not only did context again exert a differential effect on numerical ratings of loudness, but in a similar fashion context also affected direct loudness comparisons. These findings, together with Schneider and Parker's (1990), suggest that context helps determine the characteristics of equal-loudness functions.

Effects of stimulus distribution. We can also ask whether these results might depend on the subjects being able to identify the end points of the stimulus range at each sound frequency. In Condition A, for instance, it surely is obvious to the subjects that the softest low-frequency tone is softer than every one of the high-frequency tones, and symmetrically, that the loudest high-frequency tone is louder than every one of the low-frequency tones. (In part we infer this because several subjects will report something like this after a session). Might this knowledge about the extreme stimulus values matter? The answer is that such knowledge is not necessary to obtain the shifts in matching loudnesses. For it is perfectly possible to manipulate stimulus contexts without changing the actual stimulus levels used in different conditions, for example, by presenting a constant set of SPLs, but manipulating how often each tone is presented. That is, at each sound frequency we can present the low or high SPLs more or less often within a session, thereby changing the distributions and hence the mean SPLs, but not the absolute levels themselves. When this is done, essentially the same kind of changes emerge in the loudness judgments; varying the distribution of stimulus intensities acts very much like shifting to lower or higher absolute levels (Marks, 1988).

A role for critical bands? What about the choice of stimulus frequencies? It is apparent that the presence of differential context effects must somehow depend on the choice of sound frequencies. In principle, if we were to reduce the difference between low and high sound frequencies until the tones become identical, the effect of context must eventually disappear. A thought experiment suffices to make this clear: In the limit, with a single sound frequency, there is no way for the subject to distinguish the subsets of tones in a given contextual situation; consequently, any given tone -- any given SPL -- must match itself for loudness and no context effect can appear. Put another way, *with a single sound frequency, matches become "functionally" metameric.*

But systematic investigation -- through real experiments, not thought experiments -- is needed to give a complete picture. In a nutshell, the greater the difference in sound frequency between the tones, the greater are the differential effects of context. Moreover, the precise way that sound frequency enters this picture bears, I believe, important consequences for understanding the processing mechanisms underlying these curious effects of context, and by extension, for understanding how acoustic stimuli are encoded, perceived, and judged.

In a series of experiments, Marks and Warner (1991) kept the geometric-center frequency of two signals constant at 1118 Hz (this is the geometric average of 500 and 2500 Hz, the values used by Marks, 1988), but systematically varied the separation between frequencies from very small (30 Hz) to very great (over 9000 Hz). What we found was that shifting contexts had no effect at all until the frequency separation between the signals exceeded about 250 Hz, after which increasing the frequency separation still further led to increasing amounts of context-dependent change. Figure 3.8 shows how the magnitude of the differential context effect depended on frequency separation.

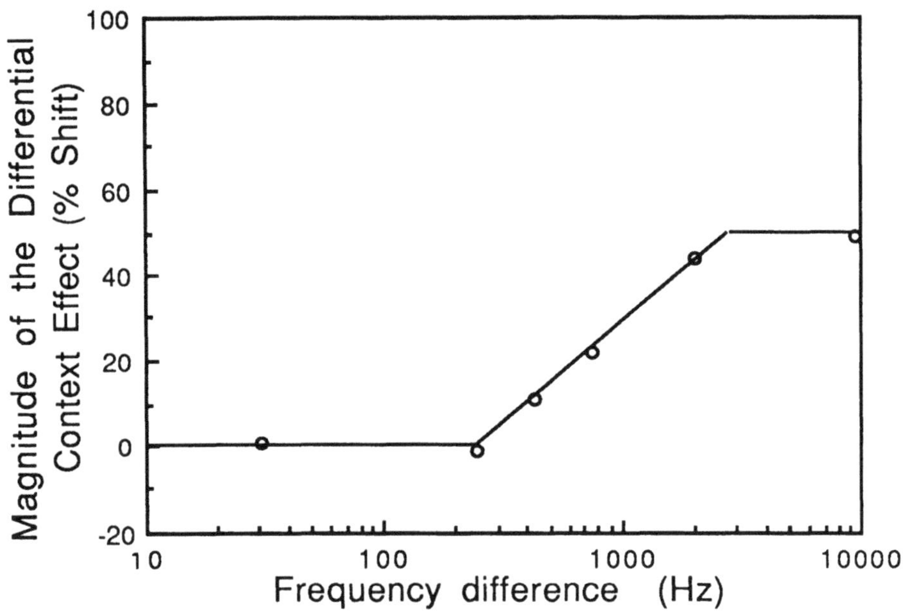

Figure 3.8: How the magnitude of the differential context effect depends on the difference in sound frequencies between the tones. Data of Marks and Warner (1991).

The value of 250 Hz is interesting because it is in the ballpark of the critical bandwidth at 1120 Hz. Critical bandwidth is a region of sound frequencies that is typically defined through paradigms of masking of tone by noise (see Scharf, 1970) or of energy summation of loudness (Zwicker, Flottorp, & Stevens, 1957). Critical bandwidth depends systematically on center frequency, and on the method of measurement, with the generally accepted values falling around 15% of center frequency (about 180 Hz at 1118 Hz). So the "bandwidth" found by Marks and Warner (1991) is about 40% greater than critical bandwidth.

Often, critical bands are conceived to represent results of imperfect mechanical filtering at the basilar membrane. But context effects like those shown in Figure 3.6 do not directly reflect such "early," front-end processes. Presumably, the present changes in relative loudnesses arise because the different contextual sets generate, implicitly, some kind of "expectations" about the possible stimulus values, with loudnesses of qualitatively different stimuli (stimuli arising from activation of different peripheral units or critical bands) in some manner "normalized" accordingly. This is to say, *the mechanism by which context acts to modify loudness starts with information that arises peripherally -- front-end information that is itself probably hard-wired and therefore cognitively impenetrable -- then incorporates that information into a central representation of loudness that is itself contextual and (perhaps thereby) cognitively penetrable.*

Context does its job automatically. Although the effects of stimulus context on loudness appear to be centrally mediated, in that they are determined by the ensemble of possible stimuli, and thus must depend on information that builds up over stimulus trials, this does not mean that the context effects are themselves under very much voluntary control. Quite to the contrary, it appears that context can operate rather automatically to modulate loudness.

Consider, for example, the question as to whether differential effects of context are related to uncertainty about the stimulus. It is conceivable that the context-based changes in loudness perception arise because the subjects are uncertain on each trial what the frequency of the signal will be, and therefore obtain incomplete or degraded information. Metaphorically speaking, the subjects may be trying to "scan" so large a region of the "sound-frequency space" that they miss some of the input deriving from peripheral nerve fibers. This is to conceive of an analogy between uncertainty of sound frequency in hearing and uncertainty of spatial location in vision. Indeed, it has long been known that the detectability of a tone can be reduced if the signal presented falls some distance, in frequency, from the signal that is expected (e.g., Greenberg & Larkin, 1968).

If stimulus uncertainty and, therefore, directed attention are important factors, we might expect the magnitude of the differential context effect to diminish or disappear when attention is focused on the signal frequency on each trial, thereby reducing or eliminating this source of uncertainty. But such an outcome does not obtain. For when subjects were cued visually before each trial as to sound frequency, the differential context effect was just as large as it was when no cue was used (Marks, in press-a). Nor was there any reduction in the effect when the stimulus sequences consisted of successive pairs of tones taking on the same frequency -- so that the first stimulus of each pair cued the frequency on the next trial (Marks, in press-a). In sum, context seems to exert its effects on loudness automatically, or preattentively. Whatever the process underlying contextual interaction may be, the result of this process is to weight the absolute, stimulus-driven information with relative or contextual information to determine the representations of loudness at different sound frequencies.

Context affects direct loudness matches. A final set of experiments sought to learn whether changes in stimulus context produce analogous effects within a very simple, more or less straightforward, direct-comparison paradigm.

To answer this question, I eliminated completely from each experimental session the numerical judgments, and simply employed a roving level, two-alternative forced-choice procedure. In each session, the stimulus ensemble comprised 15 pairs of low-frequency and high-frequency tones. I generated these by pairing each of three SPLs at the low frequency with each of five SPLs at the high frequency. On a given trial, the subjects heard one tone followed briefly by the other, and simply judged which of the two tones was louder. To produce different contextual sets, I held the SPLs of the low-frequency tone constant, but increased the SPLs of the high-frequency tones by 10 dB in Condition B relative to their values in Condition A.

Figures 3.9-3.12 show sample results obtained from individual subjects using, respectively, four different pairs of sound frequencies. It is clear that changes in the average stimulus level do effect corresponding changes in the points of subjective equality (the SPLs of the high-frequency tone judged louder than the low-frequency tone on half the trials). Which is to say, context determines direct loudness matches. Moreover, the magnitude of the context effect again shows something akin to a "critical band" -- with large, supercritical differences in sound frequency yielding large context effects, but smaller, subcritical differences yielding modest or inconsequential effects. It should be clear even this most direct and relatively simple perceptual test -- loudness comparison -- reveals a profound relativism to the perception of loudness.

Contextuality of Loudness Summation

Very briefly, let me indicate that effects of context extend into various other phenomena of intensity processing that are typically thought to take place at the "front end", and that concomitantly are often thought to be cognitively impenetrable. I am referring specifically here to various phenomena of intensity

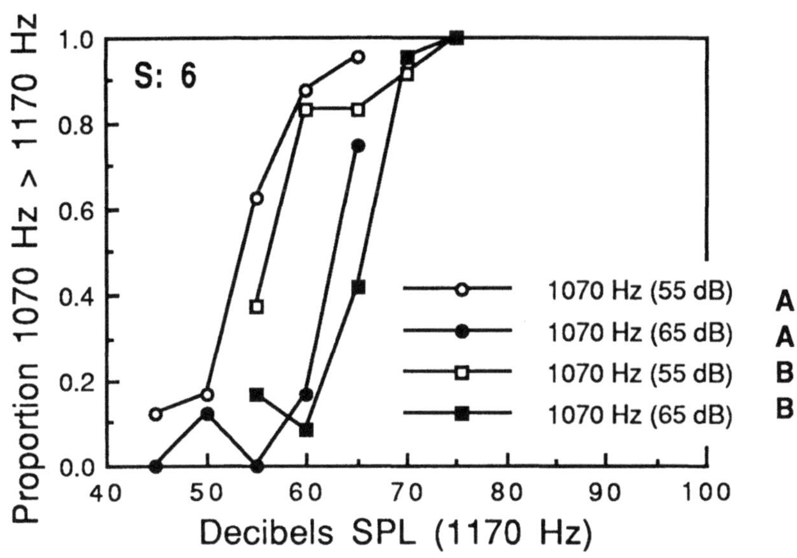

Figure 3.9: Sample data from one subject showing how the contextual set of stimuli affects direct loudness matches between 500 Hz and 2500 Hz tones.

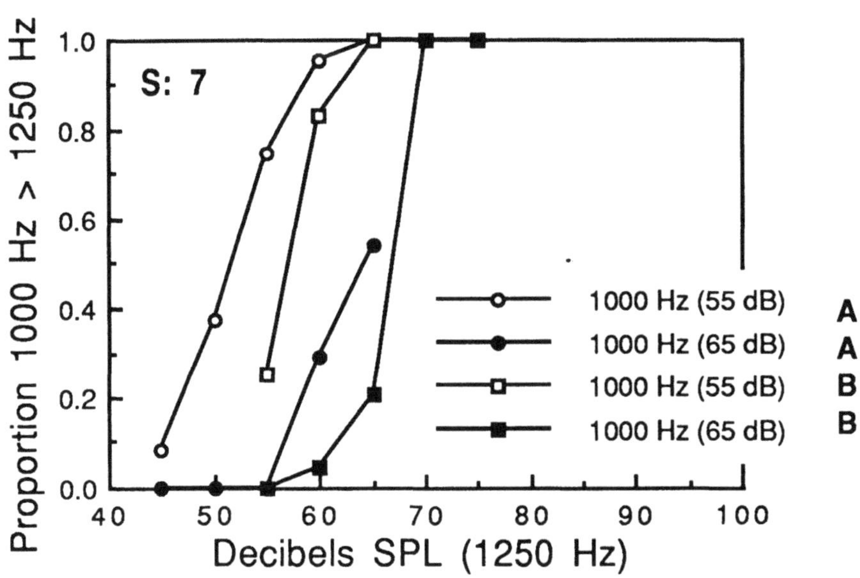

Figure 3.10: As in Figure 3.9, for tones of 1000 Hz and 1250 Hz.

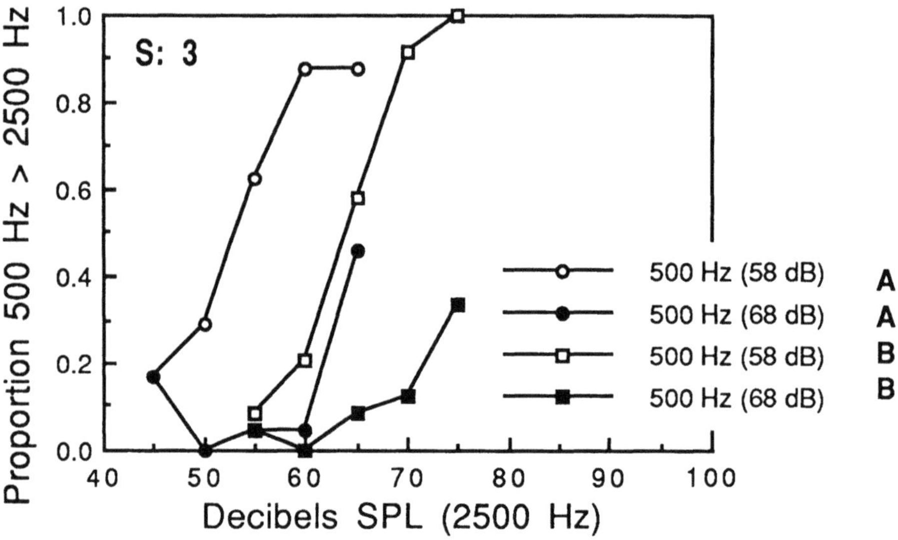

Figure 3.11: As in Figure 3.9, for tones of 1070 and 1170 Hz.

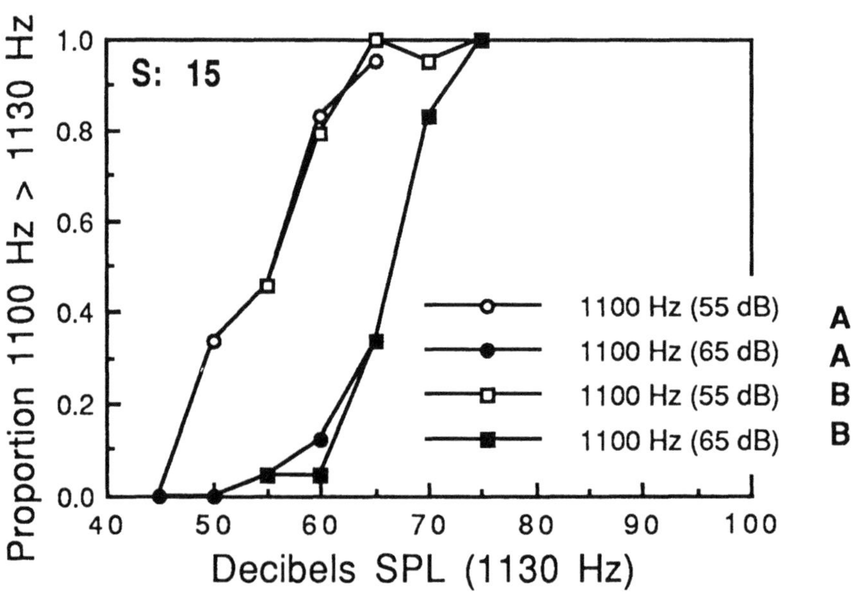

Figure 3.12: As in Figure 3.9, for tones of 1100 and 1130 Hz.

summation -- to the integration of effects of sound energy over time, to the summation of effects of multiple frequency components in a complex tone, and to the summation of effects produced by stimulating the two ears.

In a recent study, Daniel Algom and I showed that context can infiltrate the rules describing temporal integration, cross-frequency loudness summation, and binaural loudness summation (Algom & Marks, 1990). Testing all three psychoacoustic phenomena, we either manipulated the range of stimulus intensities (using wide or narrow ranges of decibels) or varied the psychophysical method (switching between magnitude estimation, where subjects assign numbers to the loudness of signals set by the experimenter, and magnitude production, where subjects adjust sound intensities to match numbers assigned by the experimenter). The goal of both kinds of manipulation was to change the overt relation between numbers and sound intensities.

Now, as I said earlier, it is tempting to think of changes wrought in stimulus-response relations as simply reflecting changes in late-stage, decisional, back-end processes, in which numbers are mapped to loudnesses -- but not to have any bearing on earlier, sensory, front-end processing itself. Unfortunately, the results suggest otherwise: Whenever the manipulation of stimulus range or psychophysical method succeeded in effecting a change in the subjects' stimulus-response mapping, it also effected a change in the invariance properties of intensity summation (equal-loudness relations). Tones judged equally loud in one testing condition of range or procedure were not judged equally loud in the other. Thus, for example, a tone heard with two ears at 60 dB was as loud as a tone heard with only one ear at either 69 dB or 67 dB, depending on whether the overall range of SPLs was large or small. Although the changes in summation were modest in size, the picture they consistently drew was one in which the effects of context extended into basic characteristics of auditory intensity processing.

Why Weren't These Experiments Done Before?

The experiments that I just recounted are really quite simple: They are simple both technically and conceptually. Indeed, although all of them date back less than half a decade, most if not all could easily have been done 30 years ago, even 60 years ago. To conceive these experiments, however, is to consider a model of perceptual information processing in which contextual factors influence perceptual responses, as in Figure 3.13. Neotitchenerianism is a hardy species.

Are There Privileged Contexts?

It is just not possible to maintain the position that loudness and other such seemingly simple dimensions of perceptual experiences are sensations that represent the outputs of an early, front-end stage, unaffected by later, back-end cognitive processes. Some revision of this position is needed. For example, if we wish to keep using the term "sensation" to refer to those front-end outputs, we may do so. But if we do, then it seems to me that we should drop the claim that loudness constitutes a sensation -- or an attribute of a sensation. If sensations are front-end outputs, then, I would argue, our perceptions never consist of sensations, and it is never sensations that subjects in psychophysical studies report on. Sensations are never directly observable, either by experimenter or by subject, but only inferred -- as intermediate outputs that are always processed further.

Alternatively, we might abandon altogether the term sensation. This solution might seem to have one distinct advantage: We then could discuss *sensory processes* without implying that these processes lead directly to sensations; instead, sensory processes could refer to the earliest stages of perceptual processing, prior to the imposition of expectations, implicit or explicit decisional processes, and so forth. But this solution -- or sleight-of-hand -- may not be wholly satisfactory. For we still would have to face the evidence that context can influence various measures of intensity summation in loudness perception, measures that are often considered sensory. Even if we drop the term "sensation," we would have to aver that context affects "sensory processing." Perhaps, therefore, it would be best to stick to the terms "perception" and "perceptual", and to drop both terms -- "sensation" and "sensory" -- altogether.

Having said this, I must confess myself to feeling some malaise about this semantic deconstruction. (As Wallace Stevens wrote, in a rather different context, "Some day they will get it right at the Sorbonne.") After all, there are various properties of perceptual processing -- for instance, the equal-loudness relations shown in Figure 3.3 -- that do seem to hold a *privileged* position.

Equal-loudness functions relating sound intensity and frequency surely have been useful, both theoretically and empirically, in various ways -- for example, in schemes for calculating the loudness of complex acoustic signals (e.g., Stevens, 1972; Zwicker & Scharf, 1969). Even if we confess that perception can be a dynamic process, especially when stimuli vary multidimensionally, and even if we accept the evidence that stimulus context can drastically modify equal-loudness relations, still, is it not possible that the curves shown in Figure 3.3 really do represent the outputs of a front-end process? Probably they do. Nevertheless, we cannot simply assume, as many sensory scientists would like to do, that by holding the constellation of variables such as stimulus set constant one thereby eliminates the effects of context. Context is not just something to eliminate. In fact, to recognize fully the implications of contextuality may be an important step in bridging the gap delimiting physics from psychology in psychophysics.

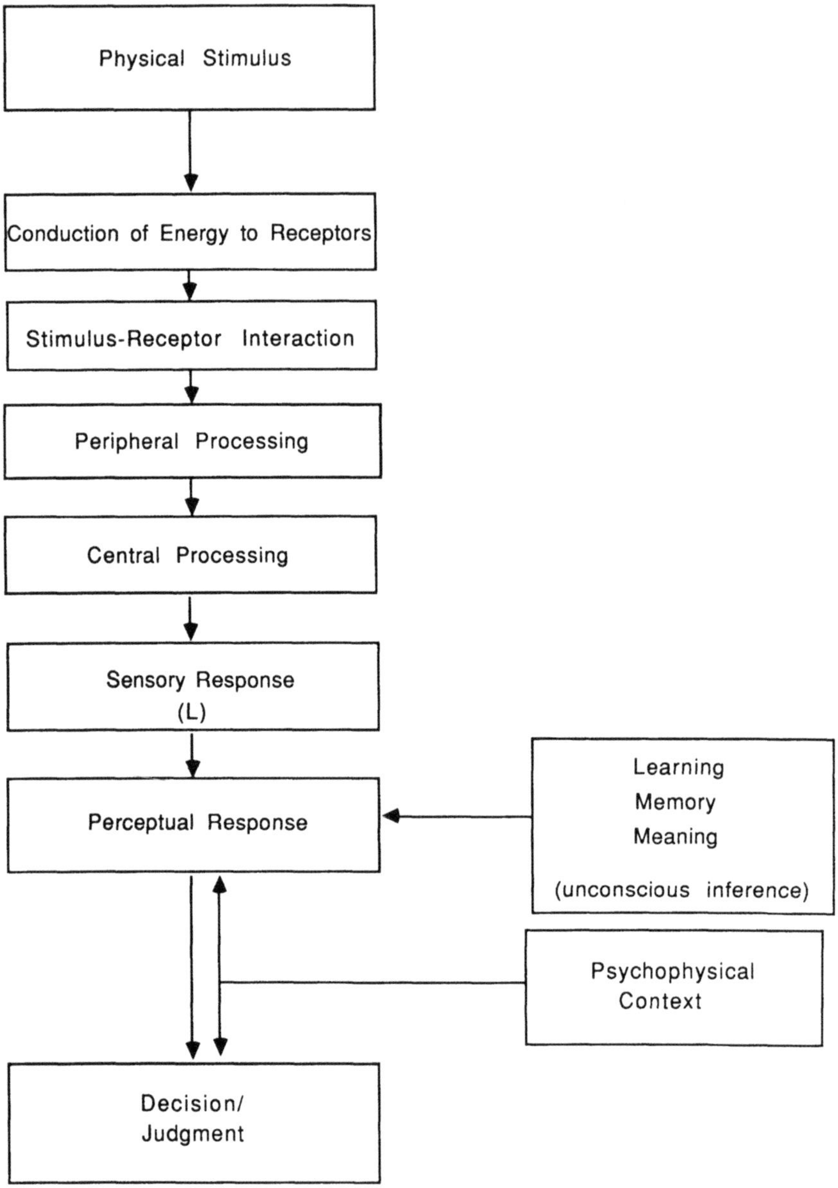

Figure 3.13: Hypothetical sequence of stages in perceptual processing of sound intensity, as in 1, but under the assumption that contextual factors affect the underlying perceptual responses, and not just overt perceptual decisions.

V. Context and Representation; the Introspective Window

Music when soft voices die,
Vibrates in the memory.
Odours when sweet violets sicken
Live within the sense they quicken.
-- Percy Bysshe Shelley

There are, I believe, two basically different ways in which we might interpret the central notion of this chapter, that is, the notion that perceptual processing is deeply and ineluctably contextual. One way is to break with much of the history of perception that I reviewed in earlier sections, and to replace the representational and causal theories with a more functional theory of perception; the other way is to revise and revamp the representational theory, maintaining its basic spirit.

The first way is more or less the way of Gibson (e.g., 1979), where perception is deemed to depend on the flow of stimulus information, and in which the temporal frame is vaguely enough defined to incorporate the kinds of contextual interactions that I have described. My own sense, however, is that such a functional model treats the problem of context mostly by ignoring the need to explain how it operates.

In order to elucidate the underlying psychological mechanisms, a more fruitful approach may be to reconsider the role of perceptual representations. As

I indicated earlier in the chapter, one way to maintain a coherent notion of "sensation" would be to reinterpret sensation as the output from a relatively early stage in perceptual processing -- but to aver that, unlike the final perceptual stage, the early sensory stage is one to which we have no phenomenal access. (The same restriction doubtless applies to various stages in perceptual processing, which are known to us only through inference, not through acquaintance.) Viewed thusly, sensation becomes a kind of hypothetical construct, not a phenomenological datum -- the substrate of perceptions analogous to the way that protein is the substrate to muscles. Accordingly, one might try to maintain the view that perceptions are constructed from sensations, conjoined to an inferential, cognitive structure, yet avoid the pitfalls of the neotitchenerian model.

Now, if sensations so defined were themselves not subject to the kinds of context effects described in the last section, we could easily interpret them as the products of hard-wired sensory-physiological mechanisms. But the evidence at hand suggests that even what many would identify as "sensory processing" is contextual and contingent. Consequently, we may be forced to conclude that sensations, like perceptions, are constructions of something else. But to follow this path leads again to the suggestion that we simply drop the term "sensations" and stick to "perceptions," conceiving the latter to be the constructions -- or representations -- of the world, as based on sensory information processed through a set of inferential and perhaps other kinds of cognitive mechanisms.

In this regard, I shall add one last word about this concept known as representation. In going from the statement "Perception can represent to us the external world" to the statement "Perception is a representation of the external world" we have turned the verb *represent* into the noun *representation*. Now, there is nothing wrong per se, in my view, with the concept of representation -- unless we begin to think of the noun as a "thing," as having some kind of quasi-corporeal existence, as being pictures inhering in the mind's eye or laying on the mind's skin, or being tape-recordings running through the mind's ear, in other words, as being some sort of mental substrate in which a whole bunch of attributes inhere. Representation is no more of a "thing" than is transportation. Although we might transport a crate of VCRs from a factory to a warehouse, transportation itself is not the factory, not the warehouse, not the VCRs, and not even the truck that carries them. Transportation is a convenient term for describing a set of relationships, a set of processes.[5] So too is perceptual representation.

By this token, perceptual representation can be taken to refer to the act by which stimulus information is interpreted within a contextual framework. Several years ago, I suggested that the very same stimulus information can give rise to different perceptual representations, depending on the task that was laid out: If the task required the identification or judgment of perceptual magnitudes, the set of representations took one mathematical form; if the task required the assessment of degree of difference or dissimilarity, the representations took a different mathematical form (roughly, the square root of the former) (Marks, 1974). Subsequent findings lent support for this dualistic model (Marks, 1979; Popper, Parker, & Galanter, 1986). The deep contextuality of loudness perception suggests that a dualistic model of representation is inadequate. The number of possible representations is potentially unlimited, or at least very great.

Such is one legacy of perception's history. Perceptual experiences are fundamentally contextual, and in part because they are so, our analysis of our own experiences -- our introspections -- often fail to provide an unfalteringly transparent window on early stimulus processing, on the mind's front end. But why expect that they should? It is sufficient, it seems to me, to give introspection its own simple due: Introspection provides the one indubitable window on phenomenal experience itself.

---

[5] This example was suggested to me many years ago by George Miller.

Consider, for instance, that sometimes we are aware of very weak stimuli and other times we are not. Now, statistical decision theory -- commonly known as signal-detection theory -- has been remarkably successful in showing, first, that the detectability of weak stimuli depends on the extent to which the stimuli are distinguished from background noise, and, second, that the level of activity aroused plus a set of decision processes act jointly to determine both the probability of correct detection and the probability of false positives (Green & Swets, 1966). One of the theory's singular successes has come in showing how stimuli that fall below a putative "threshold" nevertheless can provide usable information; yet signal-detection theory says little or nothing as to why some stimuli impact consciousness, or how for the qualitative multidimensionality of percepts. May future theories of perception account adequately for perceptual experience itself!

VI. Contextuality and Contingency: Particulars, Not Universals

I suspect that in but few of you has this problem [of 'the one and the many'] occasioned sleepless nights, and I should not be astonished if some of you told me it had never vexed you. I myself have come, by long brooding over it, to consider it the most central of all philosophic problems, central because so pregnant. I mean by this that if you know whether a man is a decided monist or a decided pluralist, you perhaps know more about the rest of his opinions than if you give him any other name ending in ist.
-- *William James*

In this chapter I have meandered rather boldly from theories of perception in pre-Classical Greece to recent data on contextuality in the perception of loudness. Now, in this final section, I shall try to join all of these threads to produce a single coherent tapestry -- and not, I hope, a patchwork quilt!

Psychology, Science, and the Search for Invariances

The quotation from William James that heads this section comes from his late work, *Pragmatism* (1907), where, as in other places, James comes down firmly in favor of pluralism as opposed to monism. I am fond of referring to the related distinction, well-known in many literary socio-political circles, that Sir Isaiah Berlin (1953) makes between what he calls the hedgehogs and the foxes -- between those monistic thinkers, who promulgate a vision of singular truth, an underlying unity to nature, and the pluralists, who relish diversity itself. Berlin's terms hinge on an aphorism ascribed to Archilochus: "The fox knows many things, but the hedgehog knows one big thing." In political thought, Karl Marx is a hedgehog and Berlin himself a fox; in philosophy, Plato sits enthroned among the royalty of hedgehogs, where Aristotle would kneel alongside the many other diligent foxes.

Although Berlin's essay concerns itself largely with Tolstoy (whom Berlin sees as a fox seeking to be a hedgehog), the main thrust and application of Berlin's distinction are to social-political thought -- to his vision of a democratic pluralism serving as an antidote to the often autocratic, totalitarian tendencies of monism; yet there is a sense in which it can apply quite well to science. For scientific thinking often displays a monistic or uniformitarian trend; this is especially notable in, say, the search by theoretical physicists for a so-called "grand unified theory," a single theoretical framework that is capable of accounting for all of the forces in the universe: electromagnetism, gravity, the strong force that binds atomic nuclei, the weak force. Mathematical formalism is often -- though not uniformly -- central to the search for invariances, the oft-cited quest to discern "unity among diversity."

Like James and like Berlin, I have brooded for many years over monism and pluralism. For it has always seemed to me that a strong strain of monism pervades not only much thinking in natural science, but especially much thinking in psychophysics. It should be apparent, for example, that the search for invariances is one variety of the general quest for uniformity amidst diversity. Near the end of his introductory chapter to the Handbook of Experimental Psychology, S.S. Stevens (1953) wrote:

> In a sense, there is only one problem of psychophysics, namely the definition of the stimulus. In this same sense, there is only one problem in all of psychology -- and that is the same problem. The definition of the stimulus is thus a bigger problem than it appears at first sight. The reason for equating psychology to the problem of defining stimuli can be stated thus: the complete definition of the stimulus to a given response involves the specification of all the transformations of the environment, both internal and external, that leave the response invariant. (pp. 31-32).

It may be hard to quarrel with a view that psychophysics should search for invariances to map its terrain -- unless that search seriously misleads the explorer. For it may be tempting to assume it is possible to take perceptual experiences and parcel out all of the rough-and-tumble, variegated, and messy effects of cognition, leaving behind a set of pristine "sensations" -- sensations of loudness and pitch, of brightness and color -- which once themselves isolated can reveal a monistic set of invariant properties. This kind of temptation is very strong indeed. It pervades the history of psychophysics and, consequently, it is deeply ingrained in the ways that many of us view perceptual processing. But that view of perceptual processing is wrong. And it is so very hard to give up monistic thinking.

Monistic thinking runs deep in psychological thought. As the quotation from Stevens (1953) suggests, monistic thinking is intimately tied to our notions of measurement, and consequently to our view of psychophysics in particular and psychology in general as a natural science, on a par with other sciences. To the extent that sensory psychophysics might yield a set of invariant properties, readily quantified, psychophysics can stand with the best of the sciences. But alas, the world does not appear quite so simple as all of that. Whatever it is that we may wish to call sensation, sensation seems to be quite contextual, and thus quite contingent.

All science, of course, is contextual and contingent. Since Kant, there have been few who look for universal principles that are independent of knowers, whether these principles be physical or psychological. Rationalism in its older forms is dead (though one may occasionally see a few zombies wandering about).

Yet physics and chemistry do not seem to be contingent in the same way that psychology does -- even if some physicists thrive in the quest for complexity (e.g., see Anderson, 1991). For so much of human behavior is culturally driven. Indeed, it has become increasingly common in recent years to see psychology as quintessentially contingent (cf. the social constructionism of Kenneth Gergen, 1985). Culture and, especially, language seem to make many of the very concepts of psychology products of their local environments, appropriate to particular places and particular times, not universal and unvarying. Psychology is a den for foxes, not a pen for hedgehogs.

It is against this backdrop that sensory psychophysics holds out its promise to be a science of Nature, not just a science of Humans, a science in which there operate quantitative and minimally contingent principles, much like the principles of chemistry and physics. But we need to recognize that all sciences are contingent, even that all sciences are historical artifacts. The principles of the physical universe may themselves have been born in the relatively brief period after the Big Bang. Certainly biology deals with processes and structures that reflect all of the historical happenstance of evolution. And even if we could ignore culture, which of course we cannot, psychology must necessarily be at least as contingent as biology. In psychology two kinds of contingency, biological and cultural, are not easily rent asunder.

But the issues go even deeper than this. The monistic view expresses the vision of a world filled with invariances, a world that will reveal its underlying uniformities only to the perspicacious scientist. It is a view with strong roots in Platonistic thought.

Plato's emphasis on essences, on the supposedly ultimate truths of mathematics and geometry, exemplifies his stance as an early hedgehog. Lurking within the domain of Platonic Forms is the notion of "commensurability," as applied to the virtues -- the notion that there is a common metric or measure that can, and should, meaningfully be applied to the assessment of possible goals, acts, needs, values, and desires.[6] In his Protagoras, Plato asserts that the very possibility of choice between two alternatives resides in their common measure, derives from the possibility that both can be weighted in the same kind of units, so that the decision rests on which alternative has the greater value. Not only choice between two valued goods, but choices between qualitative dissimilars -- say, between friendship and honor -- would demand a similar metric; in the Protagoras, though not so clearly in later essays, the universal metric is one of "pleasure," and the ultimate nature of virtue is the knowledge that permits each of us to calculate the greatest long-term pleasure.

[6] I owe much of my thinking about the issue of commensurability to the insightful and elegant writings of Martha Nussbaum; notable are her volume on *The Fragility of Goodness* (1986), and especially, the essays on "The discernment of perception: An Aristotelian conception of private and public rationality" (1990) and "Plato on commensurability and desire", both in *Love's Knowledge* (1990).

Viewed in this light, it becomes easier to understand that Plato was neither facetious nor factitious when he drew the inference, in the Republic, that the just ruler is $3^{3^{3}}$ or 729 times happier than the tyrant. For the two properties of uniformity and metricity are fundamental to Plato's theory (see Nussbaum, 1990). Furthermore, it is not too far-fetched to see an analogy between, on the one hand, Plato's notion of commensurability in the moral sphere and, on the other hand, the physical principle that the material world comprises matter and motion, quantity and its configurations. Plato's doctrine finds its elaboration, for example, in virtually all modern theories of economics, which define commodities in terms of equivalent money value or such (whether dollars, Deutschmarke, or MacDonald hamburgers), and in the psychologists' analogues of scaled utility. Common to all of these approaches is the underlying tenet that apparent differences in quality can be superseded by an intrinsic, underlying communality in quantity. And to find such universal yardsticks, or metersticks, or balance-scales, is to adhere to a particular vision of science.

Perhaps, though, we should give serious credence to an alternative to Plato's notion of commensurability, namely, to the pluralistic view that in the realm of human behavior -- in the realm of needs, goals, and, yes, even sensory perceptions -- qualities are, well, *qualitative*, are individual, are concrete and particular, not abstract and general, and that quantification, though more or less relevant depending on circumstances, will necessarily tell only part of the story (cf Nussbaum, 1986, 1990a). Partial quantitative similarity can never override qualitative dissimilarity in objects, in values, or in perceptions. (From an ethical perspective, this stance allows each virtue or act or individual to be valued on its own terms, as a concrete particular [Nussbaum, 1990].[7])

---

[7] I strongly suspect that it is the ethical sense of incommensurability that informs many a pluralism, from Aristotle to James to Berlin.

This extension of the pluralistic credo may, I believe, help explain why William James (1890) so disdained Fechner's notion that perceptual magnitudes can be quantified -- a critique that has become known as the "quantity objection." To James, every perception -- or sensation, as called it -- is qualitatively distinct. Contrary to the monists, to the uniformitarians, to the hedgehogs, James wrote

> The passion for unity and smoothness is in some minds so insatiate that, in spite of the logical clearness of these reasonings and conclusions, many will fail to be influenced by them. They establish a sort of disjointedness in things which in certain quarters will appear intolerable. They sweep away all chance of 'passing without a break' either from the material to the mental, or from the lower to the higher mental; and they thrust us back into a pluralism of consciousnesses .... (1890, Vol. 1, pp. 162-163).

James we know to be a decided pluralist, from which we may discern many of his other opinions. James never was very big on quantification.

The issue of commensurability stands at the heart of psychology's most important metatheoretical issues, for it speaks to the very nature of our discipline: Should psychology ape the science of physics, that paragon of quantification? Or must psychology also deal with those slippery notions like meaning, value, desire -- qualities not only irreducible but ultimately incommensurable?

Consider Freud's (1915/1957) quandry over the multifarious roles of the instincts (*Triebe*), that curious psychoanalytic concept conflating the biological and the mental. According to Freud, instincts lie at the frontier between the mind and the body: From the perspective of the biological needs that underlie the instincts, said Freud, all instincts are identical, in that they vary only in quantity but not in quality. Yet considered psychologically, the instincts are clearly invested in quality. Freud's short paper on "instincts and their vicissitudes" thrusts the reader directly into the two horns of a hermeneutic dilemma: How can physical processes of bodily energy, which differ from one another only in their quantities, represent differences in psychological quality? And how can a scientist of nature hurdle the gap between a language of causes or correlations and a language of meanings? For an attempt to see how Freud might have traversed at least the former frontier (with a little help from Fechner's theory of inner psychophysics), see Marks (in press-b).

If it is psychology's ultimate lot to be both intentional and intensional, to deal with goals and desires and to reflect meanings and values, then no matter how accurately psychologists may quantify -- and quantify we shall and must -- and no matter how universal the behavioral and mental principles that we establish, psychology must deal with what is unique and individual, with what is concrete and particular, whether this be a racial attitude, a rate of learning to ride a bicycle, or the relative loudness of a fife and drum on Main Street on the Fourth of July.

References

Algom, D., & Marks, L.E. (1990). Range and regression, loudness processing and loudness scales: Toward a context-bound psychophysics. *Journal of Experimental Psychology; Human Perception and Performance*, **16**, 706-727.

Anderson, P.W. (1991). Is complexity physics? Is it science? What is it? *Physics Today*, **44** (July), 9-11.

Baird, J.C. (1970a). A cognitive theory of psychophysics. I. *Scandinavian Journal of Psychology*, **11**, 35-46.

Baird, J.C. (1970b). A cognitive theory of psychophysics. II. *Scandinavian Journal of Psychology*, **11**, 89-103.

Berlin, I. (1953). *The hedgehog and the fox.* New York: Simon & Schuster.

Boring, E.G. (1957). *A history of experimental psychology* (second edition). New York:Appleton-Century-Crofts.

Boynton, R.M. (1979). *Human color vision.* New York: Holt, Rinehart, & Winston.

Brindley, G.S. (1960). *Physiology of the retina and the visual pathway.* London: Arnold.

Fechner, G. (1860). *Elemente der Psychophysik.* Leipzig: Breikopf und Härtel.

Fletcher, H., & Munson, W.A. (1933). Loudness, its measurement and calculation. *Journal of the Acoustical Society of America*, **5**, 82-108.

Fodor, J. (1981). *Representatations: Philosophical essays on the foundations of cognitive science.* Cambridge, MA: MIT Press.

Freud, S. (1957). Instincts and their vicissitudes. In J. Strachey (Ed. & Trans.), *Standard edition of the complete psychological works of Sigmund Freud* (Vol. 14, pp. 109-140).

Galileo, G. (1960). The assayer. In *The controversy on the comets of 1618* (pp. 151-336), trans. by S. Drake and C.D. O'Malley. Philadelphia: University of Pennsylvania Press. (Originally published, 1623).

Gergen, K. (1985). The social constructionist movement in modern psychology. *American Psychologist*, **40**, 266-285.

Gibson, J.J. (1979). *The senses considered as perceptual systems*. Boston: Houghton Mifflin.

Green, D.M., & Swets, J.A. (1966). *Signal detection theory and psychophysics*. New York: Wiley.

Greenberg, G.Z., & Larkin, W.D. (1968). Frequency-response characteristics of auditory observers detecting signals of a single frequency in noise: The probe-signal method. *Journal of the Acoustical Society of America*, **44**, 1513-1523.

Hartshorne, C. (1934). *The philosophy and psychology of sensation*. Chicago: University of Chicago Press.

Helmholtz, H.L.F. von (1925). *Treatise on physiological optics* (Vol. 3), trans. by J.P.C. Southall. Rochester, NY: Optical Society of America. (Originally published, 1866).

Helson, H. (1964). *Adaptation level theory: An experimental and systematic approach to behavior*. New York: Harper & Row.

Hurvich, L.M. (1981). *Color vision*. Sutherland, MA: Sinauer.

James, W. (1890). *The principles of psychology*. New York: Henry Holt.

James, W. (1907). *Pragmatism; a new name for some old ways of thinking*. New York:Longmans, Green.

James, W. (1909). *A pluralistic universe; Hibbert Lectures at Manchester College on the present situation in philosophy*. New York: Longmans, Green.

Kolers, P. (1983). Perception and representation. *Annual Review of Psychology*, **34**, 129-166.

Locke, J. (1690). *An essay concerning human understanding*. London: Basset.

Marks, L.E. (1974). On scales of sensation: Prolegomena to any future psychophysics that will be able to come forth as science. *Perception & Psychophysics*, **16**, 358-376.

Marks, L.E. (1979). A theory of loudness and loudness judgments. *Psychological Review*, **86**, 256-285.

Marks, L.E. (1988). Magnitude estimation and sensory matching. *Perception and Psychophysics*, **43**, 511-525.

Marks, L.E. (1991). Slippery context effects in psychophysics. Paper presented at the Experimental Psychology Society, April, Cambridge, England.

Marks, L.E. (in press-a). The slippery context effect in psychophysics: Intensive, extensive, and qualitative continua. *Perception & Psychophysics*.

Marks, L.E. (in press-b). Freud and Fechner, desire and energy, hermeneutics and psychophysics. In H.-G. Geissler, S.W. Link, and J.T. Townsend (Eds.), *Cognition, information processing, and psychophysics: Basic issues*. Hillsdale, NJ: Erlbaum.

Marks, L.E., & Warner, E. (1991). Slippery context effect and critical bands. *Journal of Experimental Psychology: Human Perception and Performance*, **17**, 986-996.

Müller, J. (1842). *Elements of physiology* (Vol. 2), trans. by W. Baly. London: Taylor and Walton. (Originally published, 1838).

Newton, I. (1952). *Opticks; or a treatise of the reflexions, refractions, inflexions, and colours of light* (fourth edition). New York: Dover. (Originally published, 1730).

Nussbaum, M.C. (1986). *The fragility of goodness: Luck and ethics in Greek tragedy and philosophy*. Cambridge, England: Cambridge University Press.

Nussbaum, M.C. (1990). *Love's knowledge*: Essays on philosophy and literature. Oxford, England: Oxford University Press.

Popper, R.D., Parker, S., & Galanter, E. (1986). dual loudness scales in individual subjects. *Journal of Experimental Psychology: Human Perception and Performance*, **12**, 61-69.

Pylyshyn, Z.W. (1984). *Computation and cognition: Toward a foundation for cognitive science*. Cambridge, MA: MIT Press.

Robinson, D.W., & Dadson, R.S. (1954). A re-determination of the equal-loudness relations for pure tones. *British Journal of Applied Physics*, **7**, 166-181.

Rushton, W.A.H. (1972). Review lecture. Pigments and signals in color vision. *Journal of Physiology*, **220**, 1-31P.

Scharf, B. (1970). Critical bands. In J.V. Tobias (Ed.), *Foundations of modern auditory theory* (Vol. 1, pp. 157-202). New York: Academic Press.

Scheerer, E. (1987). The unknown Fechner. *Psychological Research*, **49**, 197-202.

Schneider, B., & Parker, S. (1990). Does stimulus context affect loudness or only loudness judgment? *Perception & Psychophysics*, **48**, 409-418.

Stevens, S.S. (1953). Mathematics, measurement, and psychophysics. In S.S. Stevens (Ed.), *Handbook of experimental psychology* (pp. 1-49). New York: Wiley.

Stevens, S.S. (1972). Perceived level of noise by Mark VII and decibels (E). *Journal of the Acoustical Society of America*, **51**, 575-601.

Stratton, G.M. (1917). *Theophrastus and the Greek physiological psychology before Aristotle*. London: Allen & Unwin.

Zwicker, E., Flottorp, G., & Stevens, S.S. (1957). Critical band width in loudness summation. *Journal of the Acoustical Society of America*, **29**, 548-557.

Zwicker, E., & Scharf, B. (1969). A model of loudness summation. *Psychological Review*, **72**, 3-26.

Zwislocki, J.J. (1965). Analysis of some auditory characteristics. In R.D. Luce, R.R. Bush, and E. Galanter (Eds.), *Handbook of mathematical psychology* (Vol. 3, pp. 3-97). New York:Wiley.

Psychophysical Approaches to Cognition
D. Algom (Editor)

4

MIND IN PSYCHOPHYSICS[1]

Lawrence M. Ward

University of British Columbia

[1] This work was supported by a grant from the Natural Sciences and Engineering Research Council of Canada.

The branches of physics that deal with questions such as why iron ... is magnetic, while copper is not ... (etc) ... are called "solid-state physics," or "liquid-state physics" or "honest physics." The branch of physics that found these three simple little actions (the easiest part) is called "fundamental physics" - we stole that name in order to make the other physicists feel uncomfortable!

-----*(Feynman, 1985, p. 114)*

Minds are simply what brains do.

-----*(Minsky, 1986, p. 287)*

...the mind has a unifying power; it contracts the physical ... into a simplified appearance of itself.

-----*(Fechner, 1851/1987, p.205)*

Table of Contents

I. Caveata

This chapter represents part of the attempt by myself and other "fundamental psychophysicists" to find the "three (or n) little actions" (see above quote by Feynman) of psychophysics, i.e. a core of concepts and relations from which all the rest of psychophysics can be derived (albeit with much effort). That such a core has been found for a large part of physics (named "quantum electrodynamics" or QED) allows some hope that such a program for psychophysics is not futile. However, the quest is admittedly reminiscent of the hunting of the Snark, or perhaps of the Holy Grail, both of which have grave dangers (vanishment if the Snark be a Boojum and death if the cup be not the Grail, respectively) and seductive rewards (Snarkpelt and eternal life, respectively). The proper prolegomena to any attempt to follow this quest is a series of caveata (warnings) about what can and cannot be expected to result from the expedition.

First, it is obvious that any single paper can hope to do little more than to steer thoughts in fruitful directions. Moreover, psychophysics is vast, both empirically and conceptually (although less vast than physics). Thus, the present chapter represents a severely constrained and somewhat personal (i.e., biased) attempt to suggest candidates for the "three little actions." Second, it is not obvious that there is a consensus as to what psychophysics should in fact be about. The fundamentalist approach is necessarily very different from that of those who use psychophysical methods analogously to physiologists' electrodes ("honest" psychophysicists?), or those who use them to help solve problems of diagnosing sensory dysfunction or environmental degradation ("applied" psychophysicists?). Finally, my own inadequacy for the task at hand is amplified (to mix metaphors) by the even greater vastness of the other fields from which I wish to take direction. I necessarily had to select a biased sample of concepts and data from those fields to help inform the psychophysical task, and I have no illusions that I have mined all the gold or rejected all the iron pyrite.

One way to view psychophysics is as a scientific attack on the classical mind-body problem of philosophy. It certainly seems that Fechner saw it that way since he characterized psychophysics "... as an exact theory of the functionally dependent relations of body and soul or, more generally, of the material and the mental..." (Fechner 1860/1966, p.7). This chapter takes this view seriously, and attempts to find the basis for a core set of concepts and relations dealing with mind in psychophysics that can be linked to our emerging understanding of brain processes (inner psychophysics) as well as to our already highly developed understanding of the physical world (outer psychophysics). However, Fechner conceptualized mind and body within the 19th century Zeitgeist. There have been major developments in philosophy, neuroscience, artificial intelligence, linguistics, and cognitive psychology, as well as in psychophysics, in the 104 years since his death in 1887. It would be surprising if, in spite of the fact that Fechner anticipated many modern ideas (see Scheerer, 1987), his conceptualizations of brain and mind would serve as well at the dawn of the 21st century as they did in 1850-1887. Thus, in addition to asking what psychophysical conceptualizations of mind are necessary and sufficient (e.g., fundamental), it seems prudent to test our conclusions for consistency with the ideas of other relevant disciplines. Moreover, since several of those disciplines are expressly concerned to characterize "mind," it is possible that we can borrow fundamental concepts from them to use for our own purposes. Thus, in what follows I first describe a view of fundamental psychophysics that I have been developing for several years, including the role played in such a discipline by "mind," and then investigate several important domains in classical and contemporary psychophysics to discover the views of mind implicit in them. Following this I describe some aspects of the philosophy of mind, artificial intelligence, neuroscience, and cognitive psychology that seem relevant and suggestive. Finally, I suggest a multiple-agency view of mind and some candidates for a core set of concepts (agencies) of mind that could be fundamental for psychophysics and possibly for other disciplines as well.

II. Fundamental Psychophysics

I will take QED as the prototype of a fundamental theory in science and the conceptualization of it as arising from a distinguishable branch of physics as an indication that there might exist such a branch of psychophysics (see quote from Feynman [1985] at the beginning of this chapter). Although I cannot describe QED in detail here, there are a few aspects of it that are suggestive for any other discipline. First, it is extremely simple at the most fundamental level; there are two basic "particles," the electron and the photon, and "three little actions," electron moves from A to B in space-time, photon moves from A to B in space-time, and electron scatters photon (absorbs and then emits, or vice versa). Of course space-time and its measurement are assumed, and quite complicated equations are used to describe the "amplitude" (a complex number) for a particle to engage in relevant actions in a particular situation. Moreover, there are rules by which these amplitudes are combined to yield (real) probabilities of an action happening. However, considering the complexity of the phenomena that can be derived from the theory (all the phenomena of our world except for nuclear and gravitic, including chemistry, biochemistry, and life itself), the core of the theory is remarkably simple and elegant. All of the complexity arises from combinations and recombinations, both hierarchical and heterarchical, of the core concepts (Feynman, 1985).

It is important to remember, however, that although simple in a core sense, the application of QED to any particular situation is far from simple. It may take many physicists working for many years to develop an application, especially to calculate predictions to the number of decimal places to match the accuracy of experimental determinations. For example, the magnetic moment of an electron (its response to an external magnetic field) has been calculated to be 1.00115965246 and measured to be 1.00115965221$\pm$.00000000004 (Feynman, 1985). Because of the truly enormous number of different ways for the action "electron moves from A to B" can be accomplished (e.g., straight from A to B, from A to B but emitting a photon and then reabsorbing it along the way, something that could happen at every point in space-time between A and B, from A to B emitting and reabsorbing two photons, etc.), it took many years of effort to work out the calculations of the magnetic moment to this degree of accuracy; in fact right now a number of physicists are using supercomputers to calculate the next couple of decimal places. In an analogous psychophysical theory we wouldn't have to work this hard, since our experiments determine relevant constants only to about the first decimal place at best. Nonetheless, the point is that application of a fundamental theory is not easy, even in physics.

What form should a fundamental theory of psychophysics take? There are various dimensions along which we might attempt to characterize it. For example, we would wish to have both mechanistic (as QED) and conservation (as thermodynamics) forms of a fundamental psychophysical theory. The conservation form would most likely have to do with laws of information balance (cf. Norwich, 1981), while the mechanistic form would specify fundamental psychophysical processes. The two would need to be linked at the level of the most basic concepts, as QED and thermodynamics are linked by the concepts of motion and energy. Most psychophysicists seem to favor a nomothetic type of theory that would describe idealized psychophysical systems and would be addressed by data averaged over many subjects. However, applications, such as to sensory dysfunction, demand a theory that has reality at an idiographic level as well. Most psychophysicists also seem to agree that a formal theory is preferable to an informal one. There is some (mostly implicit) disagreement, however, as to whether such a theory should be basically a deterministic or stochastic mathematical theory (e.g., Luce, Baird, Green & Smith, 1980; M. Treisman & Williams, 1984) or a formal process theory described in a computer-programming-like formal language and mathematized only when necessary for testing (e.g., Ward, 1979; cf. Gregg & Simon, 1967), although others don't think it matters much so long as the theory is formal (e.g., Laming, 1988a). There is also (again mostly implicit) disagreement about whether the theory should be conceptualized as fundamentally dynamic (e.g., DiCarlo & Cross, 1991; Gregson, 1988; Luce et al, 1980; Ward, 1979) or static (e.g., Anderson, 1981; Green & Swets, 1966; Stevens, 1975). The static approach emphasizes laws that operate outside of time, such as the psychophysical power law, while the dynamic approach emphasizes processes that operate in time. Both can be powerful, but the dynamic approach is more general and can be "staticized" when dynamics are not important (cf. Gregson, 1988).

In addition to the above general considerations, there are some more specific aspects of a fundamental theory that should be considered. First is the relationship that should obtain between measurement theory as it is now construed (see Krantz, Luce, Suppes & Tversky, 1971) and a fundamental theory. In other fields, science does not wait for axiomatization of its procedures in a formal measurement theory before proceeding to propose and test fundamental theories. However, all fundamental theories are cast in terms of concepts (in physics, basic dimensions such as length and time) that are assumed to be measurable. Formalization of the measurement status of these concepts can reveal deep relationships between them and the elements of the fundamental theory (e.g., dimensional analysis in physics - see Krantz et al, 1971, Chapter 10). I have suggested that a necessary condition for a useful fundamental theory of psychophysics is that important axioms based on empirical results in a measurement theory for the elementary concepts be derivable in it, and that a necessary condition for a useful measurement theory is that there be some fundamental understanding of the psychophysical quantities measured (Ward, 1987). Thus, the two types of theory serve different goals but can be interlocked in the same way that fundamental physics and measurement theory have been. Falmagne (1985) develops a "modern" viewpoint on classical (especially Fechnerian) psychophysics that emphasizes such relationships.

A propos of the basic dimensions in which fundamental psychophysical concepts should be cast is my suggestion (Ward, 1989) that it be the psychological space defined by Shepard (1987). Shepard's (1987) space is based on a universal law of generalization (see *Mind in Psychophysics* section). Important here is the idea that several possibly fundamental concepts, including dissimilarity, psychological magnitude, and information in the sense of Shannon (1948) can all be defined by various metrics on this space (Ward, 1989). Interestingly, the dimensions of the space are usually considered to be physical (e.g. stimulus intensity on relevant aspects) while the *organization* of the objects within the space, as reflected by Shepard's "consequential regions" or by concepts like distance (on various metrics), are psychological (mental?). Such a relationship provides one possible fundamental connection between the physical and mental worlds of the sort we are seeking.

A final very general consideration concerns the possibility of ideal experiments in psychophysics. Again, physics serves as the prototype. Ideal experiments in physics reveal and in a sense define several aspects of fundamental physical concepts. For example, the two-slit experiment in quantum physics exemplifies and explicates wave-particle duality, the uncertainty principle, and the evolution and linear superposition of probability wave functions and their "collapse" into probabilities. Ideal experiments can be realized in several forms, but are unlike any of their realizations in that experimental details are suppressed in favor of conceptual relationships. Ideal experiments in psychophysics could be conceptualized in terms of what I have called a *fundamental psychophysical system*, consisting of one or more *sources* of energy quanta, an *afferent system* that responds to impingement by quanta from the source(s) by changing its own activity, a *mind*, an *effector system* that implements actions initiated by the mind, and a *recorder* to retain a physical record of the actions of the effector system and the source(s) for future input to another "observer" system (Ward, 1990). Figures 4.1a and 4.1b display two such idealized psychophysical experiments. Figure 4.1a describes the classical Hecht, Schlaer and Pirenne (1942) experiment in which bursts of 510 nm wavelength photons were fired at the dark-adapted eye of an observer who said "yes" whenever he saw a flash. The equations in the figure are sufficient to describe the behavior of the mind in interaction with such a physical source under ideal conditions. Figure 4.1b describes a similar experiment but with an added source (noise). The new source changes the situation in such a way that different equations must be used to describe the behavior of the mind (the equations of Signal Detection Theory). Such depictions of ideal experiments in psychophysics help to identify the irreducible minimum of concepts required for a fundamental psychophysics. They may also help to clarify the role that mind plays in fundamental psychophysics, a role that is sometimes forgotten when "honest" psychophysicists use its methods to discover laws of sensory system functioning, or applied psychophysicists use its methods to collect data that inform practical decisions.

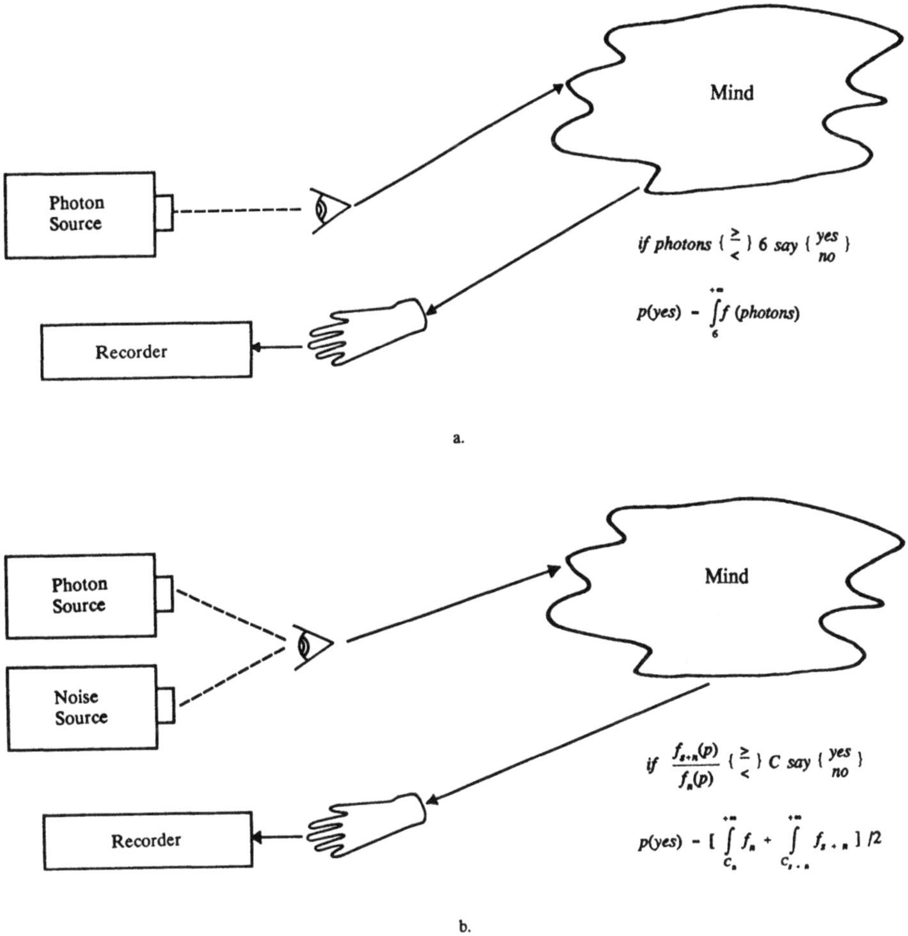

Figure 4.1: (a) An idealization of the Hecht, Schlaer, Pirenne (1942) experiment in which observers detected 100 msec, 10' visual angle, flashes of 510 nm wavelength light at 20 deg retinal eccentricity after 40 min of dark adaptation. Observers' detection behavior is limited by the statistics of the photon source. (b)An idealization of a similar experiment under much noisier conditions. Here the equations of signal detection theory describe observers' detection behavior.

III. Mind in Psychophysics

There have been several efforts to invent a fundamental theory of psychophysics, albeit somewhat different from the one I envisioned (e.g., Anderson, 1981, 1990; Green & Swets, 1966; Gregson, 1988; Laming, 1986; Norwich, 1981; Shepard, 1987). Fechner himself was obviously a fundamental psychophysicist, and S.S. Stevens (e.g., 1961, 1975) apparently also accepted most of Fechner's basic conceptualizations. I will briefly review each of these approaches, and a few others from "honest" psychophysics, to give an idea of what might someday be accomplished, with a special emphasis on where a concept of mind is important. Mind will be seen to play a central role in all of these approaches to psychophysics. Thus it is important for us to analyze this concept and provide a fundamental characterization of it that has a possibility of eliciting some consensus.

Fechner's system rested on the relations between three basic concepts, the stimulus energy (representing the "outer" physical world), the brain processes given rise to by the stimulus (representing the "inner" physical world), and the sensation (representing the mental world) (Fechner, 1860/1966). Memories, depending on the aftereffects of the psychophysical processes arising from sensations, had the same physical realization and the same mental status (Fechner, 1882/1987). For Fechner, a conscious (above threshold) sensation was apparently the unanalyzable minimum mental experience. He believed that the magnitudes of the sensations arising from all of the different modalities could be measured (possibly "experienced" - cf. Baird & Noma, 1978, p.14) on a common scale, established by counting jnd's (just noticeable differences) from the threshold of "consciousness" (expressed in physical terms) (Fechner 1860/1966, 1887/1987). This way of measuring mental phenomena was necessitated by "... the fact that as far as mental intensities are concerned we can estimate 'more' or 'less', but not 'how many'." (Fechner, 1851/1987, p.204). Thus, Fechner took as fundamental a mental phenomenon, the *conscious sensation* (above absolute threshold, which Fechner took to be the "statical" threshold of Herbart -- see Ward, 1988), and two mental operations, *detection* (because he was dealing with "conscious" sensations) and *ordinal comparison* of those conscious sensations (or equivalently, memories of them). It has been argued that Fechner's invention of the method of summated jnd's to measure sensation, which led to his logarithmic law of outer psychophysics (relation of the physical world to "sensation", the elementary concept of mind in Fechner's approach), $S=k\ ln\ (I/I_o)$, where S is sensation magnitude (summated jnd's), I/I_o represents stimulus intensity measured in relation to absolute threshold intensity, and k is proportional to the inverse of the Weber fraction, was in the service of his belief that the "true" relation between sensation (mind) and brain processes (inner psychophysics) was logarithmic (Baird & Noma, 1978; Scheerer, 1987). Since he believed that the relation of the brain to the physical world was linear (they were successive events connected by causal laws, all of which were assumed to be linear - see Scheerer, 1987), establishing a logarithmic law of outer psychophysics was tantamount to showing that the inner psychophysical law was also logarithmic. Thus, Fechner believed he had arrived at a compelling solution to the mind-body problem, in which "mind" and "brain" were complementary ways of viewing a unitary phenomenon, with the two views related by the logarithmic transformation. This approach is called *monism* and has a long tradition in philosophy (see *Mind in Philosophy* section). Interestingly, Fechner's proposed solution had little effect on philosophy, and although most philosophers now would support some form of monism, they never (to my knowledge) cite psychophysics as a reason.

Most (but of course not all) modern psychophysicists appear to accept at least Fechner's division of a person in the world into three basic "layers": the outer physical world from which stimuli arise, the brain (often construed as sensory system), and some form of "mental" or "internal" representation of the physical stimulus that may be based on brain processes but is not materialistically reducible to them, having instead a "functional reality" that must be analyzed independent of brain processes (see *Mind in Philosophy* section). They also appear to accept the fundamental quality of sensation, although they do not often comment on how it is related to consciousness (cf. Gescheider, 1988; Searle, 1990). The modern workers appear to differ dramatically, however, in how they characterize the fundamental mental operations. For example, S.S. Stevens (e.g., 1961, 1975) spent a lifetime attempting to measure sensation, conceptualized similarly to Fechner's view. However, he disagreed as to the mental operation that should be taken as fundamental, insisting that people could report directly on the magnitude of their sensations in such a way that ratio scales could be constructed from the reports. Eventually, he came to the view that *matching* was the fundamental operation of direct scaling, asserting that when people matched sensation magnitude to numbers (as in magnitude estimation) they were meaningfully reflecting ratio properties of the sensations in the numbers they emitted. Thus, Stevens believed that people could indeed judge "how much" (prothetic continua) or "where" (metathetic continua) aspects of their sensations. He did not offer a theory about how they could do this, but he apparently also believed that another operation, that of *abstraction* or *isolation* was involved: "Actually, in all human judgment the observer abstracts or isolates one feature of the situation from those other features that he might have judged if the task had been a different one." (S.S. Stevens, 1975, p.66). Thus, he conceptualized the sensation as a multidimensional experience, from which one or another aspect (sensory continuum) could be abstracted and judged. Fechner apparently took this ability for granted but it is clearly important to be explicit about it. S.S. Stevens took the exponent of the psychophysical power function, $S=aI^n$, where S is sensation magnitude as measured by a direct scaling method, I is stimulus intensity, and a and n are constants, to be the most fundamental parameter, describing the operating characteristic of the sensory transducer. Since n varied across sensory continua, the basic task was to measure it as precisely as possible. Thus, Stevens saw the sensory transducer as introducing a nonlinear transformation, reflected in sensation magnitude and preserved by at most affine transformations through the mental operation of matching.

N.H. Anderson (e.g., 1981, 1990, this book) also takes sensations in each of the sensory modalities as fundamental, unobservable mental elements (s_i) that arise from observable physical stimuli according to what he calls the valuation function, $V(S)=s$, or Psychophysical Law. To this he adds another fundamental mental element, a unitary sensation (or perception) (r) that results from the *integration* of the s_i according to the integration function, $I(s_1,s_2, ...)=r$, or Psychological Law. These mental elements and actions are linked to the final observable, a response (R) that affects the physical world, by the action function, $A(r)=R$, or Psychomotor Law. Another mental concept, the immediate *goal* of the organism, determines the forms of the valuation, integration, and action functions, since it affects "... what aspects of the sensory field are attended to and what memory storage is utilized." (Anderson, 1990, p.72). Thus, the concept of goal appears to represent a composite of "higher" mental operations that can be expressed simply by describing its influence on the transformations between the various mental elements. This is very similar to the way S.S. Stevens saw the role of the operation of abstraction, although Stevens did not think the operation affected the Psychophysical Law. Anderson's approach allows for a variety of possible valuation, integration and action function types. However, applications have stressed logarithmic valuation functions, linear action functions, and two particular integration rules, addition: $r=s_{Ai}+s_{Bj}$ and multiplication: $r=s_{Ai} \times s_{Bj}$, where A and B are two stimulus continua and i and j represent specific stimuli on those continua. In contrast to Stevens, who emphasized sensory transforms, Anderson has emphasized mental operations. He has characterized the set of possible integration rules as making up a *cognitive algebra* that describes the functioning of the mind at the most fundamental level.[2]

Laming (1986) seems at first glance to be trying to create a fundamental theory of sensory discrimination that has no place for mind. He too takes sensation as fundamental, and moreover explicitly divorces it from the level of neural activity anywhere in the system. He represents sensation by an internal state variable that, however, disappears from the calculations by choosing experimental paradigms in which "... the entire sensory machinery ... (can be considered as being) ... reflected outwards through the sense organ to operate directly on the physical stimulus." (Laming, 1988a, p.296). Laming's (1986) fundamental principles, such as *differential coupling* (sensory discrimination uses only change information), the *square law transformation* (by which small stimuli are rendered even less detectable), and the way in which these are realized in a model of a *sensory-analytic stage* that applies these and other transforms to Poisson process stimuli, and can be cascaded, all apply to "... the initial, preconscious stage of perception ..." (Laming, 1988a, p. 275). Nonetheless, Laming does require mind in the same way Fechner did: the experiments he analyses were all selected to be those that presented the subject with a "two-way decision" (Laming, 1988b), such as threshold, psychometric function, and signal detection experiments, for the purpose of allowing the "judgmental" component to be ignored. He projects a companion volume to his *Sensory Analysis* in which *sensory judgment* in experiments such as magnitude estimation and absolute identification will be treated separately. Thus, he seems to be identifying two classes of mental operations, one of which, yes/no decision making, allows fairly direct access to sensory processes, and the other of which, *judgment*, is both relative and allows no reliable inference about the underlying sensory processes

---

[2] Anderson now suggests to use the term *psychocognitive law* in place of the previous *psychological law* to designate the integration functions (Editor's note).

(Laming, 1988b). Many psychophysicists would disagree with his views about the possibility of making inferences from, e.g., magnitude estimation experiments (e.g., Marks, 1974), but many would also agree that such judgment processes are profoundly relative, and quite different in kind from yes/no decision making (e.g., Marks, 1991; Ward, 1987).

The prototypes of the yes/no experiments are probably those idealized by Ward (1990) (see *Fundamental Psychophysics section*), the absolute threshold experiment and the signal detection experiment. As Ward (1990) pointed out, the major difference between these two experiments seems to be the additional source (noise) in the signal detection experiment, which changes the observer's problem from one of ascertaining whether the source has affected the afferent system at all (number of effective quanta exceeded a fixed criterion) to one of whether a certain ratio has exceeded a variable criterion. This implies that some very different mental operations might be happening in the two cases. From the point of view of sensory analysis the equations in Figures 4.1a and 4.1b describe exactly what is "going on" in the two cases. In the opinion of some this is sufficient, viz. the statement of Laming (1988a, p. 296): "Also immaterial is the question whether the elements of the theory may be thought to have a 'real' existence." However, others are troubled by the postulation of fundamental mental processes that would seem to be impossible for ordinary people to carry out. For example, one trial in a signal detection experiment might be said to require the processes diagrammed in Figure 4.2 (cf. Baird & Noma, 1978). It would seem very unlikely that observers could know the form of the (usually Gaussian) probability density functions assumed by the theory, and even more unlikely that they could calculate $f(x_i|S+N)$ or $f(x_i|N)$, although they could probably obtain their ratio from the raw numbers (which, on the Gaussian assumption, are real numbers between about 0.0000000001 and about 0.4). Calculating β would be easier if the relevant equation were known, which it isn't if experience teaching it to students is any indication. Finally, the yes/no decision suggests that two numbers are compared,

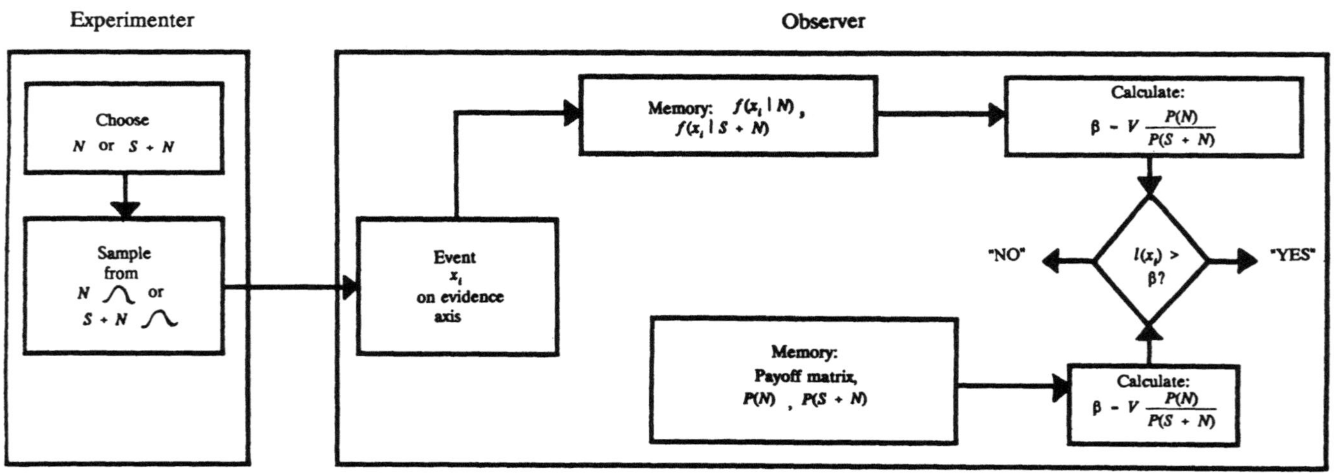

Figure 4.2: A version of a process model that takes literally the decision behavior described by signal detection theory (cf. Baird & Noma, 1978).

and yet no subject is aware of these numbers. Moreover, we know something about how numbers are compared (e.g., Besner & Grimsell, 1979; Dehaene & Dupoux, 1990), and the prevailing models are very different from those of signal detection theory even as applied to "numerical detection."

The way psychophysicists usually resolve this problem is to eschew such "process" models and simply say that people act "as if" they were (near-) ideal statistical decision makers (e.g., Laming, 1988a). Yet, some will still object that the behavior of an observer in a signal detection experiment is different in important ways from that of an experimenter doing a z-test, the similarity of the mathematics describing their decisions notwithstanding. Also, Searle (1990) pointed out in a related context the serious problems that arise when such as-if descriptions are taken literally (see also *Mind in Philosophy* section). One way to resolve this dilemma is to postulate elementary concepts that do seem somehow to describe the signal detection theory observer's behavior in a *psychologically* meaningful way (as is often done in textbooks) and then to assert that fundamental relations between these concepts give rise to the equations that are observed to handle the data to a first approximation. For example, Figure 4.3 displays one way in which the observer's behavior could be described using the classical concept of sensation, a concept of a comparator borrowed from general systems theory via MacKay (1963), and a concept of psychological magnitude suggested by Ward (1991). In Figure 4.3, the stimulus input (I_1) is converted to a sensation (S_1) that is input to a comparator (C_1) that receives its other input from a psychological "effort" generator (Ψ) and sends its mismatch signal to that same Ψ. Ψ also sends an input to C_2, which receives its other input from a "memory" of the criterial sensation that has been programmed by instructions from the experimenter but generated internally by the observer in response to those instructions. (How this comes about requires more theory, perhaps along the lines of J.R. Anderson's [1976] production systems). The mismatch signal of C_2 is directed to a response process that is also programmed by the instructions so that if the mismatch signal is positive (above background) in response to the presentation of the stimulus a "yes" response is generated, whereas if the mismatch signal is negative (below background) a "no" response is generated. The output of Ψ after it has equilibrated with C_1 is the experience of the "magnitude" of the sensation generated by the stimulus (S.S. Stevens' abstraction operation, cf. Ward, 1991). This could be different phenomenally for different people. The inputs of to C_2 from memory could be phenomenally the same as the experience of Ψ or they could be "images" that would give rise to a particular, desired, experience of Ψ when input to C_1. In either case these "criterial magnitudes" could be "minimal" (thus unadjustable) as might be appropriate for an ideal absolute threshold experiment, or a magnitude well above the minimum (thus adjustable in respect to payoffs and signal probabilities) as might be appropriate for a signal detection experiment. In the former case, under conditions of maximal sensitivity, when the input from the noise generator is near zero and the "criterial magnitude" is set to minimum, the system is dominated by the statistics of the stimulus source (e.g., as in Hecht et al, 1942). In the latter case, when the input from the noise generator is large, a different set of statistics describes the behavior of the system because of how the criterial magnitude from memory is programmed. Because the noise is always present, input to C_1 is always sufficient to necessitate balancing activity in Ψ and thus the criterial magnitude must always be higher than the minimum (low threshold theory). Because of the noise source, the mismatch signal of C_2 can occasionally be positive during the presentation interval even if the stimulus wasn't presented ("real" false alarms). Discrimination of two signals can be accomplished by programming the criterial magnitude to a level that gives above background C_2 output on some trials and below background output on others. Two-interval paradigms can be described by a system in which the memory of the activity of Ψ generated to match the first interval input is input to C_2 during the second interval in place of the criterial magnitude. Thus, the same decision mechanism, with the same fundamental mental operations programmed appropriately by the situation, can be seen to underlie behavior in several different important psychophysical experiments.

In the account just presented, the fundamental mental elements are the sensation, its magnitude (Ψ), and the memory of a criterial magnitude (or an earlier sensation magnitude), while the fundamental mental operator is the comparator (which abstracts as it compares). The picture could be (and will be) elaborated by the addition of other operations that are only implicit at this point. However, Figure 4.3 suffices to make the point that classical threshold theory and signal detection theory can be construed in similar terms with respect to fundamental mental operations, and that especially signal detection theory can be thought of in process terms different from those implied by a literal construal of statistical decision theory while retaining the power of the mathematical description of an observer's behavior within that theory.

The application of statistical decision theory to more than two stimuli is exemplified by Thurstone's Law of Categorical Judgment (Torgerson, 1961). This is a generalization of signal detection theory (although it was described much earlier than signal detection theory), and has been developed more recently by Durlach and Braida in their theory of auditory intensity resolution (e.g., Braida & Durlach, 1988) and by M. Treisman in his more general theory of criterion setting (e.g., M. Treisman & Williams, 1984). Data from absolute identification paradigms are described quite well by these theories and yet they suffer from the same lack of psychological plausibility as does signal detection theory. Because of their similar structure, however, a similar remedy is possible. The mechanism shown in Figure 4.3 can be iterated serially, or replicated in parallel, to make decisions about the locus of a sensation magnitude with respect to several different criterial magnitudes. The easiest to see is probably the serial mechanism, which would simply iterate (using a memory of Ψ as input to C_2) on a series of remembered, ever-increasing criterial magnitudes (the largest being the most intense non-painful magnitude imaginable) until there was a change in the mismatch signal from C_2 from above to below background, at which point the iteration would cease and the label of the last criterial magnitude compared would be output as the "identity" of the input stimulus. Thus, categorization, upon which both the Thurstonian treatment and information theory (as used in psychology in the 1950's and 1960's, see Garner, 1962) are based, can also be described in terms of the comparison operation.

A similar lesson can be drawn with respect to S.S. Stevens' (e.g., 1975) suggestion that matching might be a fundamental mental operation. In the context of theoretical statements about the measurement of psychological magnitude several other psychophysicists have suggested that matching is primary (Luce, 1991; Marks, 1991; J.C. Stevens, 1991; Ward, 1991; Zwislocki, 1991). In particular, I argued for a unitary concept of psychological magnitude that is abstracted, or isolated, from the composite "sensation" given rise to by a stimulus by a mechanism that uses comparators similarly to Figure 4.3 (Ward, 1991). Figure 4.4 displays how cross-modality matching might be accomplished by a cascade of comparators arranged somewhat differently from those in Figure 4.3. In Figure 4.4, the second output from Ψ goes to another comparator C_2, as in Figure 4.3, but the other input to C_2 is the input from the sensory system responding to stimuli on the response continuum, and its output is to an effector process that adjusts the stimulus magnitude on that continuum. Similarly, intra-modality matching and judgments of total intensity of several sensory stimuli can be so described. Thus, a comparison operation can be seen to be fundamental to several seemingly different mental operations that involve psychological magnitude.

Another important concept that has been argued to be fundamental is *dissimilarity* or psychological distance. Shepard (1987) suggested a universal law of (stimulus) generalization formulated with respect to a fundamental psychological

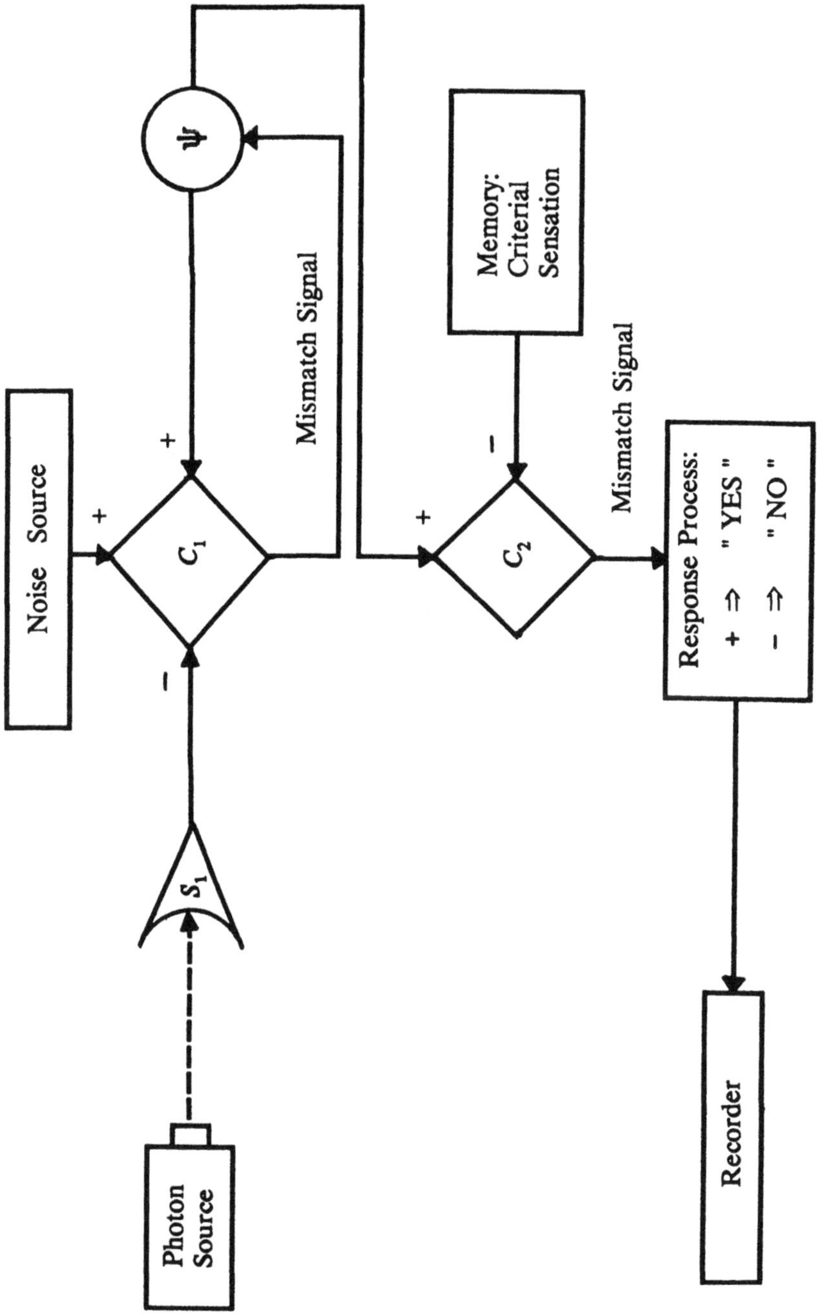

Figure 4.3: A process model that uses comparators, memory, and a psychological magnitude generator (Ψ) to accomplish the decision task of a signal detection theory experiment.

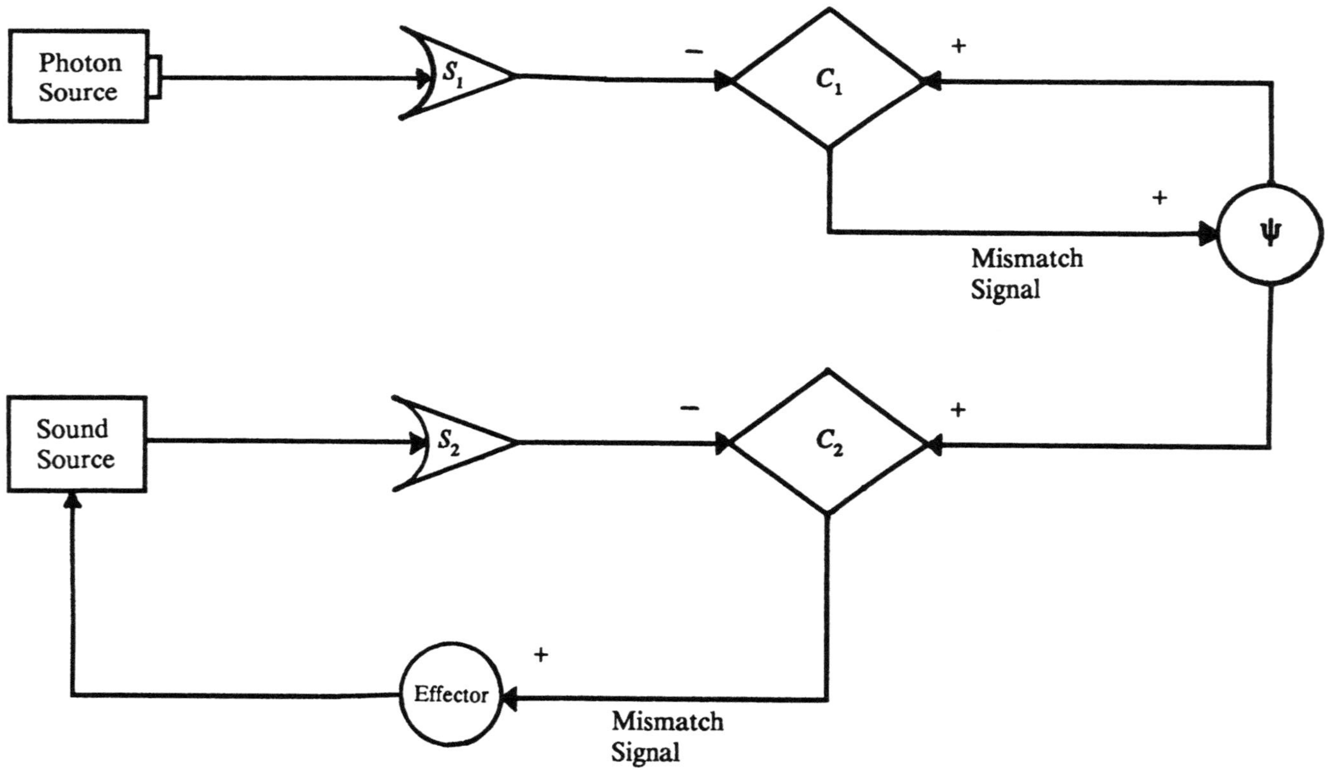

Figure 4.4: A process model that performs cross-modality matching using comparators and a psychological magnitude generator (Ψ).

space. In this space the probability that a response that has been established to a "consequential stimulus" (one that has consequences for an animal) will be given to another stimulus is an invariant monotone function of the metric distance between them in the space (their dissimilarity). If consequential regions in the space are randomly chosen by nature and are fairly regular in shape (convex and symmetrical) an exponential decay function will describe this relation. Dissimilarity (or its inverse *similarity*) has been analyzed by many authors, usually in the service of multidimensional scaling (e.g., Gregson, 1975; Shepard, Romney & Nerlove, 1972; Tversky, 1977). In all of these analyses, dissimilarity is expressed as a distance-like measure composed from the scale values of stimuli on psychological or physical dimensions or other kinds of attributes such as "features" (cf. Tversky, 1977) that are combined according to some kind of rule (the *metric*, which resembles Anderson's cognitive algebra) to yield a location in a space or some other kind of structure (e.g., a tree -- see Tversky, 1977). Thus, it seems that dissimilarity arises from even more fundamental concepts such as multidimensional sensations, abstraction, and integration, such as those already described.

S.S. Stevens' program for psychophysics consisted of seeking invariances expressed by nomothetic, algebraic expressions and measuring the constants of these expressions as accurately as possible. Judgment processes that were not linear were "biased," interfered with the attempt to measure sensation directly and validly, and were to be refined until the biases were eliminated (cf. Poulton, 1989). Many psychophysicists were and are content to follow this program, for it has yielded a wealth of important information about sensory function. However, another group of psychophysicists has taken the judgment process to be more fundamental, and its inevitable nonlinearities to be interesting and informative. Several useful models have been generated for the various psychophysical scaling procedures. Recently, I characterized some of these models in very general terms as consisting of four stages: sensory transduction, internal representation, decision mechanism, and response production (Ward, 1991). Each of the models specifies fundamental concepts relevant to each of the stages, but there is little agreement as to the nature of the concepts themselves. For example, the internal representations assumed vary from Gaussian or Poisson random variables (sometimes affected by attention) to fuzzy subsets, and the decision mechanisms vary from algebraic operations or Thurstonian categorization, to mapping and comparison, combined with various heuristics and criterion-setting processes. The kinds of process models outlined in Figures 4.3 and 4.4 above are consistent with the general character of these models but clearly there will be disagreement about the specific form such models should take. Since a lot of the diversity in the models' details arises from the varied sets of empirical facts used to inform the models, at least some of this disagreement should be resolved if we can agree on a core set of empirical laws that must be explained by a fundamental theory. This should be an important element of our program.

One of those psychophysicists who has taken nonlinearities in the judgment process to be informative is Gregson (e.g., 1988). Gregson (1988), as well as most others of this group, focuses on the dynamics of the judgment process. Thus, he treats a *time series* of observations. Unlike the others, however, he views the observer in a psychophysical experiment as a nonlinear system for which the psychophysical power law represents only a first order gain function and, as such, is relatively uninteresting, Gregson's fundamental equation is $S(\Psi_i = \Xi(\Phi_i) + N(\mu,\sigma)$, where i is the time/trials index, Ψ is the magnitude of the sensation given rise to by the physical stimulus whose magnitude is indicated by Φ, N is random noise, S is a process for assigning numbers to sensory magnitude and Ξ is a (nonlinear) function having a *chaotic attractor* (Gregson & Wiggins, 1990). A chaotic attractor is a region in the phase portrait of a recursive nonlinear function (such as Ξ) within which the behavior of the function is unpredictable but to which the value of the function is "drawn" when its parameters are in a certain range. Gregson (1988) proposes a model of psychophysical judgment (called "system Γ") in which the nonlinear function's parameters are coupled to two aspects of the stimulus input, the sensory magnitude associated with the stimulus and the first derivative of that magnitude with respect to time. The nonlinear function itself describes the behavior of a recursive loop whose output is combined with the (pure-delay-filtered) sensory magnitude to form an internal representation of the stimulus that informs the response. Thus Gregson's model resembles those discussed earlier except that there is a nonlinear, recursive loop process involved in generating the "sensation magnitude" (Ψ). This process injects "deterministic noise" or "chaos" into the representation of the sensation magnitude that is used to generate the response. This loop could be construed to be the Ψ process illustrated in Figures 4.3 and 4.4, in which case this would represent yet another suggestion as to the fundamental nature of internal representations of sensation magnitude. One especially attractive aspect of this formulation is that the nonlinearities introduced by the loop process can give rise to many of the second order properties of psychophysical data (such as the ogival form of the psychophysical function and sequential dependencies) as well as provide natural characterizations of boundary phenomena (such as thresholds).

All of the models considered above are *mechanistic* in the sense that they seek to describe mechanisms by which sensory systems operate, or psychophysical judgments are given. An alternative to such mechanistic models, of great importance in other fields and equally capable of being couched in fundamental terms, is a *conservation* theory. In physics QED is a mechanistic theory while thermodynamics is a conservation theory. Conservation laws generally state boundary conditions that any mechanistic theories must operate within but do not directly inform the mechanistic theories. Conservation theories are based on some very general "mechanisms" (e.g., the kinetic theory of heat for the laws of thermodynamics) that are only loosely related to the mechanisms of the mechanistic theories. Such theories have seldom appeared in psychology, but one has been offered in psychophysics. Norwich (e.g., 1981, 1987) assumed that an organism can perceive only when it is uncertain and that the level of uncertainty can be measured by Shannon's measure of uncertainty or *entropy:* $H = -\Sigma p_i ln\ p_i$, where p_i is the probability of stimulus i occurring. This assumption extends from the whole organism to the individual receptors and their primary neurons, where the word "perceive" means something more like "resonate to." Norwich further assumed that the phenomenon of adaptation, especially of peripheral sensory neurons, can be construed, for purposes of describing information flow through the organism, as reflecting the progressive acquisition of information as a stimulus persists in time. From these assumptions, information theory, and a few assumptions about how a receptor samples stimuli, Norwich (e.g., 1981, 1987) derived his fundamental equation for the entropy of a receptor-neuron system: $H_s = \frac{1}{2} ln(1+B/\tau)$, where τ is stimulus duration and B is a constant. By making further assumptions specific to each situation modeled, Norwich has derived the law of adaptation for sensory neurons and many psychophysical laws, including Fechner's and Stevens' Laws, Bloch's Law, Weber's Law, and the magical number 7 ± 2. This is truly a fundamental theory of the conservation type, for it makes very few assumptions at base, and has only a few concepts (entropy, sampling as a function of time) and yet from these, arranged according to each specific situation [cf. how Feynman (1985) derives Snell's Laws of reflection from a plane surface from QED] many empirical laws can be derived. A major problem for the theory is how to relate the state of the sensory receptor and its primary neuron to that of the whole organism. For example, I have shown that the whole organism acquires information much faster than the individual receptor-neuron systems, possibly because several such systems operate in parallel with respect to a given stimulus and the whole organism can combine the information from them. Nonetheless, the theory does describe the boundary conditions on how much information the whole organism can acquire. Moreover, it provides a common currency, entropy, that characterizes the stimulus, the sensory response to it, and a state of the whole organism. Norwich (1981) argues that the sensory system *calibrates* the stimulus continuum and that the whole organism is ultimately bound by this calibration. It is possible that this theory could form the foundation for a theory that is neutral to the mind-body duality in the sense required by Pribram (1986 -- see *Mind and Brain* section). At the least, entropy could be an important concept linking the mental and material worlds.

IV. Mind in Philosophy

In this section I review cryptically several of the major philosophical statements about the nature of mind and solutions to the mind-body problem that are relevant to our search for fundamental psychophysical concepts. Clearly, to do justice to the philosophical arguments is impossible here. My review follows closely that of Bechtel (1988), although I will omit most of the arguments that support Bechtel's analysis and add material from other sources. Thus, what is presented here is not the view of a philosopher but rather that of a psychophysicist. It is interesting to note that Bechtel's very competent review made no mention whatsoever of psychophysics, even of Fechner, despite Fechner's conviction that he had solved the mind-body problem and his vast writings on this topic. Apparently these writings, along with those of other scientists like Schrödinger on the same topic, had little influence on the community of philosophers, although the results of science in general have of course significantly affected their arguments.

The distinction between mind and matter in Western philosophy apparently had its origin in religious teachings in the distant past. For example, the Orphics (followers of the mythical Orpheus) made a distinction between the soul and the body, with the soul transmigrating after death and achieving either bliss or agony depending on how life on earth had been conducted (Russell, 1945). Plato (in the

Phaedo) among others supported this theory. Mind was identified with the soul, and was said to have properties such as giving life to dead matter, being infinite and self-ruled, and being the source of all motion (Anaxagoras - see Russell, 1945). The atomists argued that motion was not caused by mind but agreed with the rest of Anaxagoras' approach. In fact, for Plato, the mind was the cause of all good and fair things, the body was the corrupter of the mind. The mind gave access to the Platonic world of pure forms (especially mathematics). This view is still held today, although it is now rationalized scientifically (e.g., Penrose, 1989). For Plato, knowledge was not the same as perception. The mind was able to know the abstract forms of things, such as whether two things were the same or different, that sound and color are not alike, even that something exists, while the senses, although they perceived a rich world, could not know these other things. Interestingly, Aristotle, Plato's pupil, made a distinction between mind and soul. The mind, being that part of us that understands mathematics and philosophy, which are timeless objects, is therefore itself timeless and different from the soul, which, being the "form" of the body, perceives ordinary objects through the senses and is therefore mortal (see Bechtel, 1988 and Russell, 1945 for detailed discussions of the views of the ancients).

Many modern philosophers distinguish between mental phenomena and other phenomena of nature in terms of *intentionality*. Intentionality is the ability of a mental state to be *about something*. That is, my belief that the sky is blue is about the sky. Similarly, my belief that a sound is "loud" or a light is "red" could be construed to be about the sound or light (the stimuli) or possibly about the sensations themselves. It is an interesting question whether a sensation itself is "about" the stimulus and thus would qualify as a mental phenomenon under this definition. Some philosophers have argued that intentionality creates an essential difference between mental and other natural phenomena that denies altogether the possibility of a scientific approach to mental phenomena. For example, Brentano suggested that the important distinguishing aspect about intentionality is that the things it refers to need not be real (e.g., a child might believe that the Easter Bunny will bring candy; Bechtel, 1988). Chisholm focused on the fact that sentences that describe mental states can fail to satisfy certain logical criteria, such as truth-functionality (the truth-value of a sentence composed of other sentences can be ascertained by knowing the truth-values of the components) and extensionality (truth of an expression depends only on what it refers to, not on its meaning) (Bechtel, 1988). Others like Quine have denied the reality (usefulness?) of intentional phenomena and thus of mental states as different from other natural phenomena. Both of these approaches (using intentionality to argue that mental phenomena are essentially different from physical ones, and denying the reality of intentional, and thus mental, phenomena), if followed strictly, would exclude mind from psychophysics. The little "mind clouds" in Figures 1a and 1b would have to be deleted or replaced by a box labeled "brain". Many psychophysicists would probably not be affected by this, either in practice or attitude about psychophysics (albeit that that attitude is intentional). But others, including those I discussed earlier, would be dramatically affected, for their theories postulate mental states and mental operations.

There are two views of how a scientific account of intentionality could be developed that seem especially relevant and useful for psychophysics. One is based on what Dennett (e.g., 1978) called *"the intentional stance."* This is the perspective we adopt when we characterize a system in terms of beliefs, attitudes etc. Dennett maintained that adopting this stance gives us useful information about a certain class of complex systems, such as humans and other animals, especially when we ask "why" the system does what it does. However, Dennett also argued that we have to adopt a different stance, *"the design stance,"* in order to "... describe the mechanical activities in the system that enable it to perform as an intentional system." (Bechtel, 1988, p.71). Dennett believes that the intentional stance is necessary to understanding such systems but that no systems are "really" intentional. This is problematic for some philosophers and for psychophysics. However, there is a more useful (to us) version of Dennett's approach that treats intentional states as states of a system that are adaptive to aspects of the environment in which a system finds itself. To get around Brentano's point that intentional states can be about non-real objects, the intentional state must be interpreted from a holistic perspective, in which the entire cognitive system is related to a "notional world" (the "actual world" modified to make a person's false beliefs true and any unreasonable desires reasonable). Moreover, Bechtel (1988) suggested that we consider this relationship from the perspective of its adaptive significance, that is, from the perspective of how evolutionary processes operated to give rise to the particular relationship observed. In this view, there is an important but still somewhat indirect relationship between mind, characterized by taking the intentional stance toward human behavior, and the actual internal processing models we would use to explain those behaviors, viz. "... The intentional perspective identifies what aspects of the behavior of a system need to be explained by the processing account ..." (Bechtel, 1988, p. 75).

Bechtel's (1988) view is attractive, but it still seems to put mental states, such as the conscious sensation, in a kind of limbo in which they play no direct role in behavior in a causal sense. An alternative, or possibly complementary, view that might be useful is that of Searle (e.g., 1990) who characterizes intentional states as having *aspectual shapes*: we perceive or think about things only under some aspects of those things and not under others. For example, when we are presented with a stimulus in a yes/no experiment, we consciously experience that stimulus from a certain point of view (hopefully established by the experimenter's instructions) and with certain features (among which are those the experimenter wishes the decision to be based on). Just as a person could want a drink of water and not want a drink of H_2O (i.e., want to quench a thirst and be indifferent to the chemical properties of water), an observer in a psychophysical experiment could be set to compare the magnitude of a sound with that of a light (point of view) and would experience a particular sensation magnitude when presented with the sound. Thus, it is the aspectual shape of an intentional state that interests the psychophysicist. Searle (e.g., 1990) also argues that these intentional states can only be described completely by reference to a mental component; if we put a "brain-o-scope" (the perfect instrument of a perfect science of the brain) to a person's skull, we would not be able to divine the aspectual shape of the person's thoughts. Moreover, there can be both unconscious and conscious mental states. What distinguishes them is that in conscious mental states, the aspectual shapes are realized by the actions of neurophysiological processes while unconscious mental states consist of "... objective features of the brain capable of causing subjective conscious thoughts" (Searle, 1990, p. 588). An example of this would be a Hebbian (or Pribramian - see Pribram, 1986) cell assembly in the brain that, when active produced a conscious experience, say, that of a "red ball," but when inactive contained only the potential to produce that experience; the aspectual shape of the red ball experience is not present in the inactive cell assembly. The aspectual shapes are immanent, that is they are only present in the mind, which arises from brain activity itself, and not in the objective features of the brian that support that particular activity. This view retains the special character of mental states while arguing that mind arises directly from brain activity. Thus, it is consistent with the general view of psychophysics that mental phenomena are "real" and deeply related to brain processes.

What has philosophy had to say about the nature of the relation between minds and brains and other physical objects? Lots. The mind-body problem has been important in philosophy for far longer than psychophysics has been important in psychology. There are several major positions that have implications for psychophysics. I can only summarize them and indicate their most important implications before opting for a particular view that fits reasonably well with my own program for fundamental psychophysics. The first of these is *dualism*, which was born in ancient times and reached its sharpest exposition in Descartes' writings (e.g., *Meditations on First Philosophy* from whence came "cogito ergo sum"). Basically, dualism maintains that mind and body are different sorts of entities and that human behaviors like reasoning and language (i.e., intentional behaviors) cannot be explained by physical explanations. Mind and body can interact (in Descartes' theory through the pineal gland) but they are essentially different. This position and its more recent variants seems not to be very useful for guiding research (Bechtel, 1988), especially psychophysical research whose program it denies, since its view is basically negative: it seems to imply that a scientific understanding of the mind is impossible.

Another influential position has been *philosophical behaviorism*, which attempts to do away with the mind-body problem altogether by characterizing it as resulting from a "category mistake" (Ryle, 1949). By this, Ryle meant that we are looking for the mind to be some component of the body like the heart, brain, lungs, etc. But this is like expecting a "university" to be something like buildings, students, faculty, etc. Philosophical behaviorists deny causal efficacy to mental states. Behavior can only be explained in terms of behavioral dispositions aroused by particular stimuli (similar to probabilities in psychological behaviorism). There are several serious difficulties with this position that have led most philosophers to reject it (Bechtel, 1988). Moreover, since it seems to have no place for mind, it is inconsistent with the views of psychophysics reviewed earlier, although its emphasis on behavior is consistent with modern practice in psychophysics.

According to Bechtel (1988), most modern philosophers would endorse some form of *materialism*, in which mental states are said to be states of the brain (e.g., Searle, 1990), and so would most cognitive scientists (e.g., quote from Minsky, 1986, at the beginning of this chapter). Materialism is a form of *monism*, asserting that mind and body are not different stuff, but just different points of view (cf. Fechner's inner psychophysics and Dennett's intentional stance). Of all of the more detailed versions that have been developed, the Token Identity Theory seems to be the most useful for fundamental psychophysics, although no particular version of it seems to be just right. Token Identity Theory asserts that "... every time I am in a particular mental state, that mental state is identical to the brain state, but ... on other occasions when I am in the same mental state I may be in a different brain state" (Bechtel, 1988). The most useful version of this view suggests that mental and brain states may be categorized based on different criteria, with the mental states categorized with respect to functional criteria (vis-a-vis the environment). This position is similar to the relational approach to intentionality discussed earlier. Out of it grew the next (and) last philosophical program to be discussed here, *functionalism*.

"Functionalism maintains that mental events are classified in terms of their causal roles" (Bechtel, 1988). Several different versions of functionalism have been proposed. Folk psychological functionalism argues that knowledge about mental functions is encoded in ordinary language and that it can be cast in the form of a theory of causal relations among mental states and behavior that constitutes a functional analysis of the mind. Machine Table Functionalism appeals to an analogy between a Turning machine (a hypothetical computing device consisting of a memory tape, and execution unit, and an indicator that points to a particular place on the tape) and its program, and the brain and its mind. If the mind's functions are "computable" there will be an equivalent Turing machine (cf. J.R. Anderson, 1976). Mental states are likened to "computational states" of the Turing machine, the brain to the machine itself. A more abstract version of this proposal, in which "computational states" refer to symbolic operations that could be carried out on any of several machines (all of which could in principle be simulated by a Turing machine) is called Computational or AI (Artificial Intelligence) Functionalism. For computational functionalists (like Jackendoff, 1987; or Pylyshyn, 1984) there is a *functional architecture* of the mind that consists of symbols and algorithms that operate on them. Characterized at its most abstract, computational functionalism asserts that the mind "is" an algorithm "running" in the brain. Although this view is very popular among cognitive scientists (of whom quite a few are psychophysicists), there are several serious objections to it. First, it is apparently committed to the view that cognition consists of "symbol processing activity." The development of (non-symbolic) parallel distributed processing models for many mental functions, including perception and language, challenges the preeminence of symbolic processing (cf. Rumelhart, McClelland & the PDP Research Group, 1986). Another challenge is to the algorithmic nature of the processing. Penrose (1989) has argued that the mind's actions are not computable, although they arise in a fundamental way from the physics of the universe (which also has its noncomputable aspects in the relation between the quantum and classical levels). Finally, Searle (1980) has argued that merely carrying out an algorithm in no way implies mental phenomena such as "understanding." His Chinese Room Argument, in which he is programmed to answer questions in Chinese about a story in Chinese but does not understand either Chinese or the story, brings to our attention the importance of the biological machinery from which the mind arises, and the fact that there are many different algorithms that could equivalently accomplish a given computational task, only some of which might be involved in giving rise to consciousness (cf. also Marr, 1982).

Probably the most useful approach to functionalism for psychophysics is Teleological Homuncular Functionalism. Homuncular Functionalism postulates a hierarchy of functional levels, each with its own set of "homunculi" (classically "little men" but now just a metaphor for a particular set of mental operations) that carry out the tasks required at that level. Each homunculus at each level consists of a team of homunculi at the next lower level. This functional analysis is continued until we finally reach a level at which the task of each homunculus can be performed by a machine. At this point we have a functional explanation in which mind arises from the interactions of the homunculi doing their various tasks. None of the homunculi themselves have "mind," it is through their interactions, with each doing its own thing at its own level, that mind arises. Thus mind is not unitary but rather distributed, and its precise character at any time depends on which homunculi are active and how they are interacting. Bechtel (1988) proposed Teleological Homuncular Functionalism to include an adaptative aspect, much like the revised Dennett's intentional stance approach. The adaptive role of each homunculus (or mental process or operation) must be considered "...in order to provide a basis for deciding what kinds of causally interactive systems possess mental states ..." (Bechtel, 1988, p.135). In Bechtel's (1988) account, causal processes must be considered in terms of how they help meet the needs of the organism in terms of its survival and fitness in a given environment. One possible idea is that mental processes play a causal role in open systems (systems that can learn) in which they process information from an environment that in turn determines how the system should act to satisfy its needs. As Bechtel (1988) notes, this brings the philosophical ideas about functionalism very close to the way psychologists have been thinking for many years (since James). In the sections that follow, I will focus on viewpoints that are generally consistent with Teleological Homuncular Functionalism and with Token Identity Theory.

V. Mind in Artificial Intelligence

Computational or AI Functionalism is the program of many computer scientists. The fruits of that program have been surveyed in several places; perhaps the most accessible is the Handbook of Artificial Intelligence, especially Volumes III (Cohen & Feigenbaum, 1982) and IV (Barr, Cohen & Feigenbaum, 1989). Here I will concentrate on one particular viewpoint that is exceptionally provocative and relevant, although it might be considered to be "way out" by computer scientists and is more similar to theoretical psychology or possibly philosophy than it is to current AI practice. It is the work of one of the most creative and influential researchers in AI, Marvin Minsky (1986).

Minsky's (1986) theory is the first concrete realization of the program of teleological homuncular functionalism. He begins with specifying the "atoms" of mind, mindless parts he calls *agents*, that perform the many functions out of which the mind emerges. In his book The Society of Mind he addresses questions of function, embodiment, interaction, origins, heredity, learning, character, authority, intention, competence, selfness, meaning, sensibility, and awareness of these agents. His thesis is that mind is composed of a "society" of interacting agents that separately perform the many things minds do (functions) and in active interaction constitute "mind" (but a very different concept of mind from the older, unitary concept). Each agent is viewed as a "tiny machine" about whose activities there need be no mystery (although there may remain some in how the machine is instantiated in a particular brain). Thus, Minsky's approach can be considered to be within the Token Identity Theory camp; it is clearly monistic in approximately the same ways. Also, exactly as in the homuncular functionalist program, hierarchical (and heterarchical) causal interactions of these agents are responsible for activities at a variety of functional levels and time scales. Each agent calls upon a group of lower-level agents to do its "job," while in turn functioning as one of many agents doing the "job" of an agent at a "higher" functional level. For example, imagine a child playing with blocks. An agent called "builder" is in control of the child's behavior; its function is to make towers from blocks. In building a tower, "builder" must call upon other agents, such as "begin," "add" and "end," each of which in turn must call upon still other agents (e.g., "add" could be using "find," "get" and "put") until at last the most basic agents, those simple perceptual/motor commands that can be understood as "mechanical" brain processes, are invoked. Note also that "builder" is actually under the control of still higher agents, like "play-with-blocks." Minsky's program is to begin to specify a set of agents (actually types of agents), and the principles by which they operate and interact, that are sufficient to explain mind. Here mind is "distributed," in the sense that it consists in the activities of various agents (although perhaps not all of those active at any one time), and is constantly changing as the activities of the agents change.

Minsky's (1986) book is long and complicated and impossible to summarize succinctly. What I will do here is to select a few of the types of agents and principles of interaction he discusses that seem particularly important either for psychophysics or for the coherence of Minsky's notion. One thing that may have occurred to the reader already is that in such a society of agents there must occur conflict. In Minsky's scheme, conflict is resolved by "upward referral." For example, if conflict occurs between "builder" and "wrecker" (and knowing children it will) it will weaken the ability of the higher-level agent that involved them, "play-with-blocks," to suppress *its* rivals "play-with-dolls" and "play-with-dog," and so forth. At each level there are potential conflicts and a continual jostling for control. Whenever control fails at a lower level the conflict is referred upward until at some level firm control is again established (perhaps by a different agent, e.g., "eat" or "sleep") and control flows downward again. One powerful way for agents to gain control is to be activated by some environmental agency (e.g., an experimenter). Such outside forces can activate a cascade of agents in its service, and maintain them that way for a long time, often as long as the forces persist (the end of the experiment).

One problem that has troubled thinkers about the mind is how the mind can watch itself and still be interacting effectively with the outside world (the problem of "self-awareness"). Minsky (1986) suggested that one way this could happen is for the brain to be divided into at least two parts. One part could have inputs from and outputs to the real world (A-brain), and the other could have inputs from and outputs to the A-brain. The A-brain is then the B-brain's world. Each brain would have its own set of agents. The A-brain agents would be agents like "builder" while the B-brain agents would do jobs like "sensing" when A-brain was disordered and confused and inhibiting the currently active A-brain agents (thus allowing other higher level agents in A-brain to gain control), sensing when A-brain has done something good and making A-brain remember that, etc. Since the B-brain is "aware" of some of what is going on in A-brain, the entire system would be considered to be somewhat self-aware. However, many of A-brain's activities could be unavailable to the B-brain ("cognitively impenetrable"? - see Fodor, 1983). The B-brain could only become aware of these activities by observing their effects on the world through other, accessible A-brain agents. In order to use concepts like "mental" consistently (e.g., with the approach of Searle, 1990 - see *Mind in Philosophy* section), we might wish to think of inaccessible agents as "subconscious," inactive but accessible agents as "unconscious", and active and accessible agents as "conscious." This idea could lead to a modification of the fundamental psychophysical system such as that depicted in Figure 4.5 (cf. Figure 4.1a). There, what were labeled afferent systems, effector systems and mind have been replaced by the subconscious brain, consisting of those A-brain agents whose activities are in principle inaccessible to consciousness, the L(ower)-mind, consisting of those agents of the A-brain that interact directly with the environment but whose outputs are accessible to B-brain, and the U(pper)-mind, consisting of those B-brain agents that interact only with

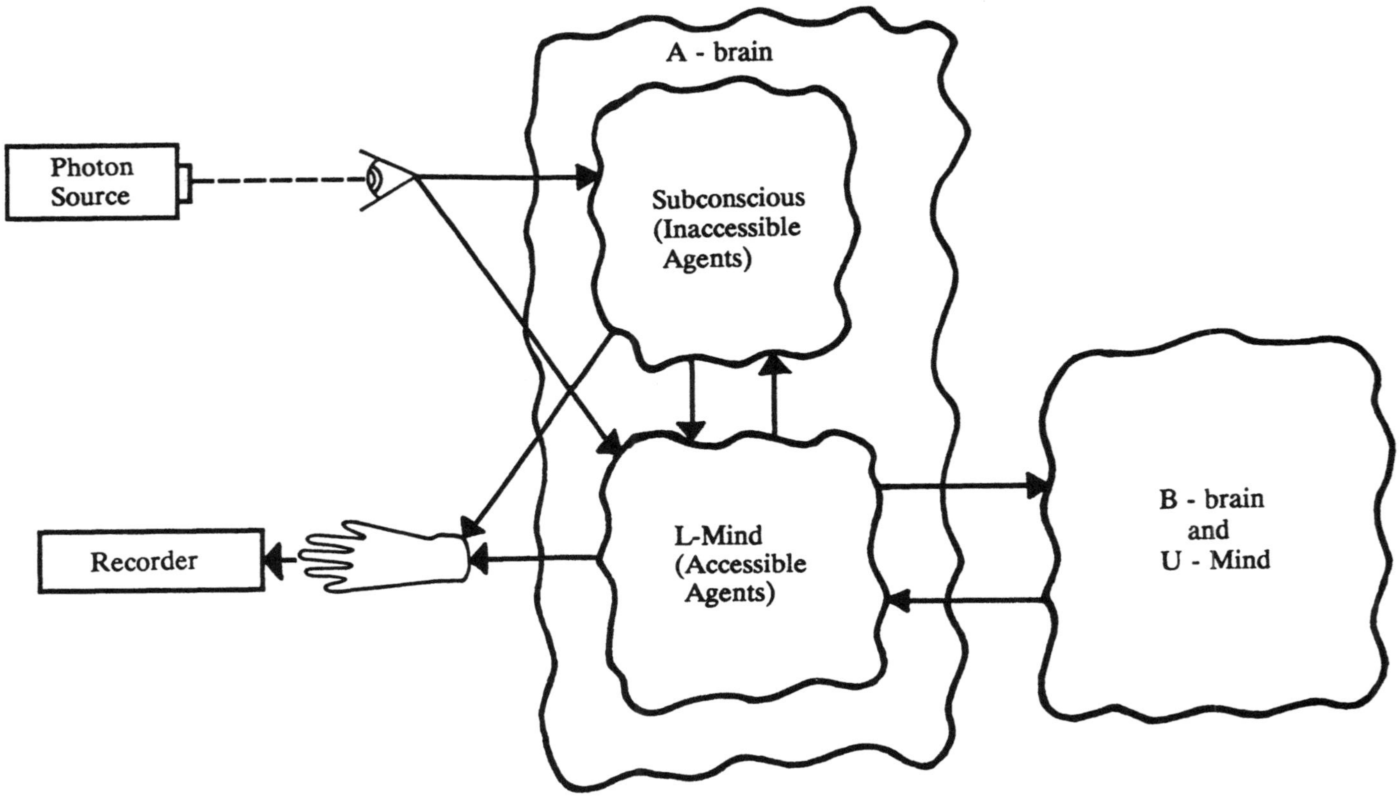

Figure 4.5: A reformulation of the fundamental psychophysical system involved in the Hecht, Schlaer & Pirenne experiment (Figure 4.1a) to reflect a functional analysis of mind.

A-brain agents and with each other. Together, L-mind and U-mind constitute the potential contents of consciousness; the active subset at any particular time *is* the conscious mind at that time. Of course there could be several such functional divisions of the brain into sub-brains, depending on the functions of the specific agents and where their inputs came from and where their outputs went.

In Minsky's scheme, consciousness is particularly concerned with the self-monitoring part of the brian, with "knowing" what we are thinking. He argues that consciousness actually is "about" (intentionality) past thoughts and thus has to do with memory. For Minsky, the awareness we call consciousness are derived from the activities of the agents that manage memories, those that learn to recognize events that are happening inside the brain. "Memories are processes that make some of our agents act in much the same way they did at various times in the past" (Minsky, 1986, p.154). He presents a detailed and plausible theory of memory, in which memories consist of a list of the agents active at the time in question (implemented by an agent connected to all of those agents and whose "job" is simply to activate all the other agents it is connected to, called a "knowledge-line" or "K-line" for short). In the future, when the K-line agent is activated by an input similar to an earlier one, all of the agents active at the earlier time will be activated, putting a person in the same state of mind as at the earlier time ("re-minding"). The theory has many interesting and important implications (and some difficulties). What is important for us here is that it is the (many) agencies that manage these memories whose activities are most closely associated with consciousness. Minsky contends that each part of the brain has several types of memory-agencies that work differently to accomplish different tasks. Thus, again, consciousness is not unitary and the same all the time, it varies with the particular memory agencies that are active at any one time. If a psychophysics experiment is tightly controlled and requires a simple decision (yes/no?) it is possible that consciousness will be similar from trial to trial. However, if a complex decision is required (matching a sensation magnitude to a number?) the agencies active may vary substantially from trial to trial. This approach is quite consistent with the tendency of some psychophysicists to emphasize the role of memory in psychophysical experiments (e.g., Braida & Durlach, 1988; Lockhead & King, 1983; Ward, 1987). It suggests that memory is fundamental because it is inextricably linked with consciousness, which is a defining feature of the concept of mind utilized informally by many psychophysicists.

An important aspect of this view for the psychophysics is that "...any self-inspecting probe is prone to change just what it's looking at" (Minsky, 1986, p. 151). This gives rise to a kind of Uncertainty Principle of Mind that asserts that there will be an irreducible minimum of uncertainty associated with any self-reflective activity. That is, in order to report on a mental experience, an agent will have to examine the memory record of the agencies that generated that experience. In so doing, the agent will perturb the record and thus introduce uncertainty as to precisely what the record was, much as physicists perturb, and thus make uncertain the various aspects of the motions of particles when they observe them (Heisenberg's Uncertainty Principle). In physics there is a tradeoff between aspects in observational precision. For example, if we wish to know the velocity of a particle more precisely we must accept less precision with respect to its position ($\Delta p \Delta \nu = kh$). Since in psychophysics we are always interested in such reports, there may be a similar tradeoff operative there. The problem is to formulate the principle for psychophysics in such a way as to indicate the relevant quantities that will trade off (the mental analogues of, e.g., position and velocity - information? magnitude? response variance?) and the minimum uncertainty (the equivalent to Planck's constant *h*). Whether this uncertainty is interpreted as trial-to-trial variability in some internal representation or external response, or as an inherent "fuzziness" to the experience of reporting on mental states is probably somewhat a matter of taste. However, such an idea is suggestive of the source of the fuzziness of internal representations of stimuli that is fundamental to my own theory of psychophysical magnitude judgment (Ward, 1979).

A final highly relevant aspect of Minsky's theory is the way he deals with magnitude and comparison. First, he points out that "real" differences can only be detected (by difference-detecting agents) if the inputs to the agent match almost perfectly, that is, if the difference to be detected is not swamped by myriad other, irrelevant differences. Psychophysicists recognize this requirement implicitly and seldom ask observers to report differences on more than a single sensory continuum in highly simplified situations (e.g., the two-interval paradigm). Minsky calls this The Duplication Problem, because it seems to require an endless duplication of agents. He avoids this problem by postulating that comparisons involve "time-blinking" a comparing agent. This consists of sending two different memories to that agent, one after another in time. Any change in the agent's output will signify a difference between the input memories *in respect of that aspect that the agent operates on*. This suggests how the comparators in Figures 3 and 4 might operate, and also suggests how a single relevant aspect of a stimulus might be judged through abstraction by directing the relevant memories into agents that operate on the relevant aspect.

Finally, Minsky (1986) argues that quantities or magnitudes are only resorted to in the brain when alternatives are so different that they can only be compared by using some kind of mental currency. This must happen all the time among the agents in the society of mind, which could use either quantities like amounts of chemicals or others that are "computed" to influence each other's activities. The point, though, is that qualitative comparison is considered to be more fundamental than quantitative comparison; the latter depends on convention (even among agents of mind) whereas the former depends on inherent aspects of the things compared. Information is always lost when quantification must be resorted to. This suggests that qualitative comparison tasks might better be taken as fundamental in psychophysics, even when the way we think about them involves quantities (such as the unidimensional strength variable in signal detection theory).

VI. Mind and Brain

Most scientists who study the brain take an explicitly monistic view of the relation between mind and brain. Their working hypothesis is that once we understand how the nervous system works we will have solved the mind-body problem, including the puzzle of self-awareness, since the mind is a phenomenon produced by the workings of the brain. There is a general principle of neuroscience, with many specific exemplars in the huge literature on the effects of brain damage or drugs on behavior, that lends strong support to this belief. It could be stated thus: *The external manifestations of consciousness are altered by changes in the structure or chemistry of the brain*. Moreover, the highly specific nature of the effects of various specifically localizable injuries (such as lesions caused by strokes) and particular drugs lend support to the functional analysis of the mind being done by cognitive psychology and AI. Any basic textbook in biological or physiological psychology contains voluminous detailed material (e.g., Carlson, 1988), although various interpretations of this material can inform very different theories of mind (cf. Brown, 1988). The monistic approach has been very fruitful and with the use of new methods of noninvasive probing of the human brain (e.g., CT, PET, and NMR) promises even more spectacular results.

One highly suggestive exemplar of this cornucopia of facts is the phenomenon called "blindsight" by Weiskrantz, Warrington, Sanders and Marshall (1974). There are really two visual systems in our brains, an evolutionarily "old" one that all of the more complex animals have (now called the tecto-pulvinar system) and a "newer" one (called the geniculo-striate system) that is characteristic of mammals. If the newer system is damaged (e.g., by a lesion in the occipital cortex) a person will not be aware of any objects present in the part of the visual field served by the damaged area. There will be a scotoma (a "hole" in the visual field) in that region. However, if the person is told that there is actually an object there, they can point to it, reach for and grasp it, and even adjust the size of their grip to the size of the object before they touch it! The person is very surprised to be touching something that apparently isn't there. This shows that there are brain processes that interact with the world without directly presenting any information to consciousness (part of Minsky's A-brain?). This suggests that some parts of the brain could play a special role in consciousness. Clearly, the geniculo-striate visual system must be such a part. Since it also is a basis for interaction with the world (receives and processes information from visual stimuli), we could speculate that it is one of the processes in the A-brain that is monitored by the B-brain and thus part of the L-mind. On the other hand, outputs from the tecto-pulvinar system, not being accessible to consciousness, form a part of the brain that would not be considered to be "mental," part of the "subconscious" in Figure 4.5.

What part(s) of the brain could possibly be candidates for the B-brain (assuming it makes any sense at all to ask that question)? Another exemplar of the general law stated above might give a clue. This is the work on "split brains" (e.g., Gazzaniga, 1970; Sperry, 1966). When the corpus callosum of the brain is cut (a last-resort operation to treat frequent epileptic seizures) the two cerebral hemispheres operate independently, no longer receiving information on each other's activity. Under these conditions, the two hemispheres are discovered to be "anisofunctional;" that is, they aren't equally good at all tasks. One hemisphere, usually the left, is especially good at language tasks, and is the only one capable of producing speech. The right hemisphere is especially good at spatial tasks but can't speak at all. Interestingly, the "person" talks as if only the things being experienced by the left hemisphere are being "consciously" experienced (of course it is the left hemisphere doing the talking). The left hemisphere literally doesn't know what the right is doing, and the right is mute. The right hemisphere often does things in conflict with the desires of the left (e.g., puts down a book held in the left hand, controlled by the right hemisphere, that "they" were reading, or making gestures with the left hand that "they" had not intended). Such phenomena resemble the "blindsight" discussed earlier and reinforce the idea that information must reach some particular part(s) of the brain before it becomes available to consciousness. The split brain results in particular suggest that the areas that control speech might be critically involved, although there is no reason to believe that they are the only ones (Minsky would say that those that control memory processes would also be involved).

One of the functions of the B-brain could be attention. In recent years our understanding of the physiology of attention has undergone dramatic revision. It is now thought that there are several brain systems that function to enhance or inhibit brain activity in various areas. For example, studies of humans with lesions in particular brain areas, as well as experimental studies with monkeys, have identified a system called the "posterior visual spatial attention system," involving a locus in the parietal lobe that disengages attention from an object in the visual field, a locus in the midbrain that moves attention to another object located somewhere else, and a locus in the thalamus (pulvinar nucleus) that engages attention with the new object (Posner, Petersen, Fox & Raichle, 1988; Posner & Petersen, 1990). At a more detailed level, the responses of cells in the prestriate area V4 and in the inferotemporal cortex (both parts of the "new" vision system) of monkeys to unattended stimuli within their receptive fields is greatly reduced compared to their responses to attended stimuli present at the same time, whereas responses of cells in more peripheral areas (e.g., V1, V2, and V3) are not affected by attention (Moran & Desimone, 1985). This attentional selectivity is enhanced on more difficult tasks that require more "effort" (Spitzer, Desimone & Moran, 1988). The new PET (positron emission tomography) techniques have extended these findings to humans. For example, Posner and his colleagues (e.g., Posner, Petersen, Fox & Raichle, 1988; Posner & Petersen, 1990) have used the subtraction method with PET (in which activation in control tasks is subtracted from activation in tasks of interest to reveal activation specific to the tasks of interest) to discover the brain areas active when, for example, observers simply fixate words (occipital cortex) versus generate various meanings of words being fixated (frontal areas involved in meaning and midbrain areas involved in attention). The same technique has revealed that, commensurate with the increased sensitivity to subtle changes in multi-attribute stimuli when attention is focused on one attribute rather than divided among several (measured psychophysically), the activity of the appropriate region of extrastriate visual cortex was increased when attention was focused on the stimulus attributes thought to be processed by those regions (Corbetta, Miezin, Dobmeyer, Shulman & Petersen, 1990). Clearly, some parts of the brain (involved with consciousness?) can and do modulate the activity of other parts that process information of special interest.

Space does not permit a review of all of the work in the brain sciences that is potentially relevant to our understanding of mind, even to its role in a fundamental psychophysics. However, a few additional ideas must be mentioned. First, there is some evidence that strange attractors and chaos (see discussion of Gregson's work in the *Mind in Psychophysics* section) play an important role in the functioning of the brain. Freeman (e.g., Freeman, 1991; Skarda & Freeman, 1987) has argued that the patterns of brain activity he has observed in the olfactory bulb and olfactory cortex in response to odors (explosive bursts of synchronous activity with a unique spatial pattern for each relevant odor) can be interpreted as shifts among the various strange attractors of complex nonlinear systems. This interpretation is consistent with the work of Gregson, and the two together indicate that sensations and other psychological experiences might profitably be viewed as transient chaotic neural activity. Since strange (chaotic) attractors are predictable in general (they occupy a bounded region of a nonlinear system's phase portrait) but not in specific (they jump in an unpredictable way among the points in the region) they are attractive candidates for descriptors of the overchanging, fuzzy, and yet somehow solid phenomena of mind.

The final two ideas I want to mention are more philosophical. First, Gazzaniga (1988) has suggested a view of how the brain and mind interact to create our conscious lives that is highly reminiscent of Minsky's A-brain and B-brain. Gazzaniga suggested that the brain interacts directly with the world, including with itself, and can be characterized by its ever-fluctuating physico-chemical state. The mind, however, can be characterized by what Gazzaniga (1988) called the "interpretive state," which senses the physico-chemical state of the brain and tries to make up a story that "explains" it. Gazzaniga postulates that the left hemisphere (usually) contains an "interpretive module" of the brain whose functioning constitutes this interpretive state. This approach helps make sense of a variety of psychological phenomena involving states of mind such as pain, love, anxiety, stress, and insanity, in which the mind tries to interpret the state of the brain and in turn affects that state. Pribram (1986) has also arrived at a view that supports Minsky's analysis, although from a completely different direction. He suggested solving the mind-body problem by assuming a pluralistic monism in which the basic components of the universe are neither mental nor physical but neutral. Mind and brain are two different realizations of the same underlying informational "structure," which is itself neutral as to any of its possible embodiments, like the structure of information in a symphony is neutral to its embodiments in a live performance, on a musical score, or recorded on a CD or tape. Pribram further suggested that "... the microcircuitry ... (of the brain) ... is encoding periodic activity, and that sensory transduction of environmental energy results in patterns of neuronal activation in the spectral domain" (Pribram, 1986). By "spectral domain" Pribram is referring to transform domains such as those described by the Fourier or Gabor transforms. Pribram also emphasized the distributed nature of these encodings into the transform domain by likening them to holograms. For Pribram (1986) both mind and brain are realizations of this more fundamental distributed spectral encoding.

VII. Mind in Cognitive Psychology

Cognitive psychology is the discipline that is engaged in the program of the homuncular functionalists, viz. the functional analysis of mind. We might expect to find among its results a characterization of elementary mental elements and operations that would be useful for a fundamental theory of psychophysics. Again the field is too enormous to survey here. And besides, psychophysicists are often cognitive psychologists as well and as such will be familiar with much of the material that could be covered. Thus, I will limit myself to bringing to the forefront of our consciousnesses a few important general ideas and a new theory of attention (Navon, 1989a, 1989b) that fit exceptionally well with the earlier discussion.

First I want to point out that the idea of a comparator as a fundamental mental operation has been suggested before in other contexts. For example, Miller, Galanter and Pribram (1960) argued that a TOTE (Test-Operate-Test-Exit) process should be taken as the basic unit ("three little actions"?) of behavior, with hierarchies of TOTE units composing the plans that guide our behavior. This unit is particularly good for describing the mind at the level of information flow, which has several times been suggested to be the most useful level at which to functionally analyze mind. The "test" operation of the TOTE unit compares an ideal state (or condition) with the current state of some agent or process; if they are the same the "exit" operation is performed, if not the "operate" process is performed on the current state, and the "test" performed again, and so forth until the test is "passed." The TOTE unit resembles a production (see J.R. Anderson,

1976). A production can be described by the following schema: {if *condition* then *action*}. Productions can be proliferated into production systems and can have both hierarchical and heterarchical relations within those systems, just like TOTE units. The "test" operation of the TOTE unit resembles closely the "condition" part of the production, and likewise for the TOTE's "operate" and the production's "action." Production systems are very useful structures with which to model mental functions (e.g., J.R. Anderson, 1976). It is especially interesting to note in this context that either TOTE systems or productions could be used to encode both the judgments of observers and the "rules" governing their behavior in a specific experiment (e.g., the instructions), as well as to describe succinctly and formally the activities of Minsky's agents of mind.

Cognitive psychology has made considerable progress in understanding what kinds of mental operations are necessary to describe human behavior. An old but still useful classification was made by Posner (1973). He identified three major types of operation: *abstraction, generation,* and *combining*. Posner identified two types of abstraction, selection of part of an input rather than another, and classifying the input into more general categories. The first type involves attention; the second involves memory. Posner used generation to refer to operations that generate or elaborate mental representations. This typically is heavily involved with memory, as when, for example, an observer is asked to imagine a mouse wearing a top hat eating a candy cane and dancing a jig. Combining operations were supposed to be operations like implicit counting, addition, conjoining, disjoining, and negating, highly reminiscent of N.H. Anderson's cognitive algebra. Comparing would of course fall into the latter category, with the comparison operation suggested in Figures 4.3 and 4.4, the "test" of TOTE units, and the test for the "condition" of a production being specific examples. As was discussed earlier (*Mind in Psychophysics* section), abstraction of both types may be implemented by specific kinds of comparisons. Another operation is implicit in the above and explicit in most discussions of memory use:

search or *retrieval*. This operation can be either inner-directed (as in memory search) or outer-directed (as in visual search). It also involves attention.

Studies of search (among others) have given rise to an important distinction in cognitive psychology. Under certain conditions (varied stimulus-response mapping, little practice, etc.) it can be determined that a series of comparison operations is being carried out, one for each object to be searched. Under other conditions, it seems that several such operations can be done in parallel. The former type of processing is called "controlled" processing and the latter "automatic" processing (see, e.g., Schneider, Dumais, & Shiffrin, 1984). This distinction has implications for the way attention interacts with mental operations: attention is presumed to be necessary for controlled processing but not for automatic processing (but see Kahneman & A. Treisman, 1984 for qualifications of this view). Moreover, automatic processing is relatively effortless and not under a person's control, while controlled processing is more effortful and, as the name implies, under a person's control at least at a gross level. In one approach, automatic processing is said to depend on evocation of remembered stimulus-response connections while controlled processing consists of carrying out a procedure (sequence of more-or-less attended mental operations; Logan, 1988). This distinction lends another kind of functional reality to Minsky's idea of brain processes that relate directly to the outside world and those that relate to other brain processes. Attention clearly seems to be an "inner" (or B-brain) process that is closely linked to consciousness.

Navon (1989a,b) has proposed a novel theory of attention that is remarkably commensurate with some of the ideas discussed so far. In order to give the flavor of this theory as briefly as possible I will quote the bulk of the abstract of Navon (1989a):

> ...The mind is likened to an anarchic intelligence system. It is assumed to comprise of a set of processing entities called modules that may be active in parallel. Their activation is externally driven, and their operation is not controlled by any other module. Cooperation among modules is often required for achieving goals. Cooperation calls for communication. Attention is assumed to regulate only the communication among modules. It exerts attentional emphasis by making the output of a to-be-attended module available for a maximal number of other modules, while limiting the ability of deemphasized modules to disseminate their output. This is achieved by a mechanism called decoupling that controls the connections among modules. The control of decoupling that is required for attentional emphasis is associated with an aversive phenomenal aspect that is usually called effort. Awareness of a piece of information amounts to the visibility of that information among various modules.

The similarity of this view to that of Minsky (1986) is obvious. It goes further in some ways, for example by suggesting that communication between modules (agents) is a major problem and that the function of attention is to decouple modules from each other. It is less extensive in others, for example it does not consider memory extensively (although it is implicit that attention could control memory by selectively decoupling [K-line] agents to manage memory), nor describe many specific modules (agents). Nonetheless it is remarkable that a highly technical and narrow approach like Navon's should be so similar to a more general and somewhat popular account like Minsky's. Such convergence suggests the broad usefulness of these ideas.

VIII. Mind in Psychophysics: Reprise

Where does all this leave us with respect to how we should begin to characterize the role of mind in fundamental psychophysics? First, the remarkable convergence of ideas from philosophy, artificial intelligence, the brain sciences and cognitive psychology suggests that a kind of pluralistic monism is the most useful working hypothesis as to the nature of mind. This view seems consistent with current practice in psychophysics and contrasts with the unitary view held in classical times. In the modern view, mind consists of many functional units (*agents*) operating at many scales of time and task and all implemented simultaneously in the brain. The lowest level units can be characterized as (mindless) tiny machines that can be usefully understood mechanically. Some agents interact directly with the world and others interact only with other agents. Mind consists of those agents that interact only with other agents and those agents that interact with the world that send outputs to them. A person's conscious mental state consists of the activities of the subset of these "agents of mind" that are currently active, and the "unconscious" consists of the potential activities of the inactive agents of the mind. The "subconscious" is a set of agents whose activities are inaccessible to the agents of mind. As this functional analysis proceeds, more precise characterizations of the actions of various agents will be obtained. For now, we can only attempt to describe in general terms which agents can be assumed to be fundamental to the simplest psychophysical situations.

What are the implications of accepting this view of a "distributed mind" for fundamental psychophysics? Given the dynamic nature of such a mind (extended operation in time), a dynamic psychophysics would seem to be required (as has been argued by some, especially Gregson, 1988). This requires explicit consideration of memory, even in the simplest situations (e.g., Figure 4.3).

Another implication is that mind will be represented in different ways in different experiments. There would seem to be no simple unitary concept of mind that will suffice in all psychophysics experiments, although some types of agents of mind, such as comparators, may prove to be ubiquitous. However, their role must be clearly specified in each situation, and the particular arrangement of interactions with other agents, as well as the specific exemplar of the type (for example auditory versus visual), will undoubtedly influence how they manifest themselves in consciousness. We must be prepared to characterize mind differently in each situation in terms of the specific agents necessary to perform the tasks required. Finally, there is an implicit requirement that we must take into account principles of mind that are fundamental and yet have not seemed directly relevant to psychophysics. For example, the principles of how different agents interact (conflict resolution, communication, competition for preeminence) and the principles of how procedures are learned and executed (creation of agents) will both be important to a complete understanding of a person's performance in a psychophysical paradigm. Even concepts psychophysicists have employed in their theories, such as attention, are much more complex than we have expected (cf. Navon, 1989a,b); in their newer incarnations they fit better with the concept of a distributed mind that with Fechner's and others' assumption of a unitary mind.

What is the minimal set of agents, or types of agents, that would suffice for the simplest psychophysical experiments? In the *Mind in Psychophysics* section I argued that even the simplest experiments, such as detection experiments, involved at least comparators, a psychological magnitude generator (somewhat mysterious - a B-brain agent that generates a kind of mental currency), a memory (for a previous psychological magnitude or a criterial one), and a response agent that interpreted the output of the final comparator into effector actions (Figure 4.3). In addition, there were (subconscious or L-mind or both) sensory system agents that presented a "sensation" to the first comparator. Finally, implicit in Figure 4.3 (and candidates for being made explicit in future models) were attention and all of the agents responsible for learning the procedures described in the instructions to the observer that resulted in the setup displayed in Figure 4.3. It seems reasonable to assert that this is a minimal necessary set; whether it is sufficient awaits more formal specification. Each of the fundamental types of agent seems necessary for more complicated experiments as well, although perhaps in different arrangements and different forms. Interestingly, it is possible that they will also be sufficient for some of the more complicated experiments as well (when arranged differently). By being explicit about what is going on in the simplest situations, albeit complicating them, we may be able to obtain a more widely applicable fundamental theory.

What are the implications of this view for the program of fundamental psychophysics? I suggest that it would be desirable to create ideal experiments that engage the minimum necessary and sufficient set of agents of mind so that we can either study them or, having characterized them, ignore them (cf. Laming, 1986). When these are thoroughly understood, more complex experiments can be analyzed as concatenations of the simpler ones, or as a simple one plus one additional agent, and so forth. Comparing ideal psychophysical experiments done with humans with those done with animals (e.g., Stebbins, 1970; Zoeke, Sarris & Hofer, 1989) would also be a good way to isolate specifically human agents, especially those having to do with language and its creations. Interspecies comparisons among nonhuman animals would be useful in characterizing the types of brains necessary to implement various kinds of mental and nonmental agents. Finally, since a formal theory is desirable, a formal language of description of the agents of mind and their operation needs to be developed, possibly along the lines of TOTE units or production systems. Since fundamental psychophysical agents are also fundamental to cognitive science, such work could be very influential.

References

Anderson, J.R. (1976). *Language, Memory and Thought.* Hillsdale, NJ: Lawrence Erlbaum Associates.

Anderson, N.H. (1981). *Foundations of Information Integration Theory.* New York: Academic Press.

Anderson, N.H. (1990). Integration psychophysics. In H.-G. Geissler (Ed.) *Psychophysical Explorations of Mental Structures* (pp.71-93). Hogrefe & Huber Publishers.

Baird, J.C. & Noma, E. (1978). *Fundamentals of Scaling and Psychophysics.* New York: Wiley.

Barr, A., Cohen, P.R., & Feigenbaum, E.A. (1989). *The Handbook of Artificial Intelligence. Vol. IV.* Reading, MA: Addison-Wesley.

Bechtel, W. (1988). *Philosophy of Mind: An Overview for Cognitive Science.* Hillsdale, NJ: Lawrence Erlbaum Associates.

Besner, D. & Grimsell, D. (1979). the mind's eye and the comparative judgement of number. *Neuropsychologia*, **17**, 373-380.

Braida, L.D. & Durlach, N.D. (1988). Peripheral and central factors in intensity perception. In G.M. Edelman, W.E. Gall & W.M. Cowan (Eds.) *Auditory Function.*

Brown, J.W. (1988). *The Life of the Mind.* Hillsdale, NJ: Lawrence Erlbaum Associates.

Carlson, N.R. (1988). *Foundations of Physiological Psychology.* Boston: Allyn and Bacon.

Cohen, P.R., & Feigenbaum, E.a. (1982). *The Handbook of Artificial Intelligence. Vol. III.* Los Altos, CA: William Kaufman, Inc.

Corbetta, M., Miezin, F.M., Dobmeyer, S., Shulman, G.L., & Petersen, S.E. (1990). Attentional modulation of neural processing of shape, color, and velocity in humans. *Science*, **248**, 1556-1559.

Dehaene, S. & Dupoux, E. (1990). Is numerical comparison digital? Analogical and symbolic effects in two-digit number comparison. *Journal of Experimental Psychology: Human Perception and Performance*, **16**, 626-641.

Dennett, D.D. (1978). *Brainstorms*. Cambridge, MA: MIT Press/Bradford Books.

Falmagne, J.-C. (1985). *Elements of Psychophysical Theory*. New York: Oxford University Press.

Fechner, G.T. (1851/1987). Outline of a new principle of mathematical psychology (1851) (E. Scheerer, Trans.). *Psychological Research*, **49**, 203-207.

Fechner, G.T. (1860/1966). *Elements of Psychophysics* (Vol. I, H.E. Adler, Trans.) New York: Holt, Rinehart & Winston.

Fechner, G.T. (1882/1987). Some thoughts on the psychophysical representation of memories (1882) (E. Scheerer, Trans.). *Psychological Research,* **49**, 209-212.

Fechner, G.T. (1887/1987). My own viewpoint on mental measurement (1887) (E. Scheerer, Trans.). *Psychological Research,* **49**, 213-219.

Feynman, R.P. (1985). *QED: The Strange Theory of Light and Matter*. Princeton, NJ: Princeton University Press.

Fodor, J.A. (1983). *Modularity of Mind*. Cambridge, MASS: MIT Press.

Freeman, W.J. (1991). The physiology of perception. *Scientific American,* **xx**, 78-85.

Garner, W.R. (1962). *Uncertainty and structure as psychological concepts*. New York: Wiley.

Gazzaniga, M.S. (1970). *The Bisected Brain*. New York: Appleton-Century-Crofts.

Gazzaniga, M.S. (1988). *Mind Matters: How the Mind and Brain Interact to Create Our Conscious Lives*. Boston: Houghton-Mifflin.

Gescheider, G.A. (1988). Psychophysical scaling. *Annual Review of Psychology,* **39**, 169-200.

Green, D.M., & Swets, T.A. (1966). *Signal detection theory and psychophysics*. Reprint. New York: Krieger, 1974.

Gregg, L.W. & Simon, H.A. (1967). Process models and stochastic theories of simple concept formation. *Journal of Mathematical Psychology,* **4**, 246-276.

Gregson, R.A.M. (1975). *Psychometrics of Similarity.* New York: Academic Press.

Gregson, R.A.M. (1988). *Nonlinear Psychophysical Dynamics.* Hillsdale, NJ: Lawrence Erlbaum Associates.

Gregson, R.A.M. & Wiggins, M.W. (1990). Nonlinear psychophysics of one output component in a ternary odour mixture: Contextual and sequential effects. In F. Muller (Ed.) *Fechner Day '90* (pp. 77-82). Wurzburg, Germany: International Society for Psychophysics.

Hecht, S., Schlaer, S. & Pirenne, M.H. (1942). Energy, quanta and vision. *Journal of General Physiology,* **25**, 819-840.

Jackendoff, R. (1987). *Consciousness and the Computational Mind.* Cambridge, MA: MIT Press (A Bradford Book).

Kahneman, D. & Treisman, A. (1984). Changing views of attention and automaticity. In R. Parasuraman & D.R. Davies (Eds.) *Varieties of Attention* (pp. 29-61). Orlando, FL: Academic Press.

Krantz, D.H., Luce, R.D., Suppes, P., & Tversky, A. (1971). *Foundations of measurement* (Vol. 1). New York: Academic Press.

Laming, D. (1986). *Sensory Analysis.* New York: Academic Press.

Laming, D. (1988a). Precis of *Sensory Analysis. Behavioral and Brain Sciences,* **11**, 275-296.

Laming, D. (1988b). A reexamination of *Sensory Analysis. Behavioral and Brain Sciences,* **11**, 316-339.

Lockhead, G.R. & King, M.C. (1983). A memory model of sequential effects in scaling tasks. *Journal of Experimental Psychology: Human Perception and Performance,* **9**, 461-473.

Logan, G.a. (1988). Toward an instance theory of automatization. *Psychological Review,* **95**, 492-527.

Luce, R.D. (1991). What is a ratio in ratio scaling? In S. Bolanowski & G. Gescheider (Eds.) *Ratio Scaling of Psychological Magnitude* (pp. 8-17). Hillsdale, NJ: Lawrence Erlbaum Associates.

Luce, R.D., Baird, J., Green, D.M., & Smith, A.F. (1980). Two classes of models for magnitude estimation. *Journal of Mathematical Psychology*, **22**, 121-148.

MacKay, D.M. (1963). Psychophysics of perceived intensity: A theoretical basis for Fechner's and Stevens' Laws. *Science*, **139**, 1213-1216.

Marks, L.E. (1974). *Sensory Processes: The New Psychophysics*. New York: Academic Press.

Marks, L.E. (1978). *The Unity of the Senses*. New York: Academic Press.

Marks, L.E. (1991). The dynamics of ratio scaling. In S. Bolanowski & G. Gescheider (Eds.) *Ratio Scaling of Psychological Magnitude* (pp. 27-42). Hillsdale, NJ: Lawrence Erlbaum Associates.

Marr, D. (1982). *Vision*. San Francisco: Freeman.

Miller, G.A., Galanter, E. & Pribram, K.H. (1960). *Plans and the Structure of Behavior*. New York: Holt, Rinehart and Winston.

Minsky, M. (1986). *The Society of Mind*. New York: Simon & Schuster.

Moran, J. & Desimone, R. (1985). Selective attention gates visual processing in the extrastriate cortex. *Science,* **229**, 782-784.

Navon, D. (1989a). The importance of being visible: On the role of attention in a mind viewed as an anarchic intelligence system. I: Basic tenets. *European Journal of Cognitive Psychology,* **1**, 191-213.

Navon, D. (1989b). The importance of being visible: On the role of attention in a mind viewed as an anarchic intelligence system. II: Application to the field of attention. *European Journal of Cognitive Psychology,* **1**, 215-238.

Norwich, K.H. (1981). The magical number 7±2: Making a 'bit' of sense. *Perception & Psychophysics,* **29**, 409-422.

Norwich, K.H. (1987). On the theory of Weber fractions. *Perception & Psychophysics,* **42**, 286-298.

Penrose, R. (1989). *The Emperor's New Mind: Concerning Computers, Minds, and the Laws of Physics.* New York: Oxford University Press.

Posner, M.I. (1973). *Cognition: An Introduction.* Glenview, IL: Scott, Foresman.

Posner, M.I. & Petersen, S.E. (1990). The attention system of the human brain. *Annual Review of Neuroscience,* **13**, 25-42.

Posner, M.I., Petersen, S.E., Fox, P.T. & Raichle, M.E. (1988). Localization of cognitive operations in the human brain. *Science,* **240**, 1627-1631.

Poulton, E.C. (1989). *Bias in Quantifying Judgments.* Hillsdale, NJ: Lawrence Erlbaum Associates.

Pribram, K.H. (1986). The cognitive revolution and mind/brain issues. *American Physiologist,* **41**, 507-520.

Pylyshyn, Z.W. (1984). *Computation and Cognition: Towards a Foundation for Cognitive Science.* Cambridge, MA: MIT Press/Bradford Books.

Rumelhart, D.E., McClelland, J.L. & The PDP Research Group. (1986). *Parallel Distributed Processing: Explorations in the Microstructure of Cognition. Vol. I. Foundations.* Cambridge, MA: MIT Press/Bradford Books.

Russel, B. (1945). *History of Western Philosophy* London: Allen & Unwin.

Ryle, G. (1949). *The Concept of Mind.* London: Hutchinson & Company.

Scheerer, E. (1987). The unknown Fechner. *Psychological Research,* **49**, 198-202.

Schneider, W., Dumais, S.T., & Shiffrin, R.M. (1984). Automatic and control processing and attention. In R. Parasuraman & D.R. Davies (Eds.) *Varieties of Attention* (pp. 1-27). Orlando, FL: Academic Press.

Searle, J.R. (1980). Minds, brains, and programs. *Behavioral and Brain Sciences,* **3**, 417-457.

Searle, J.R. (1990). Consciousness, explanatory inversion, and cognitive science. *Behavioral and Brain Sciences,* **13**, 585-596.

Shannon, C.E.A. (1948). A mathematical theory of communication. *Bell System Technical Journal,* **27**, 379-423, 623-656.

Shepard, R.N. (1987). Toward a universal law of generalization for psychological science. *Science,* **237**, 1317-1323.

Shepard, R.N., Romney, A.K., & Nerlove, S.B. (1972). *Multidimensional Scaling: Theory and Applications in the Behavioral Sciences. Volume 1: Theory*. New York: Seminar Press.

Skarda, C.A. & Freeman, W.J. (1987). How brains make chaos in order to make sense of the world. *Behavioral and Brain Sciences,* **10**, 161-173.

Sperry, R.W. (1966). Brain bisection and consciousness. In J.C. Eccles (Ed.) *Brain and Conscious Experience*. New York: Springer Verlag.

Spitzer, H., Desimone, R. & Moran, J. (1988). Increased attention enhances both behavioral and neuronal performance. *Science,* **240**, 338-340.

Stebbins, W.C. (Ed.) (1970). *Animal Psychophysics: The Design and Conduct of Sensory Experiments*. New York: Appleton-Century-Crofts.

Stevens, J.C. (1991). Magnitude matching: Application to special populations. in S. Bolanowski & G. Gescheider (Eds.) *Ratio Scaling of Psychological Magnitude* (pp. 43-56). Hillsdale, NJ: Lawrence Erlbaum Associates.

Stevens, S.S. (1961). To honor Fechner and repeal his law. *Science,* **133**, 80-86.

Stevens, S.S. (1976). *Psychophysics*. (Ed. G. Stevens). New York: Wiley.

Torgerson, W.S. (1961). Distances and ratios in psychological scaling. *Acta Psychologica*, **19**, 201-205.

Treisman, M. & Williams, T.C. (1984). A theory of criterion setting with an application to sequential dependencies. *Psychological Review,* **91**, 68-111.

Tversky, A. (1977). Features of similarity. *Psychological Review,* **84**, 327-352.

Ward, L.M. (1979). Stimulus information and sequential dependencies in magnitude estimation and cross-modality matching. *Journal of Experimental Psychology: Human Perception and Performance,* **5**, 444-459.

Ward, L.M. (1987). Remembrance of sounds past: Memory and psychophysical scaling. *Journal of Experimental Psychology: Human Perception and Performance,* **13**, 216-227.

Ward, L.M. (1988). At the threshold of fundamental psychophysics. In H.E. Ross (Ed.) *Fechner Day 88* (pp. 17-22). Stirling, Scotland: International Society for Psychophysics.

Ward, L.M. (1989). Fundamental concepts and metrics on psychological space. In G. Canavet, B. Scharf, A-M. Bonnell, & C-A. Possamai (Eds.) *Fechner Day 89* (pp. 66-71). Marseilles, France: International Society for Psychophysics.

Ward, L.M. (1990). Two-slit psychophysics. In F. Muller (Ed.) *Fechner Day 90* (pp. 261-266). Wurzburg, Germany: International Society for Psychophysics.

Ward, L.M. (1991). Associative measurement of psychological magnitude. In S. Bolanowski & G. Gescheider (Eds.) *Ratio Scaling of Psychological Magnitude* (pp. 79-100). Hillsdale, NJ: Lawrence Erlbaum Associates.

Weiskrantz, L., Warrington, E.K., Sanders, M.D., & Marshall, J.C. (1974). Visual capacity in the hemianoptic field following a restricted occipital ablation. *Brain,* **97**, 709-728.

Zoeke, B., Sarris, V. & Hofer, G. (1989-90). Comparative psychophysics: Some contextual effects in birds and humans. *The International Journal of Comparative Psychology,* **3**, 151-163.

Zwislocki, J.J. (1991). Natural measurement. In S. Bolanowski & G. Gescheider (Eds.) *Ratio Scaling of Psychological Magnitude* (pp. 18-26). Hillsdale, NJ: Lawrence Erlbaum Associates.

Psychophysical Approaches to Cognition
D. Algom (Editor)

5

INTENTIONALISM - AN EXPRESSIVE THEORY[1]

Eugene Galanter
Columbia University

[1] Portions of this research were supported by a grant from the National Aeronautics and Space Administration.

Table of Contents

I. Introduction

The aim of scientific psychology is to capture accurately multitudes of quantitative experiments while at the same time offering an image of man's nature that convincingly portrays the nuances of the human soul. Few psychological theories have attempted this double task, and none have successfully held both lay and technical adherents. In part the reason this task is difficult is that the scientific description of behavior may not be resonant with our strong intuitions about our own nature. The driving force of modern psychological theory construction is the search for mechanism. The way observable aspects of human nature unfold in behavior may be construed in two ways. In the first and most usual paradigm, environmental events stimulate an internal (i.e., invisible) structure to drive or guide the observable action. These stimuli may be either internal or external, and the structures activated by these events may have arisen either genetically or from experience or both. But the central thesis is that the person *reacts* to the stimulus. The simplest form of such a reactive model is a theory of associative connectivity that ties input to output through implicative relations: "if the stimulus is A then do response B." In some theories the strength of the association may be modulated by certain affective consequences, e.g., reinforcement or reward.

In these theories in the antecedent or stimulus is commonly represented as a signal distribution to help explain "generalization" or error. D. O. Hebb's insightful analysis invigorated this ancient theory by offering a neurology (i.e., hardware) and its psychological implications to capture these notions (1949). The experiments of Hubel and Wiesel (1963), and their colleagues added empirical support to the existence of such hardware. The recent introduction of computational ideas (Rumelhart & McClelland, 1986) supported Hebb's parallel associative functions (cell assemblies and phase sequences). The inclusion of recursion into these networks to make them sensitive to their own effects was central to Hebb's model, and was reinvigorated by the additional logical operators that modern associationism provided. There are alternatives to the connectionist model of reactive theories. Most replace the associative bond and the chaining of connections with servo systems linked hierarchically (Miller, Galanter & Pribram, 1986). This modification allows continuous modulation of activity without further stimulus input. Error could be corrected on-line by the inherent nature of the system. Neurological support for these ideas has also been forthcoming (cf. Chapter 14 in Miller, et. al., 1986).

A second mode to explain the often bewildering and autonomous behavior that seems to be an *expression* of the interior machinery rather than a reaction to stimulation is exemplified by Freud (1905/1963). He saw clearly that academic psychology was engaged in a form of "reverse engineering". From the base of behavioral data such theories search for a reactive system generator that will mimic the responses. From Freud's point of view the theoretical impetus went the other way. The first task of a satisfactory theory was to characterize the person. From the person's nature flowed the behavioral descriptions. The problem with these expressive theories is that they lack adequate analytical tools to examine the connection between the person and his acts. Freud certainly represented a dominant presence among a small professional audience as well as a following among non-scientists, but his thrall has dimmed. Sharp technical and critical analyses coupled with a falling away of the practical needs of the medical community have left only a cadre of dedicated adherents to a withering literary cult. Other theories of this expressive kind have met similar ends with even less witness. Aside from their professional origins, most of these grand overviews bear about as much current panache as the huckster offerings of Neurosemantics or Dianetics. Nevertheless, the relentless need for a deeper understanding of human nature still drives conservative scientists to speculate about and sometimes publish broad-ranging theories intended to capture and thereby illuminate the human condition.

The impetus for expressive theories penetrated academic psychology through the experimental work of the early cognitive, or more correctly, motivational theorists such as E.C. Tolman and especially Kurt Lewin. These ideas of dynamic psychology that stem from the original insights of Freud have informed some of the notions that we shall treat in the technical parts of our analysis. Both Tolman and Lewin hoped to overcome the technical limitations of Freud's theories by inventing discursive mathematical models (Lewin, 1938) or map-like simulations (Tolman, 1932). Tolman's rats made "cognitive maps" of their rodentine world and guided their behavior by following purposive paths in their brains (means-end readinesses) that were signalled by "sign-gestalts," named for the new German psychology of perception that had come to America. These structures were energized by the desires and aversions of the subject, although in his attempts to formalize these ideas he was later driven to servos and forced movements (Tolman, 1939). But Tolman's means-end readinesses came before their time, and American psychology having been bitten once by the discredited experimental method called "introspection", continued to search where the light was good and built an edifice of experimental data based on how rats learned in a maze.

But even while that work culminating in Skinner (1938) was going on, Kurt Lewin was proposing an image of the human interior which, like Tolman's, was replete with map-like structures that possessed quantitative properties of motivation he called tensions and valences. Theories such as Lewin's (1936), were praised for their attention to problems of psychological representation (Irwin, 1971), while also frequently criticized as empirically trivial (Miller, 1964). The criticism often hinged on the loose coupling between the hidden machinery of tensions, vectors, and goals and such observed behaviors as remembering and forgetting (Ebbinghaus, 1913), and choosing (Luce 1959). The current acceptance of cognitive psychology (cf. the journal *Cognitive Psychology*), and the computer metaphor in theory construction has made the use of invisible mechanisms legitimate if they can be shown to constrain observable behavior. But the point the reactivists continue to press is that human behavior must be modelled on animal experiments or we run the risk of accepting verbal reports as accurate statements about the nature of the internal machinery. We must, we are told, derive the nature of that machinery from behavior as uncontaminated by introspection as the records of the animal laboratory. That is why Fechnerian psychophysical judgments are acceptable and reports of experiential magnitudes are not (cf. Krueger, 1989).

The trouble with these reactivists ideas is that they are concerned with what serves to limit and constrain action. Their laboratory successes in liminal psychophysics or animal learning derive from the inherent simplicity or some would say triviality, of the issues they address. If the quantification of the rate or serial order of the elimination of errors in a maze is stretched to design the structure of a college curriculum, one is justified in asking to see the strong chain of causation that extends from the maze to the classroom. If acting with concern for others is simply the consequence of having received compliments that "reinforced" similar earlier actions, the layman is not being unjust when he or she demands more than the analogy of a rat pressing a lever to get food.

We begin the exposition of an *expressive* theory of intention and action that follows from Lewin's theory and offers experimental tools to implement and quantify his ideas by presenting first a schematic overview along with some examples. Then we shall connect these ideas to experimental data, and demonstrate how the theory can serve a useful purpose by imposing demands on the methods we use to organize and interpret behavioral data. We will outline some initial experimental designs that we have conducted to test the analytical power of the theory. Finally, we will speculate on its practical ramifications.

II. The Theory

We assume first that people spend most of their time laying out intentions to act. We call these internal mechanisms *ballistic intentions*. These intentions have certain properties, both structural and functional. The functional properties form three components or analytical categories of any ballistic intention. They are:

1. Scalar magnitudes of events that represent desires and aversions to reach certain internal or internally represented external states. These magnitudes can be experimentally assessed, and their values can be assigned to the psychological states of the individual. These states, which may be homeostats or schemas, and may also include temporal or spatial schematic representations of the world, constitute the "goals" or "purposes" of the ballistic intention. They are descriptive in nature but are intimately attached to the appropriate desire or aversion and may be construed as in a state of tension numerically expressible as the utility of the desire. These tensions may be quantitatively represented by "utilities". We show in the following experiments how these numbers can be estimated by psychophysical scaling methods and procedures.
2. A likelihood or expectation of attainment of the goal or purpose of the intention. Because the intention is ballistic, these expectations reflect the end state or consummation of the particular intention. Although most psychologists construe these expectations as a subjective probability, we have some evidence that demonstrates that the values are chunky, and mark discrete states such as "certainty" or "uncertainty". (Mark & Galanter, 1986).

3. A space or time or space-time metric or map that represents in a schematic way the "distance" to the goal and adjusts its topography to levels of environmental "friction" that we will describe shortly. Some properties of this map will also be described. Success in using such map-like structures (Garling, 1989) leads us to conclude that these maps can be examined as they influence behavior.

The purpose of this three part description is to give a handle to the experimenter. The ballistic intention a subject adopts in an experiment must be controlled. To do this the experimenter varies payoffs to modulate the utility of a goal (Galanter & Holman, 1967), or imposes delays to reshape the subject's space-time map (Mischel, 1958), or engages in other impositions to alter the certainty of success of the ballistic intention. These three components and their interactions must therefore be understood as a needed approximation to the actual, integral nature of the ballistic intention.

The use of the term "ballistic" may seem redundant. In common usage all intentions are ballistic. When we intend to leave the room, we convey the sense of purpose in our subsequent acts, the intent is complete in itself. However, the term "intention" has been used in some contexts (Miller, et. al., 1986) to characterize a not-yet-completed course of action. Others have used the word intention and intentional act to suggest action that is motivated as distinct from acts that are reflexive or reactive (Irwin, 1971). Finally, the notion that these ballistic intentions lack continuous monitoring, control, or modification, and are unchained by specific S-R steps, is part of the reason the prefix is used. This may explain why it is easy to underestimate how long any task will take; which suggests lines of experimentation that may permit us to study the structure of these intentions.

These ballistic intentions we postulate are outside of space and time in the usual sense. The child in the playroom who voyages to the moon and back through his ballistic intentions may, unlike the astronaut, make the trip instantaneously. The pilot who has already "landed" the plane as he crosses the outer marker inbound, needs only to monitor the various housekeeping functions, e.g., keeping the wings level and stabilizing the rate of descent. But for all its speed and satisfaction, a ballistic intention is (the child soon learns, and the pilot knows) a chimera. Without any spatial or temporal consequences the intention gets you nowhere. It must be implemented in action. This introduces the second structural concept in our theory -- the environmental *performance envelope*.

Notice that in the context of this theory the person is not simply a black box accessing information through some undefined input, but rather he or she holds information (the ballistic intentions) of overarching importance to the system parameters, i.e., the "person". Meanwhile he is moving physically through a complex environment. The nature of that environment is given to him by his sense organs and perceptual processes. It is schematically organized by the various ballistic intentions as we have seen. This metaphor is reminiscent of Gibson's "affordances" (1979) and other direct theories of perceptual processes which depend upon organismic movement as part of the set of translations that provide perceptual information. But notice that in the present theory the perceptual information serves (or disserves) the ballistic intentions of the person by imposing environmental limits on its successful execution. The person must sequester the available environmental support to translate his ballistic intention into reality. The environmental support (or lack of it) defines the perceptual envelope within which the ballistic intention may be executed.

The introduction of the performance envelope affords the opportunity to examine the structural properties of these intentional systems. When a particular ballistic intention is examined we see that it possesses a *gateway*, a state of the person or the environment that serves as a start point for the performance envelope that must be traversed to consummate the intention. The gateway may itself be one of several goals of other ballistic intentions or it may be a set of stimulating conditions that are marked by what Hull (1943) called their *stimulus intensity dynamism*. But whatever its specific nature the gateway introduces, rather than stimulates the performance envelope. The performance envelope itself represents the response-constraining environmental structures replete with barriers, detours, and other impedimenta that must be overcome by action, or perhaps a smooth downward path over which the person glides with no difficulty. We measure the transversable properties of the performance envelope by its *width*, which may offer either a narrow and therefore unique path, or a wide set of alternative actions all of which achieve the same end. Figure 5.1 is a schematic representation of such a ballistic intention.

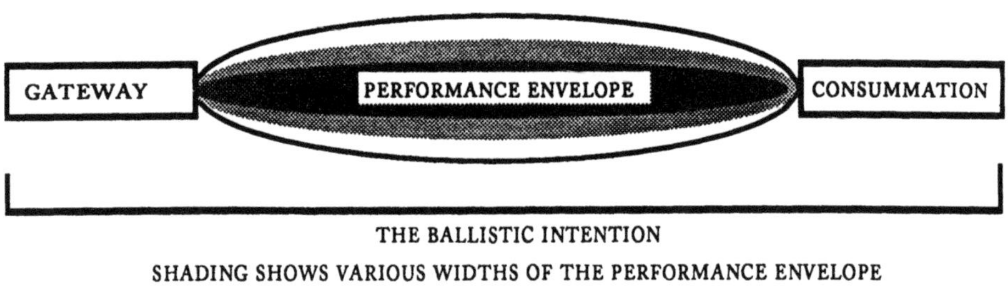

Figure 5.1: A topological representation of a ballistic intention, arranged in temporal order of execution. The magnitude of the minor axes of the elliptical performance envelopes represents the number or kinds of alternative paths available to the individual.

At any given moment several ballistic intentions may be simultaneously active and interacting. In keeping with our model of each intention as an integral unit, we describe these mutual interactions with a single parameter similar to the "Q" of a resonant circuit. Extending this analogy, we compare the ensemble of ballistic intentions to a set of resonant circuits tuned to different frequencies along a continuum. This continuum serves as a metaphor for the range of possible ballistic intentions. The expression of an intention in action is constrained by environmental bounds, and the sensory and motor limits and capacities of the person. All of these forces that limit the expression of a ballistic intention in the real world are just what we have called the performance envelope. Just as the performance envelope constrains behavior, so also does it influence the expression of any particular ballistic intention. As the environmental and internal components of the performance envelope vary, these variations tend to excite ballistic intentions that are close to the configuration of the performance envelope in much the same way that an input to a set of resonant circuits will excite those which are close in frequency to the input signal. In such a system, two resonators tuned to different frequencies may be excited by an input of a single frequency if the "Q" is low enough. Figure 5.2 shows this effect.

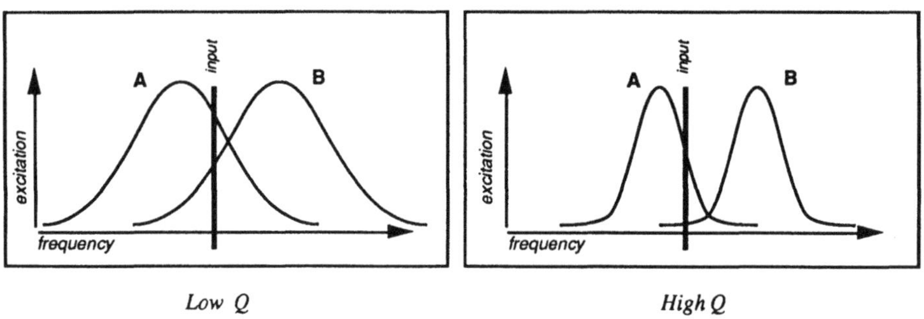

Figure 5.2: An analogy in one dimension of overlapping active intentions that may - the low Q case, or may not - the high Q case be excited simultaneously by common environmental or internal aspects of the performance envelope, represented here as the input frequency.

In the low Q circuits the input excites both A and B. In the high Q case, only A is appreciably excited. A simple relabeling of the figure makes the analogy complete. Resonators A and B represent two ballistic intentions along the continuum, while the input at frequency f represents a set of environmental and internal parameters that exist as the performance envelope at that point in time. The appeal of this interpretation of the interactions among ballistic intentions is that it allows us to describe these interactions without prior knowledge of their internal structure. It also reflects how our intentions are modulated by environmental possibilities.

Not all ballistic intentions have this consonant quality. There may be conflict among ballistic intentions. At that point we enter a well-tilled area of psychology, and it is incumbent on us to explicate our views on this time-worn topic. Conflict resolution is usually described in terms of conflict types and their behavioral representations such as approach-avoidance. We shall formulate the problem in different terms to describe how conflicts may be numerically represented, and how those representations can describe the quantitative properties of the behavioral resolutions. There are many ways of dealing with multiple or conflicting ballistic intentions, and any single formulation of the problem is bound to be incomplete. In spite of this fact, it is still useful to demonstrate how a conflict situation can be couched in terms of simultaneously present ballistic intentions, each vying with the other for control of their behavioral expression.

Consider an n-dimensional space where n is the number of ballistic intentions times the number of relevant dimensions comprising each ballistic intention. That is, each ballistic intention consists of a collection of relevant "constituent intentions", each of which can be placed somewhere along a one dimensional continuum. Two examples of such parsing of the intention into relevant intentions will make the point clear. In the first example, the subject must distinguish, and then select for action between two equilateral triangles of differing length, such as might be represented on the scope face by targets of varying distance. If these lengths are sufficiently close in value, they could be said to exist along a single continuum which refers to length. In this case, where all other aspects of the pair of stimuli are the same, the conflict can be transparently described in terms of the Q theory outlined above.

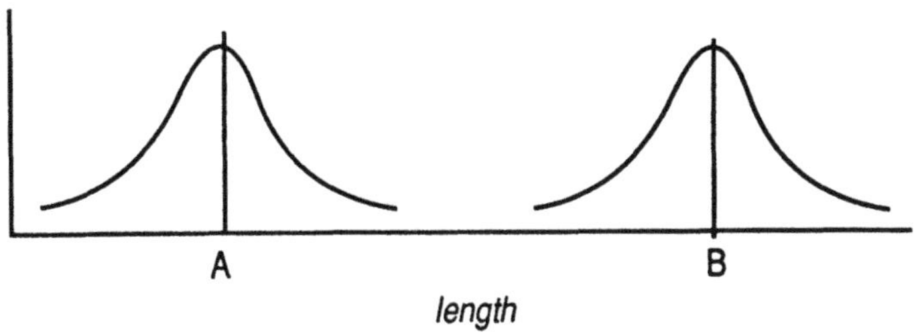

Figure 5.3: This figure along with Figures 5.4 and 5.5 show how the previous analogy of ballistic intentions to resonant circuits can break down if it purports to conceptualize variations in complexity that superficially appear sufficient to resolve the conflict. Here the difference between two intentions is sufficiently large that an alternative representation would be needed to conceptualize the task as a Q resolvable conflict.

However, if we allow the difference in length to be a very large value as in Figure 5.3, then the behavioral consequences (visual search techniques and subsequent behavior) become different in kind, not merely in degree. A theory which purports to address conflict among ballistic intentions (or stimuli) must be able to address the potential for disjoint differences.

In the second example, the subject is confronted with an equilateral triangle of length A and a square of length A. In this case, there are again, many dimensions which are trivial in the sense that those aspects of the stimulus are in both cases equal (both are the same color, the same side length, etc.). But in this case unlike the first example, there is more than one non-trivial dimension in which a difference is present. In the dimension of vertex angle, the triangle is 60 degrees and the square is 90 degrees. In the "number of vertices" dimension, the triangle is 3 whereas the square is 4. Figure 5.4 shows one analysis of this case. Since there are two non-trivial dimensions in which the ballistic intentions conflict, there is more than one way to allocate the resolution resources.

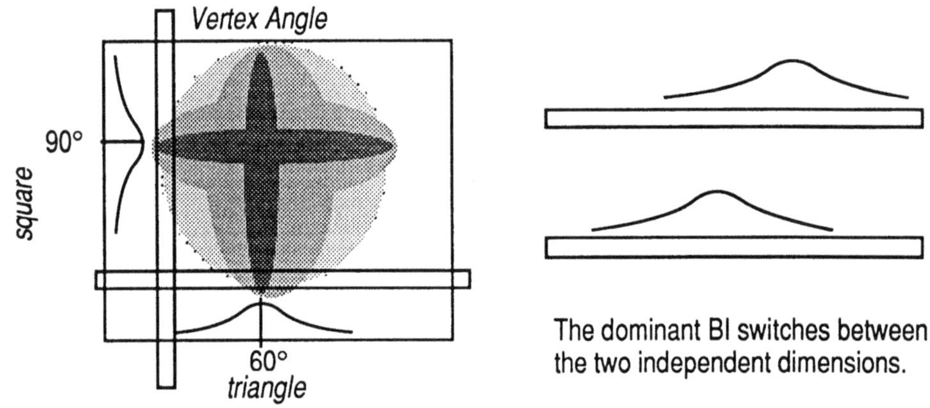

Figure 5.4: In this conflict a two-dimensional representation is needed and one solution to the conflict described in the text is shown. The Q analogy will not work here because the dimensionality of the task separates the components, just as distance in Figure 5.3 did.

One might posit a form of "time share" (Tsang & Wickens, 1988) in which the characteristic search behavior associated with square seeking is alternated with that of triangle seeking. Within this approach, conflicting aspects of ballistic intentions that are not currently of interest are ignored. Although this may happen much of the time in ecologically valid environments, it is also true that the conflicting ballistic intentions may be excited to some degree by the environmental noise present, making the pure time sharing approach less than optimal.

Another more general class of resolution mechanisms comes about when we consider the cross terms (or interaction) of the non-trivial dimensions. Attention to these cross terms quickly reveals the myriad ways in which conflict can be handled, because there are an infinite number of linear combinations of each dimension to yield the continuum along which the conflict takes place. Figure 5.5 displays an example of one such combination, in which the two dimensions have equal effect. In this conflict continuum, Q again applies, revealing the underlying coherence of the theory among the possible resolution mechanisms.

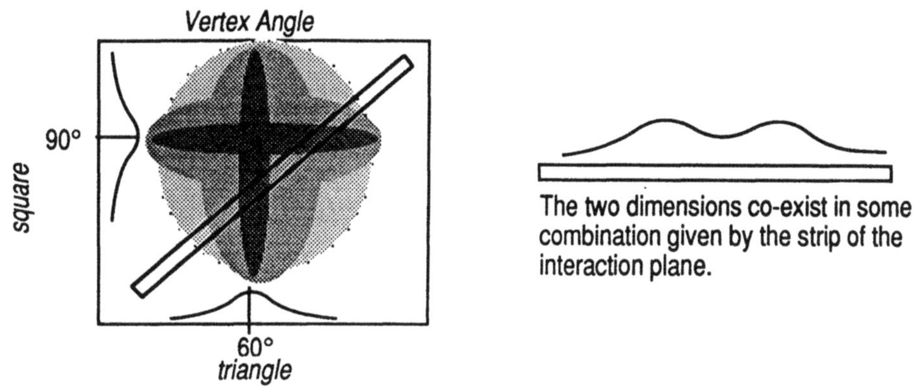

Figure 5.5: A reconceptualization of Figure 5.4 in which the correlation between the dimensions is used to imbed the conflict into the one-dimensional representation that can use the Q analogy to give a resolution.

The housekeeping demands of the performance envelope for a ballistic intention are often provided by experience of one kind or another. If your intention to leave the room includes a history of acts to accomplish the intent without using a key, you won't have the key in your hand when you get to the door. You are surprised to find the door locked. On the other hand, if you are in a security conscious environment and you have to open every door with a key, or punch in a combination, then when you get to a door that doesn't require one you behave in a totally inappropriate fashion. In the classical literature of Gestalt psychology this phenomenon was known as the "einstellung" effect or "mental set". Its experimental analysis by Luchins (1942) using a three-jar water fetching problem, was interpreted to mean that if you solved a problem routinely by a complex act, then even when the problem could be solved by a simpler one, the complicated solution was chosen. Similar findings have emerged in the area of decision making where "inappropriate", or "irrational" behavior is exhibited. In these new contexts the term mental set has been replaced by "decision frames" (Tversky & Kahneman, 1981). The present theory looks for different behavioral histories that have accompanied the current ballistic intention. We shall see shortly that these phenomena are all members of a class of events that induce what we call *friction* into the implementation of a ballistic intention within a performance envelope.

Often the performance envelope contains certain forcing functions that make ancillary demands on the system of action, and so increase what we call the *frictional* loss of efficiency in the execution of the ballistic intention. These capacity limits operate similarly to the mental set effects referred to above. The coupling functions between the ballistic intention and the performance envelope are never perfectly efficient, and therefore entail opportunity for failure. It is just in reducing this frictional component of the ballistic intention-performance envelope coupling that we may expect to enhance human performance. Notice that the width of a performance envelope and its friction may be related. On average we might expect that width = 1/friction. For example, a NASA demonstration video (NASA Langley Research Center 1981) displays the performance of a test-pilot making a series of low approaches to landing that require a transition from instrument meteorological conditions (IMC) to visual conditions (VMC). After breaking out of the overcast, the pilot has about 12 seconds of visual control during the final approach. Superimposed on the windscreen display is a point of light that shows the "look point" of the pilot during the approach. After two or three successful passes, the viewer sees that in this next approach a truck has intruded into the runway. The viewer may also note that the look point of the pilot occasionally fixes on the intrusion. However, the landing is disastrously completed. During some of these tests the pilot may -- too late -- spot the truck. Our point is that no analysis of such look-point data can inform us about the pilot's ballistic intention, which is what is guiding the approach. To use the behavioral information in these eye movement data, we must factor the glances into those that represent information acquisition for the ballistic intention (which of course is blind to runway intrusions), and those that interact with the environmental constraints -- the performance envelope.

The previous example also displays a phenomenon of some secondary importance that is illuminated by the theory. The viewer of the approach saw the intrusion clearly as soon as conditions changed to VMC. This "onlooker knowledge" had been reported by Galanter and Gerstenhaber (1956). They called it the "executive decision paradox". Subjects watching other subjects trying to predict a pattern of binary events could easily spot the pattern. The authors attributed the onlookers success to a lack of response interference. However, experiments that loaded the observer subject with response demands did not eliminate the effect. The control experiments were not sufficient to draw any strong conclusions, and consequently the effect has remained an unexplained puzzle. The present theory explains the paradox as a result of the two subjects exploiting different ballistic intentions. The check pilot in the jump seat sees things the test-pilot misses simply because his ballistic intention is concerned with the test pilots' performance and not landing the aircraft.

The executive decision paradox is similar in its effects to the paradox of performance enhancement during stress. In some situations subjects perform better under stressors such as high noise levels, continuous demanding motor control activities, (e.g., long flights or high gust loads), and other situations thought unlikely to enhance the quality of task completion. We should note that the ballistic intention in such situations may be markedly different from ones in which such forcing functions are not routine. Forcing functions may reveal discontinuities in performance quality simply because the ballistic intention is not revised to accommodate new coupling parameters in the performance envelope.

As the previous paragraphs suggest, using unconscious behavior like eye movements, requires us to know what it is about the behavior that is going to tip us to the form and structure of the ballistic intention. It was just because of this prior knowledge, or hypothesis if you like, that Hochberg and Galanter (1980) could use saccade suppression as an estimator of work load, whereas tracking the eye movements as in the NASA landing tape, provided no information. In their experiment it was not necessary to average across subjects in order to see the regularities, however those regularities were unique to the time-locked properties of the task. Generally it is difficult if not impossible to obtain repeated observations of a single event and so we settle for an average across individuals. In particular, when we collect verbal reports about a person's state of mind we often try to approximate repeated observations by asking the same question in a variety of ways -- the introspective and the psychometric approach. We begin the experimental analysis of the intentional theory by turning first to the methods and procedures that can solve some of these problems. In particular we address the question of individual subjects and their judgments, and suggest a new method to let us obtain scale values of single events without having to postulate or examine some (one-dimensional) continuum on which these events may reside.

In contexts like psychophysical scaling it is quite easy to believe that the perceived loudness of a sound grows as some regular function of the physical intensity. Consequently, if laboratory experiments yield data that uncover a neat relation between physics and subjective report, the psychophysical function with its coefficients of variation in the 90's (Galanter, 1990) validates the belief. The magnitudes reported by the hearer are generally unequivocal in meaning. The subjective judgments possess a natural (arithmetic) structure. Consequently, one is led to believe that these psychophysical functions represent a person's experiences. And to round out the quality of such data there remains the hope that a logical connection can be found to derive the parameters of these judgments from the simpler "yes/no" reports of the liminal experiment -- a hope that may justly be called "Fechner's faith".

If now we could turn these scaling techniques to our use in the present study of expressive behavior by quantifying aspects of the ballistic intentions that comprise the heart of the theory then we would have solved the preliminary problem that such a theory of the internal structures of a person demands -- quantitative experimental evidence that derives from the theory. The experiments reported below, although driven by a different set of personal scientific intentions, offer just such a technology. To see how that technology can work to provide empirical data for the current theory we must first step through the details of the procedures and the data that validate and justify these methods. Although this detour through these data involves a considerable investment of faith, a demonstration that we can assign numerical values to properties of ballistic intentions and parameters of the performance envelope, may also serve other functions for psychologists with other purposes.

In a standard magnitude estimation experiment, observers are asked to assign a numerical value to the magnitude of an "experience" associated with some particular stimulus presentation in comparison to the experience engendered by a modulus whose numerical value is assigned by the experimenter. In general these methods have averaged data across subjects. The current theory expects that different subjects may use different intentional structures even when addressing common tasks. Therefore we need assurances that such data can be extracted from one subject at a time. We have successfully revised the magnitude estimation method to obtain consistent data for a single observer using a computer-assisted ratio judgment procedure (Galanter & Wiegand, 1991). However, in the present context the demands of the theory are just the reverse -- to quantify a single state of mind, the scalar magnitude of the value of the goal of the ballistic intention, by comparison with other previously scaled stimuli. We call this variation of the magnitude estimation scaling procedure as originally explored by Stevens and Galanter (1957) "the modulus estimation" (ModEst) method (Galanter, 1987). Respondents are asked to assign a numerical value to the modulus or target event relative to a large set of other stimulus events that have been independently scaled separately. Although not yet functional, we believe that procedures similar to those developed for single subject magnitude estimates, can also be used for modulus estimation. We demonstrate the validity and robustness of the method for group data in the following experiment.

III. Experiment 1

Subjects

Thirty Columbia college undergraduates served as subjects in this experiment. They were recruited from a course in experimental psychology where they had themselves conducted magnitude estimation experiments on the loudness of noise. They participated individually.

Procedure

When a subject arrived at the laboratory he or she was given the following instructions:

> I am going to have you listen to pairs of sounds through these earphones. The first sound is the "target" sound and will always be the same loudness. The second is the comparison sound which will vary from trial-to-trial. I want you to tell me how much louder or softer the target is than the comparison sound. Do this by giving me the ratio of how much louder or softer the target sound is than the comparison. You might say "the target is one third as loud as the comparison". Or perhaps "the target is 5.7 times louder than the comparison". Give each judgment as soon as the comparison sound stops.

The data consist of a pass through fifteen pink noise stimuli that spanned 45 (relative) dB in 3 dB steps. The target stimuli for one third of the subjects was a noise of 6 dB, for the next third 21 dB and for the final third 42 dB.

Results

The magnitude (in sones) of each comparison tone was divided by its judged ratio to the target tone. If the subject "hears" sones perfectly, fifteen identical numerical judgments of the target should be obtained. The magnitudes of the target tones estimated by this procedure were converted back to deciBels. Table 5.1 shows the mean and variability of the three groups expressed in dB. Statistical support of such consistency is redundant.

Table 5.1: Means and standard deviations of judgments of the magnitude of each of fifteen stimuli relative to three standard stimuli which were converted to dB by the sone scale of loudness.

	Target Tone		
	6 dB	21 dB	42 dB
Mean (N=150)	6.07	20.17	43.22
S.D.	0.16	0.44	0.72

Discussion

This natural implementation of ModEst uses comparison stimuli from the modality of the modulus to scale the modulus. In a sense we do a cross-modality matching experiment (e.g., Stevens, 1959, 1966) with identical modalities to compare a continuum of previously scaled stimuli with the single stimulus element to be measured.

IV. Experiment 2

Introduction

In order to generalize the ModEst method to numerically characterize properties of objects and events with no particular quantitative structure, we need to construct a standardized set of scaled comparison stimuli. These comparison stimuli must vary along a dimension that has been scaled independently of the reference event being measured just as the comparison sounds in Experiment 1 were measured on the sone scale of perceived loudness. However, the "modality" of events that represent the consummation of an arbitrary ballistic intention is not clear.

Elsewhere I have proposed the use of utility as a "universal solvent" or perhaps "titre" is a better term to represent the hedonic value of mental states (Galanter, 1990). This measure has the practical advantage that it allows for the conversion of utility scale values into an equivalent utility scale for money. The utility of money has itself been cross validated in liminal psychophysical experiments (Galanter & Holman, 1967, Kornbrot, Donnelly, & Galanter, 1981), and by the use of cross modality matching methods against other sensory continua (Galanter & Pliner, 1974).

To this end a Utility Comparison Scale (UCS) of familiar events was constructed to be used as a standardized attitude measure (Galanter et. al., 1978). This instrument consists of a set of familiar items or events, for example, "You are late for an important appointment;" whose numerical utility values have been measured by magnitude estimation methods in a laboratory setting. For this experiment a set of items was used that represented a wide dynamic range on the negative or aversive limb of the utility function. The quality of these items can be judged by the high reproducibility of the scale value of money losses embedded in and among these items during their initial scaling (cf. Galanter, 1990, Experiment 2). This Utility Comparison Scale is the psychological equivalent of a standard weight, or length against which physical variables or measuring devices are calibrated. Just as the quality of such physical standards is constantly improved, we may expect that the standardized utility scale can also be updated and refined. Indeed, we currently use a newer version of the scale that was first employed in the experiments reported here.

The standardized utility scale was constructed using Columbia University students. Three groups of subjects judged the annoyance of forty seven life-familiar events (including the fifteen used in this experiment), by the method of magnitude estimation. The subjects gave numerical responses to the "annoyance" of these items as well as to eight additional items that represented various amounts of monetary loss. The results of these calibration studies indicate that the magnitude estimation scale values assigned to the "monetary loss" probe items fall on the same disutility function we have obtained in previous experiments. The power function for monetary loss has an exponent near one-half (Galanter & Pliner, 1974). The slope of the disutility function for this experiment was 0.54 (Galanter et. al., 1977). The reliability of the disutility values of the life-familiar events for all items in the original calibration experiment, and in two separate additional experiments using college students as subjects had previously been determined. The test-retest reliability of the 15 items averaged +0.96 when calculated independently for the two separate experiments.

Subjects

Four employees in the Psychophysics Laboratory served as subjects. Three were female between 17 and 50 years of age with audiometrically normal hearing. The male subject was 34, also with normal hearing.

Procedure

Subjects were tested separately in a quiet environment. They first listened to a synthesized "unpleasant" noise sample of 8 seconds duration at a level of 83 dB A, in a diffuse sound field. At the end of the stimulus exposure they were read the following instructions.

> Suppose you lived in a neighborhood where that sound occurred frequently throughout each day. I presume you would find it unpleasant. [All subjects agreed in one way or another].
>
> I want to find out how annoying such an environment would be to you. In order to compare your feelings with others, I want you to compare the annoyance of such a situation with other annoying things, like [ITEM]. Do you thing that the noisy environment would be more or less annoying than [ITEM]? Here is the noise again. [After the sense of the judgment was ascertained].
>
> Now I want you to tell me how much more/less annoying the noisy environment would be than [ITEM]; not even twice/half, twice/half, four times/one quarter, or even ten or twenty times/one tenth or one twentieth as annoying as [ITEM]. You may use any multiplier or divisor you wish just as we do in our magnitude estimation experiments.

This procedure was repeated for each of 15 non-monetary items. On three subsequent days, sometimes with a lapse of four days between sessions, the subjects were tested again with the noise level shifted to 78, 88, and 93 dB A.

Results

The subject's judgments were analyzed individually by multiplying or dividing their judgment on each of the 15 trials by the UCS scale value obtained from the standardized scale, to yield a normalized set of values. In later experiments two of the items showed ambiguities among non-college student subjects that made them unreliable. For this reason these items were removed from the present analysis. Table 5.2 shows the means and standard deviations of the 13 transformed judgments for each of the four noise levels. If the "noisy environment" was perfectly represented by the judgmental ratios, and if the scale values of the UCS were perfect reflections of their disutility, then we could anticipate that the 13 transformed judgments for each subject for each noise level would be identical. We might also conjecture that insofar as increased noise sound pressure increased annoyance, the average transformed numerical comparisons would reflect these differences. Table 5.2 verifies both of these hypotheses. The means of these judgments shift appropriately as the noise level is increased. The mean differences between the average transformed judgments foe each noise level are significant by pairwise t-tests at $p < .001$.

To get a qualitative sense of these data (based on 1974 monetary values), notice that a 78 dB noise is about as annoying as having a leaky pen. At 83 dB the annoyance reflects about the same disutility as being late for an appointment. At 88 dB the sound intensity is high enough to equate to having $40 stolen or having a check bounce, and at 93 dB we are near the disutility of being the victim of a pickpocket. This highest loudness level is close to what people living within the 40 NEF (Noise Exposure Forecast) contour near an airport experience daily, sometimes at the rate of one blast every three minutes.

Table 5.2: Means and standard deviations of the judged magnitudes of the noises at four different sound levels relative to 13 different life familiar events relative to the perceived annoyance of noises. Each of the four subjects are displayed individually.

Modulus Estimates of Utility Comparison Scale Values to Unpleasant Sounds n = 13 items per sound level					
		Sound Level			
Subject		78 dBA	83 dBA	88 dBA	93 dBA
A	Mean Std Dev	1.13 0.28	3.36 1.07	10.59 1.65	31.87 10.07
B	Mean Std Dev	1.24 0.41	3.61 1.17	12.22 4.57	33.78 10.28
C	Mean Std Dev	0.9 0.43	3.26 1.07	9.68 1.8	31.31 9.49
D	Mean Std Dev	1.55 0.34	5.27 1.8	15.73 4.18	38.21 8.66

V. Experiment 3[2]

The preceding experiments show that we can extract numerical judgments about a single object or event relative to a variety of previously scaled stimuli. Furthermore, the comparison stimulus scale can represent abstract objects of desire (or aversion) as well as the desirability of courses of action or environmental support. Consequently, we obtain for a single object (e.g., a noise in Experiment 2) a distribution of numerical values that capture the utility distribution that represents the magnitude of a vector a person has about a particular object (noise in this case) or outcome of an act whether real or imagined. The ability to scale attitudes or values of a single event or object opens a multitude of practical questions to experimental analysis. In this experiment we demonstrate the efficacy of the ModEst technique to quantify aspects of the ballistic intentions involved in the performance of a skilled task, and to study how utilities of the components of a ballistic intention in a common context may be amalgamated.

The layman can often partition complicated actions into subunits. Such analyses are routinely applied in practical contexts to aid in understanding or (re)organizing human performance. In a flight from New York to Los Angeles the pilot does a cockpit check, takeoff, enroute flight, terminal area approach, and landing, followed finally by shutdown. The more professional the analysis of the act, the finer the partition can become. At some level, however, professional analysis stops and psychological analysis must then begin.

---

[2] The computer program was designed and written by Thomas E. Wiegand; data collection and analysis was conducted by Gloria Mark.

Consider another example: A pilot may wish to deviate from his planned flight path to avoid a weather cell or frontal line. The goal is to arrive safely at the flight destination. Components of the task are selected to minimize discomfort to himself, and to the passengers and crew, as well as to minimize flight time and its associated costs. Different paths and procedures may be available to accomplish each of these goals to varying degrees. These separate paths may comprise different sequences of actions and consequently vary the parameters of the performance envelope. The variations may include frictional efficiency, width, and other as yet unidentified parameters. As a consequence, different paths may possess greater or less utility. Which is chosen?

This multipath problem is not unique, but rather is the paradigm of most human decision making and choice. The route that is selected will be influenced by factors intrinsic to the performance envelope, the different consummations, and various aspects of the pilot's general knowledge and experience. The difficulty is that we lack procedures that can parse a task into its constituents. Where we make such a division, based say on expert judgment, we have no natural scale to estimate the magnitude of the positive or negative values of the components. Even if we could assign such numbers to task parts, we have no rules for combining them into a total task cost or benefit as distinct from the costs and benefits of the task outcome. These limitations are further compounded by the strong interactions among the sub-units of the environmental envelope and the consummatory utility.

Not all parts of this complex problem are equally intractable. First, we can experimentally work around the interactions produced by different outcomes on task performance by scaling the widths or frictional efficiencies of various environmental envelopes that have a common consummation. Insofar as the final common outcome is the same regardless of the chosen path, we may plausibly argue that only the differences in psychic payoff between the routes differ. By using this indirection we can measure the same or similar task components embedded in different environmental envelopes without having to deal with the influence of final outcomes on these measurements.

The present study is a refined extension of work whose beginnings were reported in NASA Semi-Annual Progress Report No. 1, dated 15 July 1986 and in Mark (1987). In this experiment we examine the relation between utility judgments of sub-task paths and the utility of the task as a whole. This is a convergent validation procedure (von Winterfeldt & Edwards, 1986). It is based on the assumption that measurements of the same quantity done with different methods should covary. Using workload and stress ratings, Hart and Bortolussi (1984) demonstrated the robustness of their convergent validation techniques. Significant correlations occurred between the combined sub-task ratings and the total ratings in a flight scenario. Various kinds of measurements used in complex task performance that were found to be significant indicators of workload included performance on a secondary task (Ogden et. al., 1979), the event related brain potential (Israel et. al., 1980; Kramer et. al., 1983), and subjective rating techniques such as category scales (Hart et. al., 1981), magnitude estimation (Borg, 1978), and Cooper/Harper subjective ratings (Wierwille & Connor, 1983). Because the implicit precision of ratio scaling methods has been demonstrated for a variety of tasks and dimensions in laboratory experiments, and because these methods suggest combinatorial models with special constraints, we use the ModEst variant of magnitude estimation here.

The translation of ModEst scaling methods from the previous experiments with classical stimuli to the abstractions of the ballistic intention requires a steady hand on reality. It is not sufficient to measure only the magnitudes of intentional consummations under one or another set of antecedent conditions - a straightforward task. We must also demonstrate that measurements of the performance envelope parameters coordinate with measures of other aspects of the intention, and further, that predictive power resides in such coordinations. As a demonstration of such techniques we examine here the judged quality of safe traverse to well-defined behavioral goals when performance envelopes vary in their frictional efficiency.

The utility of an alternative path may be based on evaluative rather than cognitive functions. Feelings color judgment. Usually one construes the choice of sub-tasks as constrained by some overall calculus of cognitively derived utility. However, various routes to a goal may tend to derive their values from affective components weighted by cognitive calculations. If the choice between paths has little cognitive consequence, it may be fair game for feelings and desires. Consequently, predictions of task performance can err if they rely only on cognitive computations. Valuative considerations may contribute significantly to the overall evaluation of the effort. As a colleague has remarked in respect of this topic, "if the goal is to reach one's death-bed, is the life one leads to get there equivalent to any other?"

The frictional level of a performance envelope refers to its net positive and negative attributes from whatever their source which are considered in order to maximize the consummatory utility. This conceptualization accords with commonly accepted definitions of utility (Luce & Raiffa, 1957). In the case of a complex task and its corresponding sub-tasks, the assumption is that the criterion is some measure , e.g., minimum effort, for the completion of the task. At present we cannot easily distinguish on the basis of behavior alone between those utilities that contribute to the total value of the task goal that are primarily cognitive, and those that are suffused with emotive weight. In part the experiment that follows is aimed at helping to define behavioral criteria to separate these components. Additional detailed parametric studies remain to be done.

The utility measures of the sub-tasks were obtained during the performance of a simulated and simplified aircraft flight controller task. This task was divided by the experimenter into two discrete sub-tasks. On successive trials, subjects use three different paths to reach the first sub-task goal. The second sub-task, also exposed them to three different alternatives to reach that goal. Thus, there were nine possible combinations of paths all of which lead to the task goal. During each sub-task, the subject rated the utility of each path relative to an arbitrary value assigned to one or another characteristic of the performance envelope that was not part of the experimental task. This method was an early implementation of the ModEst technique. The experimenter then asked the subject to rate the utility of the combined choices relative to reaching the criterion - the task goal. Analyses helped us decide among various models of sub-task utility combination, whether the utility ratings of sub-task paths predict the whole task utility rating, and indirectly, whether judgmental models need to include the equivalent of "cognitive" noise.

Preliminary models

Based on the power function hypothesis, (Stevens & Galanter, 1957), a log transformation model of the relation of sub-task utilities to total task utility is conjectured. This model in simplest form is:

$$\log U_t \geq \sum_{n} [w_i \log(u_i)] \tag{1}$$

where U_t = The utility of the strategy used to complete the task.

u_i = The utility of the strategy used to complete sub-task i.

n = The number of tasks that the task is decomposed into.

w_i = The weight assigned to sub-task i by the combination rule.

The natural alternative is an additive model using untransformed data:

$$U_t \geq \sum_n [w_i u_i] \quad (2)$$

Both models make three assumptions. First, it is assumed that the subject is interested in maximizing some consummatory criterion. The criterion we presume that the subject is maximizing is to achieve the task goal with minimum effort and the avoidance of failure. Second, since an additive relation is proposed, the corresponding assumption of path independence is assumed. Path independence assumes that the choice made to reach the goal of sub-task i does not affect choices for subsequent sub-tasks. This assumption can be validated by testing whether the interaction between path choice utility ratings is zero. The third assumption of the model is that the combination rule should be invariant with respect to the path chosen, as long as the sub-task goals and task goals remain constant. This assumption can be tested by determining whether the fit of the model for each path combination remains invariant.

In this simulated air traffic controller task the subject must first evaluate a display method for air traffic altitude information, and then evaluate procedures for conflict resolution. The overall goal is to maintain safe traffic separation for the aircraft. The Stage 1 task includes scanning for potential collision. The Stage 2 task is to evaluate a method for changing the flight path of a target to prevent collision. The subject is told that at least one potential collision will occur on each trial.

Subjects

Five paid subjects, all students at Columbia University, participated in the experiment. Four of the subjects were male. The student ages ranged from 19 to 26. They all had vision correctable to normal.

Apparatus

Subjects were seated in a well lighted laboratory at a console containing a keyboard, a pointing device (mouse), and a color CRT. The subject was free to adopt a comfortable position facing the screen within reach of the keyboard. the subjects generally chose a position that placed their eyes slightly above and 50 cm distant from the CRT. For their control responses, subjects used the mouse and the keyboard.

Stimuli

The design of the air traffic display program was modelled to resemble the radar scopes used by air traffic controllers in 1986. Our display in particular was based on a TRACON air traffic control facility in Westbury, New York. This is a terminal radar approach installation that monitors aircraft outside a five mile radius from each of four major New York airports: Kennedy, LaGuardia, Islip, and Newark. Radar at that facility is monochrome and vector drawn, but also contains digital alphanumerics associated with the radar returns from aircraft transponders.

Aircraft: Depending on the trial, 4, 8, or 16 white dots (approximately 8 mm in diameter) representing airplanes, move across the CRT display in piecewise linear paths. The targets move within an XYZ coordinate system. The display is construed as perpendicular to the Z axis. Alongside each dot is a smaller directional dot, approximately 2 mm in diameter, which provides information on the direction of the plane's flight vector. Tracking along with each aircraft is a two letter identification code, such as "CO". At the beginning of each trial the planes start from different positions in the display. The rate of positional change varies across planes from one pixel per frame to twelve pixels per frame, but each plane moves at a constant rate. The planes blink off about every six seconds and reappear about one second later in an updated position, paralleling the timing, but not the decaying appearance, of a radar scope. The background color of the screen is dark gray.

Altitude information: Three choices are available for the display of altitude information: alphanumeric, voice, and digital meters. In the alphanumeric mode, altitude information appears beside the identification code of each aircraft. This altitude information is in the form of a one, two or three digit number which represents hundreds of feet. Voice interrogation is done by clicking the mouse over the plane in question. A synthetic computer voice responds with the plane identification code and a three digit altitude reading. The third altitude method, digital meters, displays a column of plane identifiers at the edge of the screen, beside which a three digit altitude number is displayed. The altitude displays are updated every six seconds along with the aircraft positions.

Changing flight vector: Subjects could change the course of one of the planes to avoid a collision by one of three methods: altitude change, continuous lateral direction change, or limited (12°), lateral direction change. Altitude change increased or decreased the plane's altitude by one thousand feet. Continuous lateral change changed the plane's direction, left or right, by 6° per frame. 12° lateral change changed the plane's direction, left or right, by 12° only once.

Experimental Design

The nine choice combinations were assigned to each flight scenario in a Latin Square design. Twelve flight scenarios were randomized within each cell. A trial consists of one flight scenario. The 12 flight scenarios were all different and consisted of four scenarios each of 4 planes, 8 planes, and 16 planes. The data consisted of nine cells (108 trials per subject). The experiment yielded a data matrix as follows:

		Stage 1 Choice		
		1	**2**	**3**
Stage 2 Choice	**1**	12	12	12
	2	12	12	12
	3	12	12	12

Each cell contained observations from the 12 different flight scenarios. Each observation consisted of the utility estimates reported for subtask 1, subtask 2, and the overall task. The variation in number of planes was included to make the (only) control response - change of flight path - appear to vary in its work load. Thus adding some verisimilitude and variation to the display. These data were not recorded in the present experiment.

Practice session: Subjects first read a written description of the experiment at their own pace. The altitude display and collision avoidance methods were demonstrated to the subject in the first hour. During the next three hours the subjects performed 36 practice trials to gain familiarity with the system. The standard stimuli for altitude and for collision avoidance were also demonstrated. These standard stimuli, to which the computer assigned an arbitrary magnitude, included a coincident altitude color detection system in Stage 1. In this system, any two planes at the same altitude change in color from white to red. In Stage 2, the standard format for collision avoidance was a change in velocity, which either halved or doubled the rate of pixel change per frame. We have seen that the ModEst method left the utility ratio invariant when the comparison magnitude is changed in the previous experiments. In Stage 1, the subject was asked to compare the procedure for representing altitude to the method that was currently being used. This procedure was also used when the utility reports in Stage 2 were recorded. The utility of the overall task was judged relative to the other utility judgments.

Procedure

All targets originated at different positions on the CRT display and moved in different vector paths. During the third frame (about 21 seconds) a window appeared on the display prompting the subject to implement an altitude display method. The experimenter told the subject which method to use. The subject then selected the prescribed method using the mouse. During the tenth frame (70 seconds), a window appeared requesting the (utility) estimate for that performance envelope format. The value assigned to the comparison format was also presented in this window. The subject entered his estimate based we presume, on the magnitude assigned to the standard. The subject continued to monitor the screen for a possible collision. On the 16th frame (112 seconds) a window appeared prompting the subject to select a collision avoidance method for future use. The experimenter told the subject which method to select. The subject was then free to implement the selected collision avoidance method at any time after the prompt window was closed. The subject did this by using the mouse to select a direction (e.g. right or left, increase or decrease). The subject then typed in the two letter identification code of the plane which was to be affected. The screen flashed briefly on frame 22 to alert the subject to implement collision avoidance if it had not already been done. On the 23rd frame (161 seconds) a window appeared requesting a utility estimate for this collision avoidance method. The subject typed in a response on the keyboard. If the outcome of the collision avoidance choice was successful, the planes continued on their new flight vectors. If the outcome resulted in a crash of two planes, a message flashed on the screen indicating that "a fatal air collision has occurred". On frame 24 (168 seconds) a window appeared prompting the subject for a total task (consummatory) utility judgment. The subject typed in a judgment of the overall utility of the two methods used in performing the task. The rating was made relative to how well the two procedures would have worked in completing the task.

Results

The utility estimates collected in this experiment were subjected to both a logarithmic and a linear regression analysis. However, before we performed the regressions, some preliminary transformations and tests were done to check the basic assumptions of ratio stability and path invariance. After checking that ratio stability holds, we converted the utility estimates into relative utility estimates for the sake of easy comparison across trials. This simple conversion consists of dividing the reported utility value by the comparison value.

Statistical analysis: Different events were used to compare the value of each sub-task and session in order to circumvent the bias due to past utility rating reports. By varying the values of the standard procedures we are making the assumption that the magnitude of the standard does not affect the subjects' utility estimates. This assumption was tested with the General Linear Models (GLM) procedure of SAS which handles unbalanced designs. The means for each variable were tested to see whether they differed significantly between sessions. Each session used three different comparison values. The assumption was violated for subject A whose mean utility estimates were significantly different for sub-task 1, sub-task 2, and task variables, with $p < .05$. Subject B had significantly different means for his utility estimate of sub-task 2 across sessions. The remaining subjects did not show significant differences between their utility estimates when different comparison magnitudes were used.

The mean utility estimates for subjects are shown in Table 5.3. Subjects C, D, and E usually gave utility estimates that were significantly different between the paths in sub-task 1 and 2. Subjects were generally consistent in rating voice interrogation with the lowest utility and alphanumerics as having the highest utility. In sub-task 2, subjects were generally consistent in rating 12° lateral change with the lowest utility and altitude change with the highest utility.

Table 5.3: Utility estimates made by each subject about the quality of the display using "shifty modulus" methods with different moduli for each sub-task and the combined task.

	(Entries Represent comparison ratios)						
	Sub-task 1			Sub-task 2			Total Task
Subject	**A-N**	**V-R**	**D-M**	**A-C**	**12°**	**LC**	
A	2.72	2.28	2.42	2.46	2.20	2.29	3.02
B	1.26	0.72	0.74	1.30	1.19	1.29	1.52
C	1.44	0.90	1.30	1.36	0.97	1.20	1.21
D	2.58	0.54	0.79	3.32	1.23	2.03	1.87
E	2.00	0.50	1.16	1.82	0.54	1.11	1.18

Sub-Task 1: A-N = Alphanumerics;
V-R = Voice Report;
D-M = Digital Meters
Sub-Task 2: A-C = Altitude Change;
12° = 12° Lateral Change;
LC = Continuous Lat Chg.

If the model is correct, the form of the prediction equation should be the same for all subjects, although the weights assigned to each sub-task may vary over subjects. A multiple regression analysis was performed on each subject's data. The dependent variable is the overall utility estimate of the combined path choice for both sub-tasks, and the independent variables are the sub-task 1 utility estimate and the sub-task 2 utility estimate. The model which was tested is of the form:

$$\log (Y_i) = a + b_1 \log(X_{1i}) + b_2 \log(X_{2i}) + e_i \qquad (3)$$

The results of the regression analysis are shown in Table 5.4. The asterisks refer to whether the beta coefficients of the intercept and sub-task utilities are significant.

Table 5.4: Regression analysis of the utility estimates based on a power function model to predict the utility of the total task from the sub-task utilities.

			Beta Estimates			
Subject	N	Intercept	Sub-Task 1	Sub-Task 2	p-value	R^2
A	95	0.2281	0.2829	0.7483	0.0001	0.7971
B	92	0.4118*	0.2790*	0.0324	0.0197	0.0845
C	105	0.1164*	0.0906*	0.3406*	0.0001	0.3343
D	99	0.1174*	0.5176*	0.9215*	0.0001	0.8211
E	59	0.1675*	0.1707	0.5379*	0.0001	0.7751
* Significant at $p<0.05$ Mean R^2 = 0.5624						

Four out of the five subjects gave subtask utility estimates that were predictive of the overall utility according to the model specified in equation 3. Subject B's utility estimate for the paths used in sub-task 2 was not significant.

The percentage of variance explained in the total task judgment, R^2, ranged from values of .08 to .82. Models fit for three subjects, A, D, and E explained more than 77% of the variance of the holistic task judgment. Subject B's model shows an R^2 close to zero, and subject C a moderate value R^2 value, explaining 33% of the variance of the holistic task judgment. The residuals plotted against the predicted values for each subject show the residuals to be evenly distributed around zero indicating that the equal variance assumption of the error terms for the model appears to be met. They also indicate that the fit of the log-log model is appropriate.

Table 5.5: Regression analysis of the utility estimates based on a linear additive model to predict the utility of the total task from the sub-task utilities.

			Beta Estimates			
Subject	N	Intercept	Sub-Task 1	Sub-Task 2	p-value	R^2
A	95	0.0841	0.2096*	1.0516*	0.0001	0.7770
B	92	0.6953*	0.4399*	0.3343*	0.0015	0.1368
C	105	0.5868*	0.1655*	0.3559*	0.0001	0.2872
D	99	0.5286*	0.6868*	0.7156*	0.0001	0.8013
E	59	0.0248	0.5146*	0.5483*	0.0001	0.8456
* Significant at $p<0.05$ Mean R^2 = 0.5695						

Next, a strictly additive model was tested to compare the fit with the fit obtained in the log transformed model. This type of model is of the form:

$$Y_i = a_i + b_1X_1 + b_2X_2 + e_i \tag{4}$$

The level of significance of beta parameters for the stage utility estimates are shown in Table 5.5. Subjects A, D, and E show that the model explains more than 77% of the variance of the total task judgment. All beta estimates for the slopes are significant for both variables. In order to explain certain anomalies in these data it will be useful to have the range of utility estimates available, as shown in Table 5.6.

Table 5.6: The range of utility estimates used by each subject in judging the utility of the sub-tasks and the total task.

Subject	Subtask 1			Subtask 2			Whole Task		
	Min	Max	Range	Min	Max	Range	Min	Max	Range
A	0.75	6.00	5.25	0.38	4.50	4.19	0.67	6.50	5.83
B	0.50	1.70	1.20	0.02	1.93	1.50	0.75	2.25	1.50
C	0.03	2.50	2.47	0.40	2.50	2.10	0.71	2.50	1.79
D	0.13	4.00	3.88	0.50	4.00	3.50	0.25	4.44	4.19
E	0.01	2.00	2.00	0.10	2.00	1.90	0.20	2.40	2.20
All	0.01	6.00		0.02	4.50		0.20	6.50	

The largest range in utility estimates for any individual subject is 5.83. The average range over all subjects for all estimates is 2.90 with a standard deviation of 1.46. The ranges suggest that subjects imposed reasonable upper and lower bounds on their estimates. In order to validate the assumption of path independence, the interaction between the subtask utility estimates was tested for significance. A third alternative model was tested of the form:

$$\log Y_i = a_i + b_1 \log X_1 + b_2 \log X_2 + b_3 \log X_1 * \log X_2 + e_i \qquad (5)$$

When a partial F test was performed, placing the first two terms in the model, the interaction term was not found to be significant for four subjects. For subject D, the interaction term was significant with $p<.01$. When an overall F test (simultaneous test) was performed, the interaction term was not significant for all subjects except D. It follows from the prediction equation that the inter-subject difference would exceed the intra-subject difference. The form of the prediction equation should be the same for all subjects but the parameters could be different. Using a dummy variable model, the additive model shows significant differences between subjects with $p<.0001$.

The third assumption of the model stated that the combination rule for sub-task utilities should be invariant with respect to the choices made. The model was tested for significant differences for each of the path combinations. Nine different path combinations were used. Approximately twelve ratings were made for each of the nine path combinations. Subject D did show a significantly different model over path choices, as shown in the slope estimate for his sub-task 1 utility, with $p<.01$. All other subjects satisfied the assumption.

Discussion

Notice first that this experiment, although decked out in fancy dress, was a classical psychophysical experiment. The variations in the task were not *chosen* by our subjects, they were *displayed* by the experimenter. The occasional interactions between the subject and the task were actually part of the "stimulus" display. In effect subjects were passive observers of a set of possible procedures an air traffic controller might employ in his work.

A second important limitation on the analysis is the relatively narrow dynamic range of the judgments as discussed below. This makes any test of a power function against a linear model quite weak. The experiment failed to provide displays that would elicit ratings to show differing levels of difficulty. None of the subjects experienced difficulty in providing a numerical estimate of their utility relative to the standards. In general, all subjects reported that their utility estimates closely reflected the utility of their choices. However, our intent is not to ensure optimum conditions for a scaling experiment, but rather to start applying judgments of magnitude in contexts where these numbers may have predictive behavioral consequences. This experiment must be recognized as a step in the direction of extending psychological theory, not as a test of one or another scaling procedure.

The important result is the general consistency of the subject's judgments to hang together, and to conform to modest demands of reliability, consistency within subjects, and observance of plausible restrictions on any model such as path independence, and ratio preservation. Four of the five subjects showed an invariant model over path choices. This phenomenon shows the robustness of the internal consistency. Subjects generally applied the same weighting regardless of whether the choice is good or bad. In order to test this assumption of the model, we had to assign choices to the subject; otherwise, the subject may never have picked a path of low utility. This requirement as noted above makes the experiment less than we would have liked it to be. Current efforts with a new display and simulation program will permit us to fix this limitation. The model is also robust with respect to success or failure of the outcome. This result may indicate that in the case of failure, the subject may assign responsibility to extrinsic factors.

Four of the five subjects' data showed a significant relation between their judgments of the utility of the component sub-tasks and overall utility judgments. Unfortunately, only two of the subjects used the ratio judgement procedure in reporting the utility of the various choices. Because of this, conclusive evidence showing the validity of the double log model was not obtained. The mean R^2 of .5695 is about the same for both the double log model and the simple additive model. One reason for the similar fit of both models is that the range of the utility estimates is not very large (Table 5.6). It is not possible to tell whether a power function or linear function provides a better fit based on the data obtained in this experiment. Within the narrow range of values of the data, the power function appears close to being linear. The log transformed data in an additive model cannot be argued for merely on statistical grounds, but it can be supported on theoretical grounds. The way to provide a stronger test of the proposed model would be to collect data on subjective utility estimates that extend over a larger range of values. The path choices in this experiment were not regarded as significantly different by two subjects. This may have resulted in a low range of utility estimates.

The result showing that subjects B and C have different models over sessions (where each session has different modulus values) is quite significant. This outcome could explain why subjects B and C have low R^2 values. Subjects B and C could have the potential to be consistent in component-to-task ratings but may be influenced by the different modulus values. The evidence to back up this claim is that subject C had models from three sessions that accounted for over 63% of the variance and subject B showed two models that accounted for over 35% of the variance. More subjects are needed to determine whether subject B, whose R^2 was 0.08, is an anomaly. It is possible that subjects B and C were internally consistent yet performed poorly because they were confused by one path choice. Models were fit for the three levels of sub-task 1 choices, over all levels of sub-task 2. Models were also fit for three levels of sub-task 2 choices over all levels of sub-task 1. Models for subject B did not yield an R^2 higher than 0.20 for any of the six path choices. Subject C did not show an R^2 for any path choice higher than 0.37. Thus, it is unlikely that confusion about a path choice would be the cause of a low R^2. If we eliminate subjects B and C from the mean

R^2, since they are inconsistent over sessions, we find that the mean R^2 for the additive model is now 0.81. Because of several sources of variance that exist in the nature of this experiment, this mean R^2 of 0.81 is quite good.

The air traffic controller's (ATC) goal is to work within the capacity of his information processing resources so as to maximize decision making performance. If this capacity is exceeded, poor decision making can result. In terms of this study, we predict that one of the consequences of exceeding capacity limitations could be a decrease in the internal consistency, or predictive quality, of the utility ratings. Danahar (1980) discusses two air collisions due to poor decisions by ATC. A crash of two commercial carriers over Carlton, Michigan in November, 1975 occurred due to ATC decision not to take immediate action. In another case study, ATC failed to maintain vertical or lateral separation resulting in the collision of a commercial and private aircraft near San Diego in September, 1978. Finkelman and Kirschner, in 1980, proposed that decision failure is due to ATC working for an extended period of time using "reserve capacity". The overworked ATC is thus unable to process information adequately when an emergency arises. An alternate model by Sperandio (1978) proposes that the strategy of the ATC changes as more information is introduced. As more aircrafts appear on the screen, fewer variables per aircraft are processed. In studying memory errors in the ATC-pilot communication, Loftus et. al. (1979) showed that memory load and retention interval were significant factors.

VI. Conclusion

A scaling technique - *modulus estimation* - is described, and three experiments are reported that demonstrate its robustness, and its applicability to represent quantitative properties of ballistic intentions. The ModEst procedure permits multiple estimates of an internal or external event or object by comparing it to a set of previously scaled or standardized items. The final experiment departs from the usual psychophysical format of most scaling experiments to let us examine the quantitative interaction among the components of the ballistic intention. This application scaled the magnitudes of aspects of the performance envelope of a ballistic intention that required subjects to guide aircraft safely across a radar screen without collision. The gross effects tested here should not be construed as a reflection of the limits of discrimination of these methods. Indeed, it is the fine distinctions that ModEst may make possible that justifies its quite general application wherever desires, aversions, attitudes, interest, or other internal expressive states must be quantified. The natural applicability of this scaling method to social, political, and personal questions opens many avenues for quantitative exploration. The calibrated (utility) scales that should be used for these purposes can determine accurately the absolute magnitudes, of e.g., (dis)utility and its money equivalent or with an appropriately calibrated scale -- political vigor, social attitudes, market decisions, or personal health.

The numerical procedures that we currently use to quantify an expressive state *(S)* that represents the frictional aspects of the performance envelope or the utility of the consummation of a ballistic intention can be represented as follows. We want to establish the value of *S*, symbolized $u(S)$ as a function of the known values of a set n of familiar events E, each of which has a value $u(E_i)$, $i=1$ to n. We train subjects in ratio judgment procedures with a computerized task that involves estimating the lengths of lines (cf. Galanter & Wiegand 1991). If they meet the skill criterion built into that task they continue the evaluation by being given a statement of the event, E_i together with an arbitrary but constrained numerical value generated by the machine $u'(E_i)$ and are asked to assign a number $u'(S)$ to the state being evaluated. The numerical ratio $u'(S)/u'(E_i)$ is then normalized by $u(E_i)$ (which leaves it dimensionally accurate) to yield a value of $u_i(S)$ for every E_i. That distribution of numbers, which ideally should be constant valued, can then be summarized by one or another descriptive statistic to yield the measure of S. The nature of the distribution of $u_i(S)$ is also a proper topic of study; different states give rise to widely varying distributions of the state metrics. Exactly which parameters are of psychological interest remains to be seen, as does the identification of these parameters with experimentally manipulated conditions superimposed on some standard set of experimentally created ballistic intentions.

References

Borg, G. (1978) Subjective aspects of physical and mental load. *Ergonomics*, **21**(3), 215-220.

Danahar, J.W. (1980) Human error in ATC system operations. *Human Factors*, **22**(5), 535-545.

Ebbinghaus, H. (1913) *Memory: a contribution to experimental psychology*, New York: Teachers College.

Freud, S. (1963) *Three contributions to the theory of sex*, New York: Basic Books.

Galanter, E. (1987) *Modulus estimation: Quantification of single events*, Columbia University, NASA 87:2.

Galanter, E. (1990) Utility scales of monetary and non-monetary events, *American Journal of Psychology*, **103**, 4, 449-470.

Galanter, E. & Gerstenhaber, M. (1956) On thought: the extrinsic theory. *Psychological Review*, **63**, 218-227.

Galanter, E. & Holman, G.L. (1967) Some invariances of the isosensitivity function and their implications for the utility function of money. *Journal of Experimental Psychology*, **73**, 333-339.

Galanter, E. & Pliner, P. (1974) Crossmodality matching of money against other continua. In H.R. Moskowitz et. al., *Sensation and Measurement*, Dordrecht Holland: D. Reidel, 65-76.

Galanter, E. & Wiegand, T. (1991) Multiple moduli and payoff functions in psychophysical scaling, Chapter 10 in *Ratio Scaling of Psychological Magnitude*, S.J. Bolanowski & G.A. Gescheider (Eds.) Hillsdale NJ:LEA.

Galanter, E., Golding, N., & Haber, N. (1978) *A new scaling method to quantify individual attitudes during social surveys*. Columbia University, NASA-5.

Galanter, E., Popper, R., & Perera, T. (1977) Annoyance scales for simulated VTOL and CTOL overflights. *Journal of the Acoustical Society of America*, **S8**(A), 1.

Garling, T. (1989) The role of cognitive maps in spatial decisions. *Journal of environmental psychology*, **9**(4), 269-278.

Gibson, J.J. (1979) *The ecological approach to visual perception*, Boston: Houghton Mifflin.

Hart, S.G., Childress, M.E., & Bortolussi, M. (1981) Defining the subjective experience of workload. Proceedings of the Human Factors Society, 25th annual meeting, 527531.

Hart, S.G., & Bortolussi, M.R. (1984) Pilot errors as a source of workload. *Human Factors*, **26**(5), 545-556.

Hebb, D.O. (1949) *The organization of behavior*, New York:Wiley.

Hochberg, J. and Galanter, E. (1980) *Acoustically induced visualization interrupts visual information acquisition*, Columbia University, PPL 80/5.

Hubel, D.H. & Wiesel, T.N. (1963) Receptive fields of cells in striate cortex of very young, visually inexperienced kittens. *Journal of Neurophysiology*, **26**, 994-1002.

Hull, C.L., *Principles of behavior*, (1943), New York:Appleton-Century.

Irwin, F.W. (1971) *Intentional behavior and motivation: a cognitive theory*, Philadelphia:Lippincott.

Israel, J.B., Wickens, C.D., Chesney, G.L. & Donchin, E. (1980) The event related brain potential as an index of display monitoring workload. *Human Factors*, **22**(2), 211-224.

Kornbrot, D., Donnely, M., & Galanter, E. (1981) Estimates of utility function parameters from signal detection experiments. *Journal of Experimental Psychology: Human Perception and Performance*, **7**(2), 441-458.

Kramer, .F., Wickens, C.D. & Donchin, E. (1983) An analysis of the processing requirements of a complex perceptual motor task. *Human Factors*, **25**(6), 597-621.

Krueger, L. (1989) Reconciling Fechner and Stevens: Toward a unified psychophysical law. *Behavioral and Brain Sciences*, **12**, 251-320.

Lewin, K. (1936) *Principles of topological psychology*, New York:McGraw-Hill.

Lewin, K. (1938) The conceptual representation and measurement of psychological forces. *Contributions to psychological theory*, Durham NC:Duke University Press.

Loftus, G.R., Dark, V.J. & Williams, D. (1979) Short term memory factors in ground controller/pilot communication. *Human Factors*, **21**(2), 169-181.

Luce, R.D. (1959) *Individual choice behavior: a theoretical analysis*, New York:Wiley.

Luce, R.D. and Raiffa, H. (1957) *Games and decisions*, New York:Wiley.

Luchins, A.S. (1942) Mechanization in problem-solving: The effect of Einstellung. *Psychological Monographs*, **54** (Whole No. 248).

Mark, G. (1987) *The prediction of complex task utility on subtask utility*. M.A. Thesis, Columbia University.

Mark, G. & Galanter, E. (1986) Chunking uncertainty: psychophysical studies of expected utility, Eastern Psychological Association.

Miller, G.A. (1964) *Mathematics and psychology*, New York:Wiley.

Miller, G.A., Galanter, E. & Pribram, K. (1986) *Plans and the structure of behavior*, New York:Adams-Bannister-Cox.

Mischel, W. (1958) Preference for delayed reinforcement: An experimental study of a cultural observation. *Journal of abnormal and social psychology*, **56**, 57-61.

Ogden, G.D., Levine, J.M. & Eisner, E.J. (1979) Measurement of workload by secondary tasks. *Human Factors*, **2**(5), 529-548.

Rumelhart, D.E. & McClelland, J.L. (1986) *Parallel distributed processing: Explorations in the microstructure of cognition*, Volume I. Cambridge, MA:MIT Press.

Skinner, B.F. (1938) *The behavior of organisms: an experimental analysis*, New York:Appleton-Century.

Smith, J.d., Ellis, S.R. & Lee, E.C. (1984) Perceived threat and avoidance maneuvers in response to cockpit traffic displays. *Human Factors*, **26**(1), 33-48.

Sperandio, J.C. (1978) The regulation of working methods as a function of workload among air traffic controllers. *Ergonomics*, **21**, 195-202.

Stevens, S.S. & Galanter, E. (1957) Ratio scales and category scales for a dozen perceptual continua. *Journal of Experimental Psychology*, **54**, 377-411.

Stevens, S.S. (1959) Cross modality validation of subjective scales for loudness, vibration and electric shock. *Journal of Experimental Psychology*, **57**,201-209.

Stevens, S.S. (1966) Matching functions between loudness and ten other continua. *Perception and Psychophysics*, **1**, 5-8.

Tolman, E.C. (1939) Prediction of vicarious trial and error by means of the schematic sow-bug. *Psychological Review*, **46**, 318-336.

Tolman, E.C. (1932) *Purposive behavior in animals and men*, New York:Appleton-Century.

Tsang, P.S. & Wickens, C.D. (1988) The structural constraints and strategic control of resource allocation. *Human Performance*, **1**(1), 45-72.

Tversky, A. & Kahneman, D. (1981) The framing of decisions and the psychology of choice. *Science*, **211**, 453-458.

von Winterfeldt, D. & Edwards, W. (1986) *Decision Analysis and Behavioral Research*. Cambridge: Cambridge University Press.

Wierwille, W.W. & Connor, S.A. (1983) Evaluation of 20 workload measures using a psychomotor task in a moving base aircraft simulator. *Human Factors*, **25**(1), 116.

Psychophysical Approaches to Cognition
D. Algom (Editor)

6

THE CONCEPT OF PERCEPTUAL SIMILARITY: FROM PSYCHOPHYSICS TO COGNITIVE PSYCHOLOGY[1]

Robert D. Melara

Purdue University

[1] Preparation of this chapter was supported in part by National Institutes of Health Grant NS28617 to Robert D. Melara. Thanks go to Daniel Algom, Duncan Day, Jeffrey Mounts, Randall Robison, and Jonathan Bullock for their comments, suggestions, and assistance in preparation. Address all correspondence to Robert D. Melara, Department of Psychological Sciences, Purdue University, West Lafayette, Indiana, 47907.

Table of Contents

I. Introduction

A 1600-Hz 75-dB (A) pure tone seems a great deal like a 1605-Hz 75-dB (A) pure tone. Cars resemble trucks. One can compare an electron orbiting its nucleus with a planet orbiting the sun. If psychology has any claim to being a unique science (if a science at all), the concept of similarity must, in my view, occupy its center. Humans, like all other animals, are masters at identifying whether two events are the same or different. Perceptual and cognitive acts depend on this ability: distinguishing between the telephone ringing and the doorbell buzzing; noting how a current problem is structurally identical to an earlier one; recognizing shared traits between yourself and your father. We also excel at ordering events in similarity: Mahler might remind us more of Brahms than of Beethoven; a red circle might seem more like a red ellipse than like a green circle. And, as these examples make clear, the concept of similarity spans human experience, from the most mundane acts of sensation to creative acts of metaphor and analogy. To understand such diverse similarity relations, I think that psychologists should begin with perception; this is my personal bias. Perceptual relations are, to my mind, the ground that humans use to build the richness and complexity of their experience. Hence, this chapter is mostly about perceptual similarity.

In this chapter, I shall discuss psychologists' struggle, from the beginnings of the discipline, with the issue of perceptual similarity. These beginnings were dominated by psychophysicists, like Fechner, who attempted to create a science of psychology by relating physical changes in, say, sound intensity, to psychological changes in, say, perceived loudness. Currently, the dominant force in experimental psychology is the study of human cognition. Modern topics of inquiry include humans' ability to categorize, to recognize, and to solve problems.

The goals and the levels of theoretical sophistication have changed greatly from then to now. Contemporary cognitive theories, for example, encompass a wider range of human experiences and provide a fuller account of those experiences. Yet, curiously, psychologists have characterized perceptual similarity in comparable terms for over 100 years.

This review is chronological and, by necessity and choice, highly selective. Much that could be included about this vast topic is ignored along my historical journey. Instead, I focus on a set of themes that appear ubiquitous. My aim is to demonstrate how the history of ideas and their development provide insight into how best to characterize the concept of similarity today. At the close of this review, I summarize the important historical messages, using these to detail a personal view of the nature of perceptual similarity.

II. Fechnerian Psychophysics

As any introduction to psychology's history will describe, psychophysics, and so the science of psychology, began with Gustav Fechner (1860). On October 22, 1850, Fechner claims to have dreamt the solution to the problem of how physical changes relate to corresponding psychological experiences. At the core of this relationship is the first measure of dissimilarity: the "just noticeable difference" or jnd. The jnd -- the average of the 1st and 3rd quartiles of a cumulative density function -- is a classical threshold measure because it is that amount of difference between two psychological events that the perceiver notices 50% (or some other arbitrary value) of the time. It forms the basis for the first ruler or "scale" of psychological experience, jnd being the scale's fundamental unit. The conviction among psychologists that it is possible to measure precisely the experience of similarity among events has remained central to this day. Fechner sought to identify the axioms that characterized his scale. Both his successes and his failures in this regard have influenced later theorists.

Fechner presumed that physical quantities and psychological experiences were related mathematically, his so-called "outer psychophysics." He focused on the specifics of this relationship. For any point on a physical scale, Fechner wished to determine what physical increment was needed to make a psychological difference. This increment, as noted earlier by Fechner's colleague at the University of Leipzig, Ernst Heinrich Weber, depended on the absolute physical point: As physical quantities, like sound pressure, grow more intense, physical differences must increase to maintain constant psychological differences. In particular, Fechner discovered that a *logarithmic* relationship held between physical magnitude and sensation magnitude: as shown in Figure 6.1, arithmetic increases in perceived intensity are associated with geometric increases in physical intensity. In other words, when intensities are weak, only a small physical change is needed to notice a change; however, when intensities are strong, the same psychological change requires a relatively large physical change. The perception of intensity thus grows quickly for weak stimuli, but more slowly as stimuli become stronger.

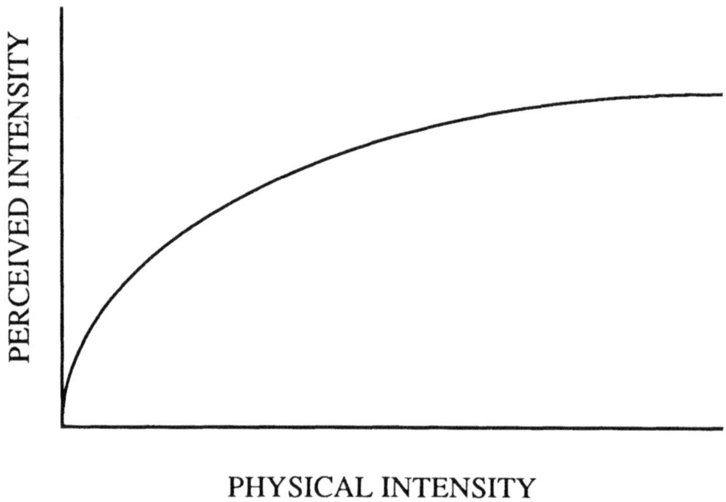

Figure 6.1: Graphic representation of Fechner's law showing the claimed logarithmic relationship between physical intensity and perceived intensity.

Fechner derived this logarithmic relationship mathematically by exploring the formal properties of the smallest psychological difference, the jnd. He assumed a "mathematical auxiliary principle," stating that whatever relationships hold between physical and psychological at the level of human experience -- that is, at the unit of the jnd -- should also hold when differences are made infinitesimally small, and so are outside human experience. Through this principle, Fechner integrated a differential equation called the "fundamental formula",

$$ds = K(di/i) \quad , \tag{1}$$

where i is stimulus intensity, di is a very small intensity increment, ds is a very small sensation increment, and K is a constant. Integration showed that the simplest relation that holds between S(ensation) and I(ntensity) is a logarithmic one:

$$S = \log I \quad . \tag{2}$$

In the years following Fechner's discovery, now known as *Fechner's law*, psychologists have debated its validity: Do changes in sensation really relate logarithmically to changes in physical quantities? Fechner's work was based on "indirect" scaling techniques. One example is the method of constant stimuli, in which subjects compare a test stimulus with a standard stimulus, judging whether the test is more or less intense (i.e., "heavier," "louder," "brighter," and so forth) than the standard. Unfortunately, more direct scaling techniques have not supported the logarithmic law. S.S. Stevens (e.g., 1975), for example, popularized the technique known as magnitude estimation, which requires subjects to estimate sensory quantities directly (e.g., assigning each loudness a particular value). Although the original impetus behind Stevens' technique was to lend additional support for Fechner's law, Stevens soon discovered that the relationship between the sensory experience and physical magnitude was expressed best not by a logarithmic function, but by a power function:

$$S = b\,I^a \quad , \qquad (3)$$

where a, the exponent of the function, depends on the particular sensory dimension being judged. The reason for the discrepancy between Stevens' function and Fechner's function is still unknown (see Krueger, 1989). As Marks (1974) has argued, it may be that the functions (and the techniques that produced them) reflect different, but equally valid, aspects of sensory experience.

For our purposes, the importance of Fechner's jnd lies in it representing the first scientifically plausible attempt to scale psychological differences. Fechner was satisfied to relate the physical to the psychological along just one dimension of experience (e.g., loudness). In his system, the psychophysical dissimilarity between two sensations is the cumulative number of jnds that separate two physical quantities. One can sum the jnds either by using the logarithmic function, or else by actually measuring experimentally the jnds separating two events. A 65-dB tone might be separated from a 60-dB tone, for example, by 10 jnds. Thus, the concept of the jnd was, in essence, a model of similarity relations. It stated that these relations could be scaled into a ruler that distinguished the different psychological experiences of, say, tonal loudness. Moreover, Fechner, and later psychophysicists in this tradition, believed that (1) the jnd unit is *absolute* -- it remains the same, in principle, whenever it is measured -- and (2) the jnd unit is psychologically *constant* -- it reflects basically the same psychological experience wherever on the scale it is measured.

III. Thurstone's Law of Comparative Judgment

Fechner's model of similarity -- the concept of the jnd as described above -- was challenged in 1927 when Louis Leon Thurstone detailed an entirely different approach to the measure of psychological experiences in a brief but influential paper in *Psychological Review*. The target of Thurstone's challenge was Fechner's idea that the jnd unit is a fixed entity. Thurstone pointed out that in comparative judgment tasks -- such as Fechner's method of constant stimuli -- identical stimulus pairs will often lead to different responses. Thurstone was convinced that such response "aberrations," from the point of view of Fechner's law at least, could conceivably reflect a lawful process of similarity. According to Thurstone, presenting an observer with a stimulus activates one value along a psychological continuum. As shown in Figure 6.2, Thurstone presumed that the values were distributed normally on the continuum. The experience of each value is created through what Thurstone dubbed the *discriminal process*. So, for example, presenting a sound activates a value on a loudness continuum. On different occasions this same sound will yield different discriminal processes, that is, different loudness values; but the probability that a particular value is activated corresponds to expectations derived from the normal distribution. Consequently, the psychological value most likely to be experienced corresponds to the mode of the distribution, or what Thurstone called the *modal discriminal process*. The difference between the mode and some other value from the normal distribution, the latter experienced each time the stimulus is repeated, is called the *discriminal dispersion*. This difference corresponds to the standard deviation of the normal distribution.

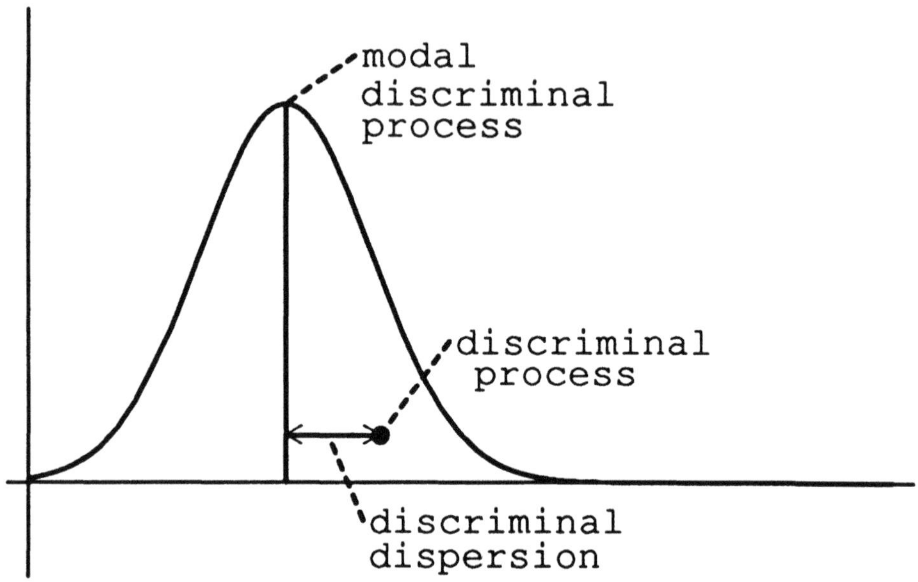

Figure 6.2: Representation of a value created along a psychological dimension through the activity of a discriminal process, as hypothesized by Thurstone (1927). A set of such processes forms a normal distribution whose central tendency is called the modal discriminal process, and whose standard deviation is called the discriminal dispersion.

Thurstone's *Law of Comparative Judgment* is based on the *discriminal differences* that result when subjects compare one stimulus with another. A discriminal difference is a distance-based measure of dissimilarity, corresponding to the separation along the psychological scale between the discriminal processes associated with each stimulus presented. Thus, if a subject was asked to judge the louder of two sounds, X and Y, each sound would give rise to a discriminal process along a psychological scale, x and y, respectively, as shown in the top two panels of Figure 6.3. x and y are normal deviates -- that is, they correspond to values sampled from a normal distribution -- and so they vary from trial to trial in accordance with that probability distribution. The difference between x and y on any given trial is the discriminal difference. Over many trials, a distribution of

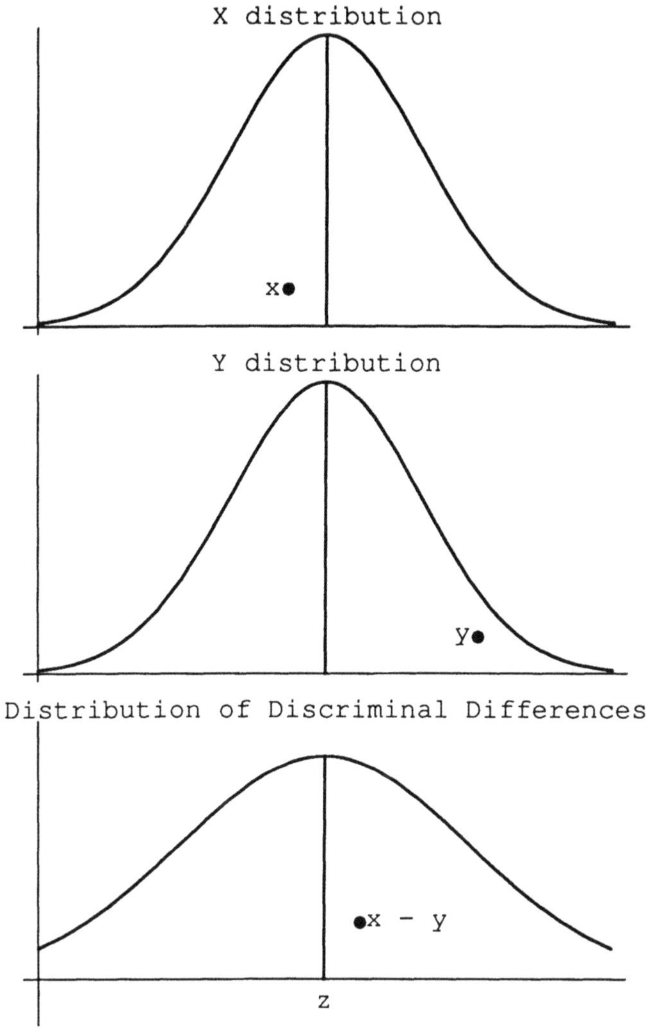

Figure 6.3: Graphic representation of a discriminal difference. The top two panels are discriminal processes x (first panel) and y (second panel), corresponding to Stimuli X and Y, respectively. The bottom panel represents a distribution of discriminal differences between X and Y, having a mean of z, and twice the dispersion of X and Y.

discriminal differences is formed, which has a mean of z, as illustrated in the bottom panel of Figure 6.3. The Law of Comparative Judgment, then, states that when subjects judge the dissimilarity between X and Y,

$$x - y = z\sqrt{\sigma_x^2 + \sigma_y^2 - 2r\sigma_x\sigma_y} \quad , \qquad (4)$$

where z is the mean discriminal difference expressed in standard score form, σ_x (σ_y) is the discriminal dispersion associated with X (Y), and r is the correlation between the X and Y discriminal dispersions.

Unfortunately, the Law of Comparative Judgment cannot be solved in the form given above because it will always yield more unknowns than equations. To deal with this, Thurstone proposed a number of restrictive situations, which he called "Cases," that would permit the law to be usable in practice. For example, in the simplest Case, Thurstone's Case V, he assumed that the discriminal dispersions for different distributions were equal ($\sigma_x = \sigma_y$), and that there was no correlation between dispersions ($r = 0$). Here, the Law of Comparative Judgment reduces to

$$x - y = z\sigma\sqrt{2} \quad , \qquad (5)$$

where the dispersion, σ, is a constant.

Thurstone's law is important for students of similarity because it conceptualizes similarity relations as fundamentally probabilistic. At the least, the law permits one to evaluate Fechner's assumption that units of dissimilarity (i.e., summed jnds) remain constant psychologically. Thurstone believed that the variability in judgments that classical psychophysicists attributed to measurement error was actually an intrinsic part of the judgment process. The full impact of Thurstone's ideas were only realized several decades later when the theory of signal detectability (Green & Swets, 1966) was developed. Nonetheless, two aspects of Thurstone's approach, which themselves were borrowed from Fechner, strongly influenced the next development in the study of similarity, namely, *multidimensional scaling:* (1) that similarity relations are scale-able values and, as such, can be conceptualized as distances in a psychological space, and (2) that it is best to measure similarity relations indirectly, using variations of the method of constant stimuli, by asking subjects to compare psychological magnitudes between (or among) pairs (or triads) of stimuli.

IV. Multidimensional Scaling

Both the classical approach to psychophysics, epitomized by Fechner, and the Thurstonian approach, examined the psychological properties of a single dimension of experience. The goal of developing psychophysical scales -- defined technically as psychological rulers that meet the central axioms of measurement theory (see Krantz, Luce, Suppes, & Tversky, 1971; Suppes, Krantz, Luce, & Tversky, 1989) -- had been confined to mapping one physical dimension (e.g., intensity) onto one psychological dimension (e.g., unidimensional *distance* between points). By mid-century, the more interesting cognitive question -- How do organisms integrate information from separate psychological dimensions? -- had been largely ignored.

A shift to this question began in 1938 when Richardson described a method to analyze judgments of "triadic combinations." Subjects were presented with three stimuli at a time and were asked which pair was most similar and which pair was most dissimilar. The technique Richardson used to analyze these data, called multidimensional scaling, was a geometric version of factor analysis. A data set having N x N dimensionality, where N is the number of stimuli being rated, was decomposed into some smaller number of "factors," where each factor was a dimension. Multidimensional scaling thus allowed an investigator to determine how many psychological dimensions subjects used when judging similarity among a set of complex stimuli. Unlike factor analysis, which has a similar goal, multidimensional scaling is inherently geometric, representing stimuli as points in a real space, and representing similarity relations as the psychological distances among the points. Thus, in its original form, the technique was a natural extension of the unidimensional approach to similarity espoused by Fechner and then Thurstone.

The popularity of multidimensional scaling did not begin in earnest until the 1950's with the publication of a landmark paper by Attneave, which I describe later in detail, and with the publication of Warren Torgerson's book in 1958, Theory and Methods of Scaling. In the book, Torgerson detailed the quantitative properties of multidimensional scaling. To obtain similarity judgments, he advocated the "method of triads," an extension of Richardson's triadic combinations, where subjects determine whether Stimulus A of the triad is more similar to Stimulus B or C. Like Fechner's indirect methods of scaling, this procedure yields proportions: How often, for example, is Stimulus A judged more similar to B than C? The first step in multidimensional scaling is to transform these judgments into distances. Torgerson assumed that the judgment data were scaled by subjects at an interval or ratio level of measurement. To obtain distances, Torgerson transformed the original data using a normal distribution function:

$$ {}_{A}p_{BC} = \int_{-\infty}^{d_{AB}-d_{AC}} \frac{1}{\sqrt{2\pi}} e^{-\frac{1}{2}x^2} dx \quad , \qquad (6) $$

where ${}_{A}p_{BC}$ is the proportion of times Stimulus A was judged more similar to Stimulus B than Stimulus C, and d_{AB} is the distance from Stimulus A to Stimulus B.

Knowing distances, however, is not the same as knowing values on a scale. In multidimensional scaling, scale values are equivalent to the projections of points in the space onto a set of reference axes. The problem for techniques of multidimensional scaling, then, is to determine scale values from knowledge of distances. The problem contains three parts: (1) determining whether the points can be represented in a (Euclidean) space; (2) determining the minimum number of dimensions in that space; (3) determining the projections on axes in the space. All of these issues were solved in an important paper by Young and Householder (1938). They showed that by constructing a symmetric matrix B, whose elements,

b_{YZ}, are the scalar product of vectors from arbitrary origin X to points Y and Z,

$$b_{YZ} = \frac{1}{2}(d_{XY}^2 + d_{XZ}^2 + d_{YZ}^2) \quad , \tag{7}$$

one could (1) identify the space as real and Euclidean by obtaining only positive (or zero) eigenvalues; (2) determine the dimensionality of the space from the rank of the matrix; (3) determine projections onto an arbitrary set of axes by factoring matrix B into a matrix A of spatial coordinates. As in factor analysis, the orientation of the axes in Euclidean space could be rotated to enhance psychological meaningfulness.

Multidimensional scaling, at least in its earliest versions, was thus a two-stage process, where the first stage transformed interval- or ratio-level similarity data into distances, and the second stage used the Young-Householder procedure to determine the location of points in a space having a minimum number of dimensions. Unlike the Thurstone model, many early versions of multidimensional scaling considered each point as fixed in space (but see Richardson, 1938). In this sense, the early models maintained a classical psychophysics approach to the problem of similarity relations.

The attractiveness of multidimensional scaling to psychologists derived not from its power as a data reduction device, but from the presumed properties of the space formed by the dimensions it extracted. Two fundamental characteristics are associated with this space: (1) it serves as a psychological model and (2) it is metric. As a model, psychological similarity is captured in the spatial relations among stimuli, with each stimulus occupying a point in that space and each axis reflecting a potential dimension of comparison. Multidimensional scaling provided an intuitive way to conceptualize similarity relations: Two stimuli are similar psychologically if they share a circumscribed region of the similarity space.

The conception alone would have been less valuable perhaps had it not been accompanied by powerful mathematical properties. The assumption is made that similarity ratings have their origin in a space that inheres metric properties. A metric is a scale that assigns a distance to any pair of points such that three conditions are satisfied (Beals, Krantz, & Tversky, 1968):

1. *Symmetry*: the distance between two points does not depend on order; the distance from X to Y is the same as from Y to X.
2. *Positivity*: distances can never be negative. The distance between a point and itself is zero; the distance between any two distinct points is always positive.
3. *Triangle Inequality*: the sum of distances among three points (X to Y plus Y to Z) can never be less than that between any two of the points (X to Z).

By satisfying these three conditions, called the *metric axioms*, in the context of a model of similarity, excitement lay in the hope that one could understand formally the nature of a psychological event. Of course, this hope harks back to the earliest days of psychophysics, in which the goal was to identify a valid and precise psychological ruler based on knowledge of physical properties of the stimulus. Just as the summed jnds served for Fechner as a measure of psychological "distance" in one dimension, so did multidimensional scaling promise to model dissimilarity as distance among experiences comprised of multiple dimensions of change. The best example of a psychologist who exploited these mathematical properties was Attneave (1950), whose work I describe next.

V. Attneave's Seminal Paper

Multiple dimensions raises a central psychological issue never faced by Fechner. One is forced to identify the nature of distance between two points in the space. In other words, what rule do subjects use to combine psychological discrepancies along each of the dimensions? This problem was addressed early on by Attneave (1950) in a very influential paper. Here he explored humans' emphasis on the *dimensions* of experience when making judgments of similarity. In the course of experiencing their world, humans discern colors, shapes, sizes, pitches, loudnesses, and a host of other psychological dimensions. The dimensional approach to complex stimuli is one long emphasized in psychology, especially by Boring and Titchener (see Boring, 1933). Attneave recognized that to combine a set of separate dimensions into our usual full and coherent perception of the environment, we can choose from an infinite variety of geometries (i.e., combination rules). Attneave thought it reasonable to restrict his analysis, however, to two kinds of rules (called metrics) found in the Minkowski family of geometries. The first kind, the Euclidean metric, is the basis of the usual layperson definition of distance: Points X and Y can be identified as corners of a right triangle, with the distance between them as the hypotenuse of the triangle as given by the Pythagorean theorem,

$$d = \sqrt{A^2 + B^2} \ , \tag{8}$$

where A and B refer to the lengths of the triangle's perpendicular sides. Attneave remarked that if psychological distances are Euclidean in nature it implies that humans attach little importance to the underlying dimensions -- that is, to the orientation of the reference axes in the space -- because, unlike most geometries,

Euclidean distance is invariant to rotation of axes. In other words, the hypotenuse (i.e., the distance between X and Y) remains the same no matter what reference axes are used to create the right triangle (i.e., despite changes in the lengths A and B). Thus, "within a space of given dimensionality, one set of axes or one frame of reference is as good as any other" (p. 521).

Attneave contrasted this metric to the Householder-Landahl metric, in which distance between two stimuli is the sum of the separations between stimuli along each of the component dimensions in the space. Thus, in a two-dimensional space,

$$d = A + B \quad . \tag{9}$$

This metric is commonly referred to as the "city-block" or "Manhattan" metric, because distance is covered in the same way that one navigates between two points in Manhattan: up an avenue and across a street. Like most metrics, but unlike the Euclidean metric, the city-block rule emphasizes the underlying psychological dimensions when computing distance. In other words, city-block distance is not invariant: The city-block distance between points X and Y depends on what reference axes are used to create the right triangle because A and B, and thus their sum, change with the reference axes. Thus, as a model of psychological similarity, it states that perceivers are aware of and take into account the psychological dimensions that compose complex stimuli.

Attneave asked subjects to judge similarity among different sets of simple stimuli, including parallelograms varying in size and tilt, squares varying in size and brightness, and triangles varying in base and altitude. In each case, the raw similarity ratings were considered distances, which were used to locate the stimuli in a two-dimensional space. To regard ratings as distances in a Minkowski space, the ratings must meet the distance axioms. In addition to satisfying the three general axioms, all Minkowski geometries must also satisfy the axiom of *segmental additivity* (Beals, Krantz, & Tversky, 1968): Given three points on a line, X, Y, and Z, with X and Z as end points, the distance between end points must equal the sum of the segments (X to Y and Y to Z). Attneave found, however, that ratings from his subjects were consistently sub-additive: The distance from X to Z was greater than the sum of X to Y and Y to Z. Because of this, Attneave decided to subtract an additive constant from each of the ratings in order that he "might obtain quantities which would display, at least over a considerable range, the properties of distance" (p.524).

When comparing the two different combination rules, Euclidean and city-block, Attneave found that the city-block metric provided much better fits to his observed dissimilarities. This result suggested that underlying dimensions may serve as unique reference systems, and so cannot be rotated in space without psychological consequences. As we shall see, Attneave's restriction to the Minkowski family, specifically his comparison of the Euclidean metric with the city-block metric, was to influence profoundly the future study of similarity relations.

Attneave also found that stimulus dissimilarity was well predicted by the difference between physical values transformed logarithmically. This nonlinear relationship implicates Fechner's law, and Attneave recognized this. But several later experiments in his study yielded another, more interesting nonlinear relationship. In these experiments, Attneave used an *absolute identification* procedure; he trained subjects to associate a three-letter word to each of the stimuli. The errors in training served as his measure of similarity. In other words, subjects often confused the name of one stimulus with another's, presumably because the stimuli were perceived as similar. Attneave examined how these confusions related to the judged distance separating stimuli. His results are depicted in Figure 6.4. As one can see, a nonlinear relationship obtained that, in some sense, is not unlike Fechner's function. Attneave called relations like these "second-order Weber-Fechner functions." He also acknowledged the link between his functions and those obtained by Hull's student Hovland in the context of conditioned responses, research that we will describe later. The importance of these nonlinear functions lies in the fact that stimulus confusability diminishes appreciably as one changes the stimulus pair from identical to nonidentical. At larger distances, however, confusability changes much less with changes in stimulus difference. As we shall see, modern theorists have made much of this relation.

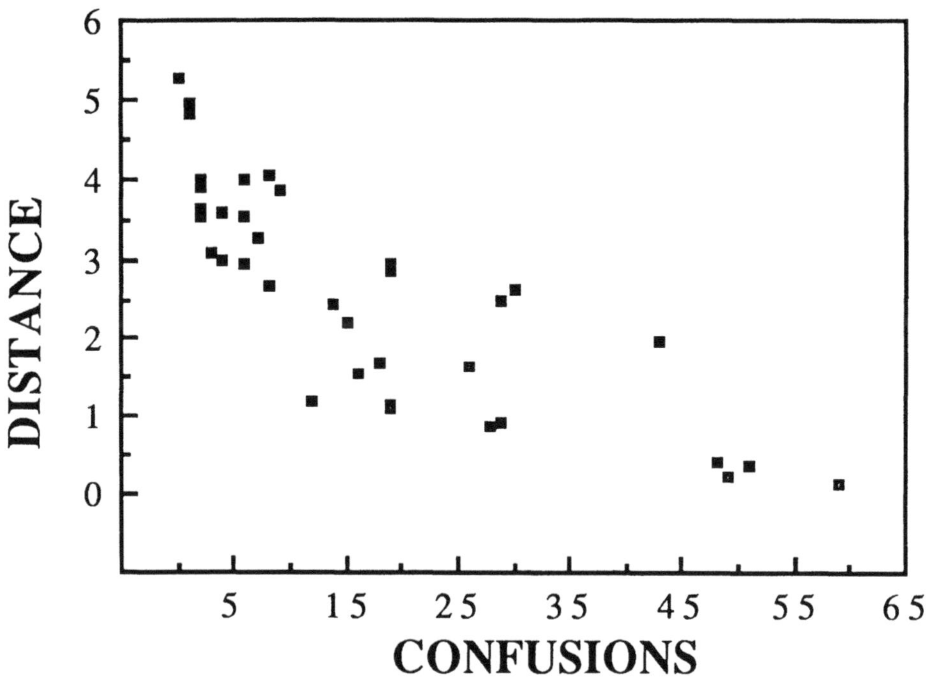

Figure 6.4: Decreasing decay relation between distance and confusability among simple geometric stimuli from data reported by Attneave (1950).

Attneave noted that nonlinearity will seem more or less pronounced depending upon the *weight* subjects attach to the component dimensions of a multidimensional stimulus. Indeed, he found that the weight assigned to a dimension can change as a function of the kind of judgment subjects make. For example, Attneave's subjects assigned greater weight to area than to form when making unidimensional judgments of triangles. But area received much less weight in the context of multidimensional judgments. Moreover, these differences in weighting were more extreme in the confusion data than in the similarity data. As we shall see, the notion of differential weighting of dimensions takes on prominence in subsequent work on similarity.

Finally, Attneave recognized a serious limitation in conceiving of similarity in metric terms: It is trivial to think of examples of similarity relations that violate the metric axioms. Attneave was particularly interested in validity of the axiom of triangle inequality. The example he used came originally from William James (1890): The moon is similar to a lamp (in providing light); the moon is similar to a soccer ball (in shape); but a lamp is not similar to a soccer ball. These relations violate the triangle inequality: The distance from lamp to soccer ball is greater than the sum of distances from lamp to moon and from moon to soccer ball. Attneave suggested that many forms of similarity may not be described well by distance, at least in its formal sense. As we shall see, this criticism has become central to recent critiques of distance models of similarity.

In summary, then, this small paper published in 1950 captured most of the central themes in similarity research for the next 40 years. First, Attneave conceived of similarity among stimuli as distance in space. Second, he considered the space to be organized around psychological dimensions which he believed, in accord with his data, were oriented uniquely in space. Third, he argued that psychological spaces were likely to be either Euclidean or city-block in structure. Fourth, he found that the relationship between distance and confusions was nonlinear, such that similarity asymptotes as distance increases. Fifth, he suggested that subjects differentially weight component dimensions when making similarity judgments. Sixth, he identified problems with the spatial model, most prominent being the failure of the metric axioms, especially with non-perceptual stimuli. In what follows, I describe the important developments in the study of similarity since Attneave and how these developments were foreshadowed, in large measure, by his seminal work. I believe that Attneave's six contributions also provide important hints about where future progress in the field may be found.

VI. Interacting and Separable Dimensions

The nature of the combination rule has been central to most discussions of similarity among multidimensional stimuli. Most of this effort has been spent evaluating the two rules emphasized by Attneave, namely, Euclidean and city-block. In his 1958 book, Torgerson suggested casually that characteristics of the dimensions themselves may play a role in how perceivers combine information. After reviewing previous work on multidimensional scaling, Torgerson noted that the city-block metric appears to fit the data best when the dimensions being evaluated are "simple, obvious and compelling" to the perceiver. Thus, Attneave's success with this metric may lie in the fact that the dimensions he tested -- form, size, hue -- are easily identified and distinguished by subjects. On the other hand, dimensions tested by Torgerson that were fit best by a Euclidean space -- the saturation and brightness of color chips -- are not as distinct to most perceivers. Torgerson concluded that, as a general spatial model, subjects' behavior was described well by the generalized Minkowski equation,

$$d = [\sum_{k=1}^{N} |x_{ik} - x_{jk}|^r]^{\frac{1}{r}} \qquad r \geq 1 \ , \qquad (10)$$

where x_{ik} is the value of Stimulus i on dimension k, N is the number of dimensions of difference, and the exponent r equals 1 when the space is city-block and 2 when the space is Euclidean.

The Minkowski family of metrics, also called the power metrics, are particularly appealing as models of similarity. This is because they require segmental additivity which, in turn, is the basis of psychological maps, scales, and other multidimensional representations (Tversky & Gati, 1982). Tversky and Krantz (1970) proved that segmental additivity, when juxtaposed with certain other axioms and assumptions, dictate a Minkowski metric. Torgerson believed that in many experimental situations, the best-fitting Minkowski metric will fall between city block ($r = 1$) and Euclidean ($r = 2$).

More than any other investigator, it was Garner (1974) who picked up on Torgerson's comment, and attempted to understand more fully how different pairs of dimensions lead to different combination rules (see also Shepard, 1964, 1987). Garner argued that certain pairs of psychological dimensions, which he called "integral" or "interacting" dimensions, are combined immediately and effortlessly by perceptual systems. Saturation and brightness of colors was Garner's favorite example of such dimensions; pitch and loudness exemplify auditory interacting dimensions. He argued that perceptual integration of interacting dimensions was so powerful that perceivers cannot even distinguish the two dimensions, at least initially. Conversely, Garner argued that other pairs of psychological dimensions, which he called "separable" dimensions, are processed independently by perceptual systems, and are therefore easily distinguished by perceivers. Attneave's dimensions, such as size and color, exemplify a separable pair of dimensions.

Garner discovered that interacting pairs could be distinguished empirically from separable pairs through a set of "converging operations" (Garner, Hake, & Eriksen, 1956): procedures that yield one pattern of results when interacting dimensions are tested, and a different pattern of results when separable dimensions are tested. One member of Garner's set asked what combination rule obtains in multidimensional scaling. Garner argued persuasively that existing studies of scaling dictate the city-block metric for separable dimensions and the

Euclidean metric for interacting dimensions (e.g., Handel & Imai, 1972; Hyman & Well, 1967, 1968; Indow & Kanazawa, 1960; Melara, 1989b; Torgerson, 1958).

The distinction between separable and interacting was bolstered by a second member of Garner's set: the pattern of choice reaction times (and accuracies) that obtain when either two interacting or two separable dimensions are paired (e.g., Garner & Felfoldy, 1970; Melara, 1989a). With separable dimensions, speeded performance to one dimension is unaffected by changes in the other dimension. However, with interacting dimensions, speed to classify one dimension depends greatly on how the other dimension is varied; subjects respond relatively fast when relevant and irrelevant dimensions are correlated across trials. But subjects respond relatively slow when two interacting dimensions are varied orthogonally, a phenomenon that was later dubbed *Garner interference* (Pomerantz, 1983, 1986). Garner (1974) mentioned several other operations that identify two dimensions as either interacting or separable. The important point is that a conceptual distinction noticed first in similarity relations could be generalized to a cadre of information-processing tasks.

Although Garner's analysis led to a new understanding of how humans organize multidimensional experiences -- these certainly being the most common kinds of experiences -- it also caused new problems and anomalies. Let us examine a problem that has been recognized only recently. If one considers strictly the geometric relations obtained in multidimensional scaling of separable dimensions, on the one hand, or interacting dimensions, on the other, then one accepts a particular model about how perceptual systems integrate information. Take Euclidean-defined space as a model of interacting dimensions. This metric implies that, perceptually, no dimensions in the similarity space are unique psychologically or, stated another way, that any reference axes in the space are as real psychologically as any other. In fact, Garner and his colleagues have actually maintained an even stronger position, namely, that two integral dimensions are not distinguished at all in early perception (see Garner, 1974, p. 119; Lockhead, 1972, 1979). Clearly, this stronger view emphasizes the connotative sense of "integral." What is not recognized explicitly by these authors is that the strong view implies a unidimensional, rather than a Euclidean, psychological space. For our purposes, it is sufficient to focus on the Euclidean model per se.

The central premise of this model -- that interacting dimensions correspond to arbitrary axes in Euclidean space -- has not stood up well to empirical scrutiny. Marks and I (Melara & Marks, 1990), for example, evaluated the model with the auditory interacting dimensions of pitch and loudness (see also Grau & Kemler-Nelson, 1988). We had subjects classify stimulus sets constructed according to axes oriented in one of three ways in psychological space, as depicted in Panel A of Figure 6.5. If axes are indeed arbitrary for such dimensions, classification performance should not vary by orientation. In contrast to this hypothesis, we found, as shown in Panel B, that performance was greatly affected by orientation of axes: Subjects performed best (i.e., suffered the least Garner interference) when the reference axes corresponded to pitch and loudness, and performed worse the farther axes were rotated away from that orientation. These results suggest that Euclidean models of similarity, at least in their strictest sense, are inappropriate for understanding how perceivers combine information from separate dimensions. Below I review other, more general arguments against spatial models.

VII. Shepard's Contributions

Shepard, in a series of papers in the late 1950's and early 1960's, extended in important ways the research on similarity relations begun by his predecessors. Particularly noteworthy are three of his contributions. First, Shepard, in concert with the earlier work of Hull, hypothesized that psychological distance relates to

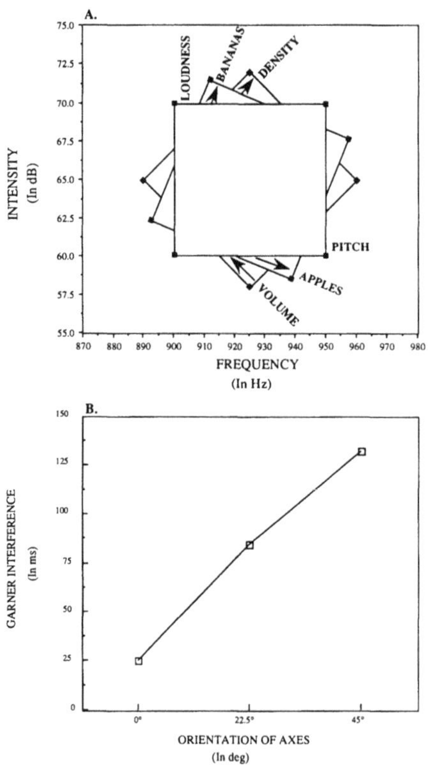

Figure 6.5: Panel A: Representation of three stimulus sets used in auditory classification experiment of Melara and Marks (1990), each created from one of three different orientations of frequency-intensity axes: 0° (pitch loudness), 22.5° (apples-bananas), and 45° (volume-density). The direction toward the positive pole of each dimension is specified by arrow. Panel B: Garner interference (mean difference between selective attention and baseline performance in milliseconds) at each of three orientations of frequency-intensity axes (0°, 22.5°, 45°).

degree of judged or experienced dissimilarity by a particular nonlinear function, no matter what the dimension being tested. Second, extending the work of Torgerson (1958) and Coombs (1964), Shepard showed that the scale of measurement for similarity judgments need not reach interval level to derive spatial relations. Indeed, such distances are possible even when extremely weak assumptions are made about the original judgment data. Third, Shepard suggested that changes in spatial relations may be attributable to how subjects attend to each of the component dimensions. He argued, in fact, that attentional processes could alter the best-fitting metric of the similarity space. I review each of Shepard's contributions in turn.

Contribution #1: The Exponential Decay Function

In 1943, Clark Hull published his monumental Principles of Behavior where he introduced an innovative mathematical approach to the study of how animals learn. Among the various learning phenomena that Hull addressed in this book was stimulus generalization, brought to the attention of experimental psychologists by Pavlov (1927). Pavlov showed that behaviors elicited by one stimulus can also be elicited (will generalize to) other, physically similar stimuli. Thus, a dog conditioned to a 1000 Hz tone may, following learning, also salivate to a 990 Hz or 1010 Hz tone.

Hull reviewed the dissertation results of his student Hovland (1937a, 1937b) on the conditioning of the human galvanic skin response to sounds varying in pitch or in loudness. Hull reasoned that the degree of generalization experienced by Hovland's subjects was some decreasing function of the psychological difference from the conditioned stimulus. As his measure of psychological difference, Hull used a Fechnerian measure, namely, the number of jnd units separating the conditioned stimulus from the test stimulus. He then re-examined

Hovland's data, plotting this independent variable against degree of generalization. Figure 6.6 depicts the results for test stimuli varying in pitch. Not surprisingly, the more jnds separating the test stimulus from the conditioned stimulus, the less the stimulus generalized (i.e., the smaller the galvanic skin response). Most important, Figure 6.6 makes clear that the relationship between psychological difference and generalization is nonlinear, not unlike the function reported by Attneave (1950; see Figure 6.4): Loss in generalization was greatest to test stimuli most similar to the conditioned stimulus. Hull hypothesized that generalization and similarity are related by negative growth: an exponential decay function.

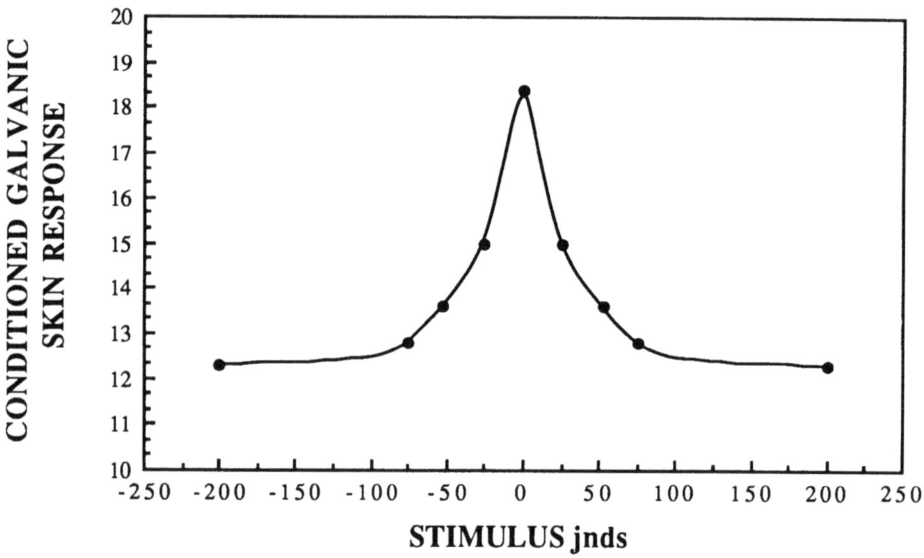

<u>Figure 6.6:</u> Decreasing decay relation between generalization of conditioned responses (i.e., galvanic skin response conditioned to tones of varied pitch) and number of jnds from the point of conditioning (represented on the abscissa), adapted from Hull's (1943) re-analysis of Hovland's (1937a) original data.

Shepard (1957) began his analysis by considering generalization in absolute identification situations, like Attneave's, where subjects associate a specific response to each member of a set of stimuli. One can construct stimulus generalization gradients by plotting the relative frequency with which a given stimulus receives each possible response. These frequencies translate directly into confusion probabilities, and Shepard was interested in how these probabilities can be transformed into distances in a metric psychological space. Shepard, like Hull before him, assumed a negative exponential transformation function.

Shepard's rationale for using the exponential function has evolved over the years. In his 1957 paper, Shepard argued that the exponential function derives naturally once assuming that the transformation is differentiable. The assumption implies that straight lines in physical space are transformed into smooth curves in psychological space. Thus, with extremely small psychological distances on one dimension, segments form a straight line, and so distances are additive (i.e., segmental additivity holds). The exponential decay function is just such a differentiable function. Shepard concluded that because physical distances are additive, an exponential transformation leads to additive psychological distances. Unfortunately, Krantz (1967) discovered a logical difficulty with Shepard's analysis: If ratios of physical distance equal corresponding ratios of psychological distance, then the two types of distance must be related linearly and hence are indistinguishable, a situation that is known to be untrue (see also Gregson, 1975).

In 1958, Shepard derived the exponential function through a trace model of generalization. In this model, each stimulus presented in an absolute identification experiment creates its own internal representation or trace. With a time delay, and in the absence of a stimulus, each stimuli's trace begins to diffuse to other nearby traces along a continuum. Thus, if the continuum is one of pitch, the trace corresponding to 1000 Hz begins to diffuse over time to other adjacent frequencies along that psychophysical dimension. The diffusion is hypothesized to follow a normal distribution; thus, from a normal density function one can derive the probability that a trace corresponding to one pitch was associated inadvertently with a different pitch. Time acts to increase the variability of this normal distribution. In absolute identification, training to associate each stimulus with a specific response causes a *decrease* in the variability of each trace distribution, relative to that same distribution earlier in the experiment. As is shown in Figure 6.7, each point of time in training leads to its own normal distribution, with more variability in those distributions further in the past (i.e., earlier in training). The usual generalization gradient can therefore be viewed as the sum of normal distributions across time. This composite distribution, included in Figure 6.7, is negative exponential in form.

Recently, Shepard (1987) provided yet another defense for the exponential function. Now touted as a "Universal Law for Psychological Science", Shepard argued that an exponential function arises when organisms seek regions of psychological space that will lead to reinforcing consequences. If an organism is reinforced for responding to Stimulus X, for example, it must decide whether it will also be reinforced by responding similarly to Stimulus Y. Generalization, according to Shepard, is thus a search for the size of a "consequential region," that is, the set of stimuli represented in a region of psychological space that lead to similar reinforcing outcomes. Shepard discovered that the conditional probability that Stimulus Y comes from the consequential region that led to reinforcement from Stimulus X is closely approximated by the negative exponential (see also Shepard, 1986; cf. Ennis, 1988).

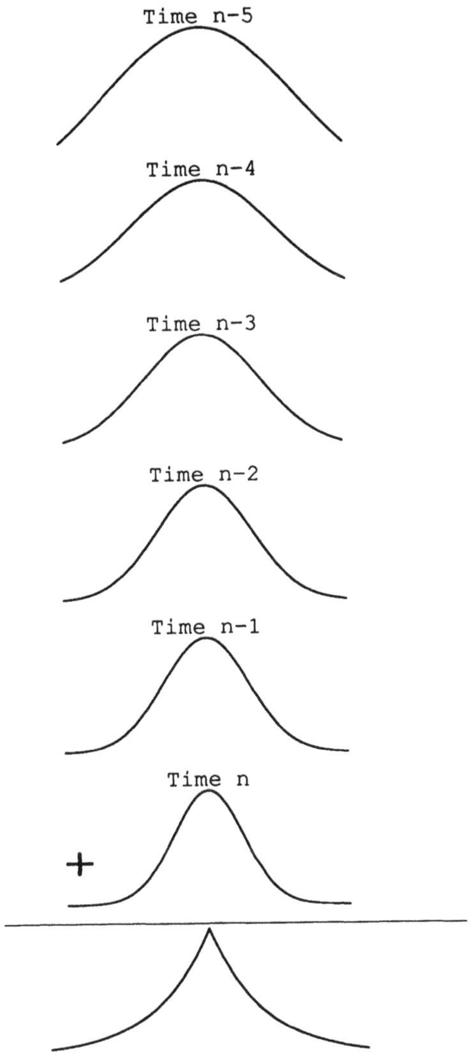

Figure 6.7: Representation of Shepard's (1958a,b) trace model of generalization with each distribution representing a particular point in absolute identification training. Over the course of training, with the trace for each of several points in time represented by a normal distribution, trace variance is proposed to decrease. Shepard described the entire course of training as the integration (represented by plus sign) of individual trace distributions, that composite distribution being negative exponential in form, as shown in the bottom panel of the figure.

The Exponential Function Reconsidered: Confusability Versus Intradimensional Similarity

One might observe that Shepard's explanations speak more to the psychology of creativity than to the psychology of similarity relations. Theoretical originality notwithstanding, Shepard has provided compelling empirical support for the notion that, independent of the stimulus domain being tested, a decreasing decay function relates psychological distance to degree of generalization or confusability. Importantly, such a general relationship probably does *not* exist between distance and a construct that I shall refer to as *intradimensional similarity*. I define the latter as the phenomenal similarities that exist among values on a single dimension of experience. For convenience, I shall assume that similarity judged directly (e.g., by rating techniques) comes closest to being a strict measure of this construct, although these conventional judgments may be influenced by non-perceptual effects of context (e.g., Anderson, 1975; Birnbaum, 1974; Birnbaum, Parducci, & Gifford, 1971; Parducci, 1965). My claims here are (1) that intradimensional similarity is not the same as confusability and (2) that, consistent with suggestions from previous research (e.g., Indow, 1988; see also Shepard, 1962a), intradimensional similarity is related to distance *linearly*, not curvilinearly. I shall defend these claims now, and use them at the end of the chapter to inform a new approach to the study of similarity.

The claim that there is a difference between confusability in absolute identification and similarity judged directly is hardly surprising. In the former, one measures how often a subject confuses a reference stimulus with each of several test stimuli. Within a limited range of stimuli, such confusions are probably due largely to intradimensional similarity: The more phenomenally similar a test stimulus is to the referent, the more likely the two stimuli are to be confused. But, beyond that range, as the generalization gradient flattens, subjects experience the same minimal number of confusions to many different stimuli. Reference Stimulus

A, for example, may not be confused any more with Test Stimulus Z than with Test Stimuli W, X, or Y. When rating stimulus similarity, on the other hand, Reference Stimulus A may be judged as more similar to W, X, and Y than to Z, despite equal confusability in absolute identification. It is conceivable that rated dissimilarity becomes progressively smaller at greater distances from the reference stimulus, although, to the best of my knowledge, this function has not been studied systematically (but see Shepard, 1962a, p.127). Nonetheless, the function relating dissimilarity to distance is almost certainly unlike that obtained in generalization experiments. Thus, it seems clear that confusability is conceptually distinct from intradimensional similarity, especially when the range of stimuli is great.

Unfortunately, as we shall see, many modern theories of similarity (e.g., Ashby & Perrin, 1988; Nosofsky, 1991; Smith, 1989) treat these two concepts synonymously, either implicitly or explicitly. In my view, the terms confusability and intradimensional similarity need to be kept separate. Confusability is a performance measure; a subject is attempting to avoid interference from incorrect items when performing an identification or categorization task. Intradimensional similarity, on the other hand, is a phenomenal measure; a subject gauges his or her subjective experience of how one item relates to another. It seems clear that, for some selected range between a reference item and a test item in a set, similarity determines confusability: The more similar the two items, the more likely they are to be confused. At some point, however, the similarity of a reference item to a test item no longer determines the confusability between the items simply because, outside the limited range, confusability is minimal. Thus, confusability is some nonlinear function of similarity,

$$C_{ij} = e^{s_{ij}^{\alpha}} \quad , \qquad (11)$$

where C_{ij} is the confusability of Stimulus i with Stimulus j, S_{ij} is their intradimensional similarity, and α determines a family of nonlinear functions, with $\alpha = 1$ being the Hull-Shepard function (cf. Ennis, Palen, & Mullen, 1988). In addition, confusability, as measured in absolute identification tasks, is often affected by how stimuli are ordered in the set, fewer confusions being made to values at the extremes of a set (e.g., of line lengths) compared with middle values (see Bower, 1971; Johnson, 1975, 1991). This latter notion will need to be included in any complete account of confusability. Moreover, the right side of Equation 11 may also describe the relation between intradimensional similarity and a second performance measure of difference, namely, reaction time in a same-different paradigm (see Melara, 1989b; Podgorny & Garner, 1979).

In similarity rating experiments, subjects are typically introduced to the entire range of stimuli that they will be asked to rate, and are encouraged to spread out their ratings along the entire range of the rating scale. Perhaps owing to these procedural traditions, the evidence suggests that distance in multidimensional space is, for a large range of stimuli in the set, some linear function of judged similarity:

$$d_{ij} = a + b\, D_{ij} \quad , \qquad (12)$$

where d_{ij} is the scale distance between Stimulus i and Stimulus j, D_{ij} is their intradimensional dissimilarity measured by direct judgments, $D_{ij} = -S_{ij}$, a is the intercept and b is a positive slope. This relationship implies that confusability and distance are related non-linearly:

$$C_{ij} = e^{\left(\frac{a-d_{ij}}{b}\right)^{\alpha}} \quad . \qquad (13)$$

Although many different measures of judged similarity will probably relate linearly to distance, similarity judgments may, as a general rule, be influenced easily by context effects such as the range and frequency of stimuli (e.g., Anderson, 1975; Birnbaum, 1974; Parducci, 1965). Nonetheless, it seems valuable to search for a measure of intradimensional similarity that is as free as possible from effects of context. Greater independence from context might be claimed to characterize many performance measures (e.g., absolute identification), because subjects are motivated to avoid errors in performance no matter what stimulus set is tested. Unfortunately, context effects have been reported with these measures (e.g., Gravetter & Lockhead, 1973). Moreover, as I have argued, the range of intradimensional similarity measured by these instruments is severely limited. At the end of this chapter, I shall discuss how a context-free measure of intradimensional similarity might be used to understand similarity relations among multidimensional stimuli.

Contribution #2: Non-Metric Multidimensional Scaling

One of the advantages of multidimensional scaling is that different dependent variables that all purport to measure some aspect of similarity relations -- be they similarity ratings, generalized conditioned responses, absolute identification confusions, or same-different reaction times -- can be addressed in the common terms of scaled distance. Unfortunately, these different *proximity measures* may not all operate at the same level of measurement: some may be ratio-level measures, but most are at an ordinal or, at best interval level of measurement. And, importantly, early techniques of multidimensional scaling assumed that the original data matrix reflected interval level or better measurements. Thus, many of the more interesting analyses that use multidimensional scaling would apparently violate this basic measurement assumption.

It is with respect to this problem that Shepard made his second contribution to the study of similarity. Shepard (1962a, 1962b) discovered that one could recover metric (i.e., distance) properties in a set of similarity data from non-metric (i.e., ordinal) properties of the data. The problem Shepard addressed is that of the so-called "distance function." The distance function is that transformation in multidimensional scaling that changes the proximity measure into a distance measure. To accomplish this, earlier techniques exploited the assumed metric properties of the data; hence, the transformation -- be it linear (Indow, 1988), logarithmic (Shepard, 1958a,b), or Gaussian (Torgerson, 1958) -- assumed that proximities could be assigned uniquely to another scale (i.e., one of distance) up to multiplication and addition by a constant, what are called the "affine" group of transformations (Krantz, Luce, Suppes, & Tversky, 1971). This metric assumption is strong, and Shepard's success resides in his efforts to weaken it.

Shepard claimed that distances could be recovered through a function that depended only on rank order relations in the original data. In other words, the proximities need only be related monotonically to distances: As dissimilarities increase, so should distances. Shepard designed a computer program to perform this "analysis of proximities," which was later improved by Kruskal (1964a, 1964b). The program basically discovers which monotonic transformation from proximities to distances minimizes the number of dimensions needed to describe the original set of data. Kruskal's improvements on Shepard's approach include an explicitly defined loss function -- that is, a measure of fit between the data and the spatial solution -- and a general procedure, namely, gradient descent, for minimizing the loss (see also Shepard, 1974). In any case, the simple requirements of Shepard's approach -- identifying a monotonic distance function and achieving minimum dimensionality -- were sufficient to yield unique and quantitative (i.e., metric) solutions in multidimensional scaling.

Problems with Spatial Models

Nonmetric scaling provided a workable way to analyze diverse kinds of proximity data with a single technique. Yet the technique for achieving this goal -- transforming the data matrix monotonically -- has not gone without criticism. Schönemann and his colleagues (Schönemann, 1990, Schönemann, Dorcey, & Kienapple, 1985; Schönemann & Lazarte, 1987) have argued forcefully that such transformations cannot be justified psychologically and that, in any case, transformations disrupt important similarity relations present in the original data:

> ... we should not lose sight of the fact that the intervening monotone transformations are completely ad hoc, psychologically unexplained, and a priori unknown. Their sole purpose is to enhance the appearance of a good fit. In invoking monotone transformations, the investigator voluntarily and often quite unnecessarily restricts his range of admissible inferences severely, because, strictly speaking, any claims about the fit would always have to be qualified with a reference to this large class of transformations: instead of speaking of a "best fit with the city-block metric," it would be more appropriate to speak of a "best fit of the city-block metric cum unexplained ad hoc monotone transformation" (Schönemann, Dorcey, & Kienapple, 1985, p.5).

Schönemann also claims that, generally speaking, similarity relations obtained through multidimensional scaling (metric or nonmetric) often violate the metric axioms that they must satisfy to be Minkowski spatial models. In particular, Schönemann finds evidence for violations of segmental additivity, that is, the requirement that a line in space is comprised of segments that can be added together. His research indicates that the sum of the segments of the line are typically longer than the line itself, a phenomenon he calls "sub-additive concatenation." As an example, a subject might be asked to judge the similarity between equi-pitched sounds taken in pairs: a 50 dB sound versus a 60 dB sound, a 60 dB sound versus a 70 dB sound, and a 50 dB versus a 70 dB sound. According to the segmental additivity axiom satisfied by Minkowski metrics, the distances between the first two pairs should sum to equal the distance between the last pair. Schönemann argues, however, that the first two pairs consistently sum to a distance greater than that of the last pair. On this basis, he claims that all members of the Minkowski family of metrics are inappropriate models of similarity.

Tversky and his colleagues (Tversky, 1977; Tversky & Gati, 1978, 1982) have made an even more extreme claim, namely, that *no* spatial models are adequate for similarity data. Their claim rests mainly on the assertion that similarity data violate the axiom of triangle inequality, which must be satisfied by all distance metrics, irrespective of the particular family of geometries. To remind, the triangle inequality axiom states that the distance between two points via an indirect path (X to Y to Z) must be at least as long as the distance between points via a direct path (X to Z). Tversky contends that, with proximity data, distance along the indirect path is consistently *shorter* than that along the direct path. The reader will recall that Attneave (1950) raised this same point earlier: The distance from lamp to soccer ball is probably much greater than the distances from lamp to moon and from moon to soccer ball.

To deal with this problem, Tversky recommends dispensing with geometric models as explanations of psychological similarity. In their place, Tversky (1977) proposed a set theory of similarity, an elaborated version of the theory offered by Restle (1961). According to Tversky's version, which he calls the *contrast theory*, similarity between two objects, x and y, is a function of the attributes shared by x and y, minus functions of the attributes distinctive to x or y. In formal terms,

$$S(x,y) = \theta f(x \cap y) - [\alpha f(x - y) + \beta f(y - x)] \qquad \alpha,\beta,\theta \geq 0 \,, \tag{14}$$

where S is similarity, x and y are sets of attributes corresponding to the objects being compared, α, β, and θ weight the importance of commonality or distinctiveness, and f refers to a nonnegative scale. By treating each object as a set of constituent features, Tversky's model can accommodate the traditional scaling approach to similarity by assuming that a dimension is represented in either of two ways, intensively (prothetic) or qualitatively (metathetic). Intensive dimensions, like loudness, are represented by nested sets: Louder sounds, for example, include all the features of softer sounds, the latter set being embedded in the former set. Qualitative dimensions, like pitch, are represented by chained sets: A higher pitched sound may share properties of a lower pitched sound, but may also have its own distinctive properties. Graphic depictions of nested and chained sets are given in Figure 6.8.

Figure 6.8: Examples of nested and chained sets, used in Tversky's (1977) contrast model to represent prothetic and metathetic continua, respectively.

Contrast theory is a powerful alternative to geometric models, dramatizing possible causes of violations to assumptions of those models. To explain violations of the triangle inequality, for example, consider the triangle shown in Panel A of Figure 6.9. Each point has two letters, and each letter represents a set, as represented in Panel B. The first letters -- here a, b, and c -- are three intersecting sets, as are the last three letters -- x, y, and z. According to the triangle inequality axiom, the indirect path -- ax to cx to cz -- must be at least as long as the direct path -- ax to by to cz. However, according to Tversky's contrast theory, this need not be true. Points corresponding to the indirect path may share sets: Points ax to cx along the indirect path have set x in common; points cx to cz have set c in common. No sets coincide along the direct path. Thus, contrast

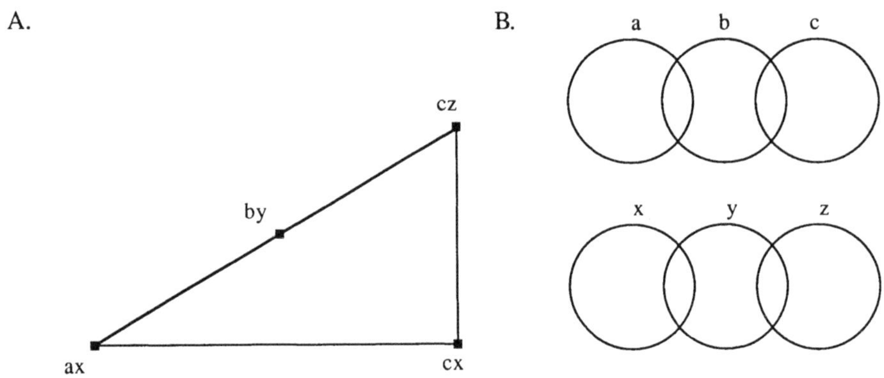

Figure 6.9: Panel A is a set-theoretic representation of the distance between points ax and cz, adapted from Tversky and Gati's (1982) study where it was used to explain violations of the triangle inequality axiom through the coincidence hypothesis. Each pair of letters represents two sets selected from two groups of three intersecting sets, as represented in Panel B.

theory predicts that dissimilarity along the indirect path should be *less* than that along the direct path. Because it is based on the coincidence of sets, Tversky and Gati (1982) call this predicted violation of the triangle inequality the *coincidence hypothesis*.

Tversky and Gati (1982) obtained good support for the coincidence hypothesis when testing simple two-dimensional stimuli in similarity rating tasks, classification tasks, and recognition tasks. Note, however, that Tversky's results present a conundrum when juxtaposed with Schönemann's. The latter claimed that the triangle inequality is typically satisfied; the problem is rather that the indirect path is *greater* than expected by this axiom. According to Schönemann, this causes a violation of the segmental additivity axiom, where segments sum to a length greater than the line they constitute. Thus, Tversky's coincidence hypothesis is opposite Schönemann's subadditive concatenation hypothesis. Both investigators report data with similar stimuli and judgment tasks that are compatible with their respective hypotheses. The reason for the discrepancies remains a mystery.

Tversky's model dispenses with some of the more problematic aspects of spatial accounts. For example, all geometric models assume symmetry: The distance from X to Y equals that from Y to X. This is not assumed in contrast theory; symmetry holds only if the distinctive features or their weights are equal. Otherwise, one would not expect symmetry in similarity. In real life, of course, asymmetries abound. As Tversky (1977) points out, for example, one says "the son resembles the father" not "the father resembles the son", indicating a fundamental asymmetry in this similarity relation.

Contrast theory also distinguishes between similarity and dissimilarity. In distance models dissimilarity is typically defined as the opposite of similarity, so that data using either measure are equivalent. Equivalence is not presumed in the contrast model. Indeed, in this model it is reasonable to suppose that subjects will place more weight on common features when judging similarity, and more weight on distinctive features when judging dissimilarity. Differential weighting makes the contrast model flexible in handling asymmetries between similarity and difference. That such asymmetries exist was shown by Tversky and Gati (1978) who asked subjects to judge countries either in terms of their similarity or dissimilarity. Subjects in the similarity group judged East Germany and West Germany to be more similar to each other than Sri Lanka and Nepal; but subjects in the dissimilarity group judged East Germany and West Germany to be more different from each other than Sri Lanka and Nepal. The contrast model accounts for these results by assuming that common features were weighted more when making similarity judgments than when making dissimilarity judgments. Later, we will see that contrast theory is limited in its ability to account for asymmetries between similarity and difference.

Krumhansl (1978) has defended geometric models by suggesting that the violations of metric axioms reported by Tversky could be explained by the different densities of psychological space. The basic idea is that, if stimuli are represented as points in space, two points from a crowded (dense) region of space will be judged less similar than two points from a relatively open region. In other words, density in space causes perceivers to make finer stimulus discriminations, leading to greater judged dissimilarity. In formal terms, Krumhansl proposes that

$$\bar{d}(x,y) = d(x,y) + \alpha\delta(x) + \beta\delta(y) \quad , \tag{15}$$

where $\bar{d}(x,y)$ is the spatial distance between points x and y, $\delta(x)$ [$\delta(y)$] measures the density of the region surrounding point x (y), and α (β) represents a weighting of x (y) density.

Krumhansl argues that although d(x,y) must satisfy the metric axioms, d(x,y) need not. In fact, Krumhansl claims that her *distance-density* model predicts certain violations of the metric axioms. Violations of the symmetry axiom -- that the distance from x to y equals that from y to x -- are expected if the local densities and density weights are unequal. In particular, Krumhansl found empirical support for the idea that the similarity of x to y is greater than the similarity of y to x if (1) $\alpha > \beta$: the subject attaches greater attentional weight to x than to y; and (2) δ(x) < δ(y): the region surrounding x is less dense than that surrounding y.

Although Krumhansl's model does predict violations of certain metric axioms, it also assumes that the triangle inequality axiom is satisfied. To deal with apparent violations in this axiom, Krumhansl contends that in any given judgment task perceivers may consider one dimension (of a multidimensional stimulus) more important than another dimension. This has the effect of altering similarity relations across judgment tasks. When comparing a lamp with the moon, the luminance dimension may be emphasized. When comparing a soccer ball with the moon, however, the roundness dimension may be emphasized. This differential weighting would cause certain anomalies in distance to appear, as when one is asked to compare a lamp with a soccer ball.

Tversky and Gati (1982) have retorted that the distance-density model is insufficient to salvage geometric models of similarity. Nonetheless, Tversky's admonitions have done little to diminish the appeal or popularity of these models, at least among cognitive psychologists studying relations among perceptual stimuli. At the same time, Tversky's model has suffered from several criticisms, as summarized by Ashby and Perrin (1988), including (a) the problem of deciding what counts as a feature, (b) the elusiveness of defining feature salience, and (c) the relatively poor ability of the model to predict subjects' performance in identification and categorization tasks. The latter criticism has recently become central as models of similarity have been used to understand and predict certain higher-level cognitive behaviors. As I describe in the next section, the success of multidimensional scaling models to account for performance in identification and categorization tasks has added to their continued appeal.

A further reason that scaling models are attractive, as I have argued in this chapter, may be their link to the scaling tradition begun by Fechner. Experimental psychologists are invariably drawn to the promise that a precise ruler can be constructed, like those of the physicist, for the purpose of measuring substantive psychological phenomena. It remains to be seen whether the physicist, or any natural scientist for that matter, is an appropriate role model for the psychologist. In any case, psychological phenomena are usually quite complex, requiring various modifications of the rulers. I alluded to one of these modifications above in describing how Krumhansl included a mechanism for weighting dimensions differentially. This mechanism was actually proposed originally by Shepard (1964). I describe Shepard's contribution next, and the influence it has had on recent approaches to the study of similarity.

Contribution #3: Similarity as Underlying Identification and Classification

In what I consider his third important contribution to the study of similarity, Shepard suggested that a subject's state of attention dictates the similarity relations that inhere in multidimensional space. Shepard's (1964) study had as its goal simply to identify the best-fitting of the two traditional Minkowski metrics -- Euclidean and city-block -- to similarity judgments of circles with radial lines that varied in either circle size or line angle. Shepard found that the averaged proximity data were not described well by a Euclidean or a city-block combination rule. The reason, according to Shepard, was that some subjects attended to the size dimension and ignored the angle dimension, other subjects did the opposite, and still other subjects attempted to balance the contribution of the two dimensions. Shepard concluded that spatial models are appropriate for conceptualizing similarity relations. Nonetheless, they must be augmented by a mechanism that weights dimensions according to subjects' changing states of attention.

Recent developments in multidimensional scaling attempt to do just that. In the individual differences scaling procedure, INDSCAL, introduced by Carroll and Chang (1970; Carroll & Wish, 1974), proximity data are not averaged across subjects, but are held separate in individual subject matrices. The procedure derives a spatial solution that applies to the group as a whole. But it also computes a matrix of weights, with each element corresponding to how salient a particular dimension is to a particular subject. Thus, by differentially weighting dimensions for each subject, INDSCAL incorporates into a scaling procedure Shepard's ideas about differences in attentional state.

Cognitive psychologists have capitalized on this development in their efforts to understand what processes underlay identification and classification learning. The tack is to predict how well subjects will perform in identification or classification tasks by knowing the weighted similarity relations among stimuli. A seminal contribution to this effort was provided by Getty and his colleagues (Getty, Swets, Swets, & Green, 1979; Getty, Swets, & Swets, 1980). They sought to predict training errors in a task of absolute identification. Subjects first rated the similarity between all n(n-1)/2 pairs of stimuli. These proximities were used as input to an INDSCAL analysis, which provided inter-stimulus distances and dimensional weights for each subject. Getty et al. then used the INDSCAL weights to define subject-specific stimulus distances in Euclidean space:

$$d_{ij} = [\sum_{k=1}^{N} w_k \mid x_{ik} - x_{jk} \mid^2]^{\frac{1}{2}} \quad , \tag{16}$$

where d_{ij} is the distance between Stimulus i and Stimulus j, x_{ik} is the coordinate of Stimulus i on Dimension k, and w_k is the salience or attentional weight that subjects assign to Dimension k. The resulting distances were then converted into predicted confusabilities in the identification task using the Hull-Shepard exponential decay function,

$$C_{ij} = e^{-ad_{ij}} \quad , \tag{17}$$

where C_{ij} is how confusable Stimulus i is with Stimulus j, and a is a sensitivity constant specified for each subject. After making similarity ratings, subjects performed 150 trials of absolute identification to the same stimuli, receiving feedback after each response. Transformed similarity ratings (C_{ij}) were used to predict performance in this task.

To determine the conditional probability of making an error in the identification task -- that is, of responding R_j to Stimulus S_i -- Getty and his colleagues used a model of biased choice proposed originally by Luce (1963):

$$P(Rj \mid Si) = \frac{b_j C_{ij}}{\sum_{k=1}^{N} b_k C_{ik}} \quad , \tag{18}$$

where k refers to the set of stimuli, and b_j gauges the relative bias toward making response R_j. The complete model -- transformed similarities combined with biased choice -- was able to predict 97% of the variance across all identification responses, although it did considerably worse when predicting only the errors of identification. The important contribution of the Getty et al. model lies in using a spatial model of similarity, together with Shepard's ideas about the role of attention in similarity relations, to understand subjects' ability to label a set of unfamiliar stimuli.

Nosofsky (1984, 1986, 1987, 1991) has used the Getty approach extensively, expanding it to account for performance in categorization tasks, where many stimuli are mapped onto fewer responses. To make categorization predictions, Nosofsky substituted "categories" for "stimuli" in estimating Luce's biased-choice model, index k in Equation 18. As Nosofsky points out, this substitution creates a model that is equivalent to Medin and Schaffer's (1978) context exemplar theory of categorization. Accordingly, Nosofsky labels his hybrid model the Generalized Context Model. Unlike the Getty model, Nosofsky does not assume Euclidean distance, but instead fits the proximity data to different values of r in the general Minkowski equation (Equation 10). The Generalized Context Model has been very successful at predicting performance in both simple and relatively complex categorization tasks, using both integral and separable pairs of dimensions. Let us review it now in greater detail, beginning with the context exemplar theory.

According to Medin and Schaffer's (1978) theory, the similarity of a test stimulus to a reference stimulus is based on an attribute-by-attribute comparison along the stimuli's constituent dimensions. For example, suppose we wish to know the similarity between a large, green triangle and a small, green square. We would estimate a similarity parameter, s_k, between values on each of j dimensions. In this example, j equals 3, namely, size, hue, and shape. The similarity estimate equals 1 if the attributes match, as occurs with the hue dimension in our example.

Otherwise, the estimate takes on a value between 0 and 1 inclusive. Unique to the Medin-Schaffer model is how similarity is determined between two stimuli. The model uses a multiplicative rule in which the similarity between stimuli in the pair, S_{ij}, is the product of the individual similarity estimates on each of the j dimensions (see also Nosofsky, 1984):

$$S_{ij} = \prod_{k=1}^{j} s_k \quad . \tag{19}$$

To then determine the probability that Stimulus i is placed into Category x, Medin and Schaffer determine overall similarity, S_{ix}, between Stimulus i and each stimulus in Category x, sum those similarities, and divide that sum by the sum of similarities between Stimulus i and each stimulus used in the m categories of the experiment (see also Nosofsky, 1986):

$$P(i|x) = \frac{\sum_{x \in c_x} S_{ix}}{\sum_{y=1}^{m} (\sum_{y \in c_y} S_{iy})} \quad . \tag{20}$$

In order to accomplish the effects of Medin and Schaffer's multiplicative rule, Nosofsky (1986) defined similarity, S_{ix}, through a nonlinear transformation of distance:

$$S_{ix} = e^{-d_{ix}^{\alpha}} \quad , \tag{21}$$

where $\alpha = 1$ (Hull-Shepard function) or $\alpha = 2$ ("Gaussian" function), assuming a Minkowski combination rule to calculate d_{ix}.

It will prove instructive to review Nosofsky's procedure for predicting classification performance from similarity data. Nosofsky (1986) tested the stimuli used by Shepard (1964), circles varying in size and radial angle. In order to determine d_{ix}, Nosofsky collected a matrix of confusions from subjects' errors in absolute identification. These confusions were then used as input to a multidimensional scaling analysis. Distances, computed by, say, a Euclidean combination rule, were then transformed into "similarities" according to Equation 21. The "similarities" were then used to predict how well subjects categorized these same stimuli, using a biased-choice version (Luce, 1963) of Equation 20 (see Equation 18). As mentioned above, Nosofsky's model has been outstanding at yielding accurate predictions in each of an impressive number of recent tests (see Nosofsky, 1984, 1986, 1987, 1991).

Based on our earlier analysis of similarity and generalization, it seems clear that what Nosofsky calls "similarity" is better regarded as the performance measure confusability (see Equation 13). Because the distances were transformed non-linearly, and because confusion data usually are related non-linearly to distances, there seems to be little psychological reason for not using the original confusion data in the first place. Presumably, by transforming the confusion data into distances, and transforming the distance data into "similarities," Nosofsky achieved a more stable set of data. Nonetheless, it is important to keep in mind the distinctions among distance, intradimensional similarity, and confusability, if only to keep track of the various transformations that are exacted on the original data set.

A certain lack of logical consistency with these transformations has become evident recently in a study (Nosofsky, 1991) that replaced confusion data with similarity ratings. Like the confusion measures, Nosofsky used the similarity ratings as input to multidimensional scaling, and then transformed those distances non-linearly through Equation 21 to derive measures of "similarity." Now, if ratings are related linearly to distances, as we suggested earlier, then the motivation for performing this set of transformations becomes dubious. Indeed, according to our earlier analysis, Nosofsky's "similarity" is related non-linearly to similarity! The only motivations for the transformations appear to be (a) as a way of maintaining the Medin-Schaffer multiplicative rule and (b) because such transformations provide a reasonable fit to the categorization data. Unfortunately, in my view these transformations have also clouded our understanding of how intradimensional similarity affects categorization.

VIII. Eliminating Similarity from Models of Categorization

Several recent approaches to categorization have stressed a limited role for similarity. Medin (1989) contends that when constructing many kinds of real-world categories humans may rely minimally on similarity per se. One kind is exemplified by Barsalou's (1983) investigations into "ad-hoc" categories, that is, categories that humans use for some special purpose. An oft-used example is the ad-hoc category "things to take out of one's house in case of fire." The category members may include children, photo albums, money, and pets: items that would not be considered particularly similar in other contexts. Medin and others claim that such categorizations are explained better by appealing to the knowledge subjects bring to bear in order to maintain the category's coherence. In this view, categorizers operate on implicit theories of the world; they attempt to fit incoming data to these theories. Murphy and Medin (1985) offer the example of a person diving into a swimming pool with all his clothes on. Our classification of this event is really an attempt to explain it coherently in light of our knowledge of the world. The category that we finally select, such as "example of a party drunk", reflects our attempts to maintain coherence.

Modern theories of categorization have not excluded similarity completely, however. Medin notes that many of people's naive theories depend on similarity relations. The principle of homeopathic medicine, for example, in which one assumes that the cure to a disease will resemble its symptoms, is one case in which similarity plays a role in new theory-based models of similarity. But similarity in these models rarely follows from the psychophysical tradition of Fechner that we have traced in this chapter. Many cognitive psychologists have taken seriously the caveats of Tversky and his colleagues regarding the problems inherent in metric approaches to similarity. Moreover, these psychologists believe that many of the relations of interest to them -- the similarities among complex stimuli like countries (e.g., Tversky, 1977), or among stimuli comprised of nominal or conceptual features (e.g., Barsalou, 1983; Torgerson, 1965), or the effects of context on similarity (e.g., Rips, 1989) -- are not addressed well by geometric approaches. Among these psychologists, Tversky's contrast theory has been enormously influential because it addresses the non-perceptual relations that are the focus of much current work in similarity and categorization.

But even Tversky's model has become unsatisfactory to some. Medin (1989) contends that a feature-based model of similarity must be able to accommodate the fact that features may or may not be independent and may or may not be at the same level of abstraction. In the category, "substitutes for hammer," for example, the features "made of metal," "of medium size," and "easy to grasp" can be summed to provide better evidence for a good fit to the category, because the more of these features, the better for hammering. On the other hand, the category "ways to avoid predation" may include features that are not additive such as "lives in trees" and "is armored," because having more than one of these features does not necessarily enhance an animal's chances of not being eaten.

Medin, Goldstone, and Gentner (1990) report evidence that they believe is incompatible with contrast theory. Here they distinguish between similarity among attributes and similarity among relations. If one stimulus is a red square paired with a red circle, and a second stimulus is a blue circle paired with a blue triangle, then the stimuli share the attribute "circle" and the relation "same color." Medin and his colleagues found that attributes and relations differ in how they affect judgments of similarity and difference. In particular, they found that subjects stress relations when judging similarity, but stress attributes when judging difference. The consequence of this asymmetry can be seen in Figure 6.10. When subjects were asked whether B or C was more similar to the standard A, they chose C because it is relationally similar; both are colored uniformly. But when asked which was more different from A, subjects also chose C because it differed most at the level of attributes.

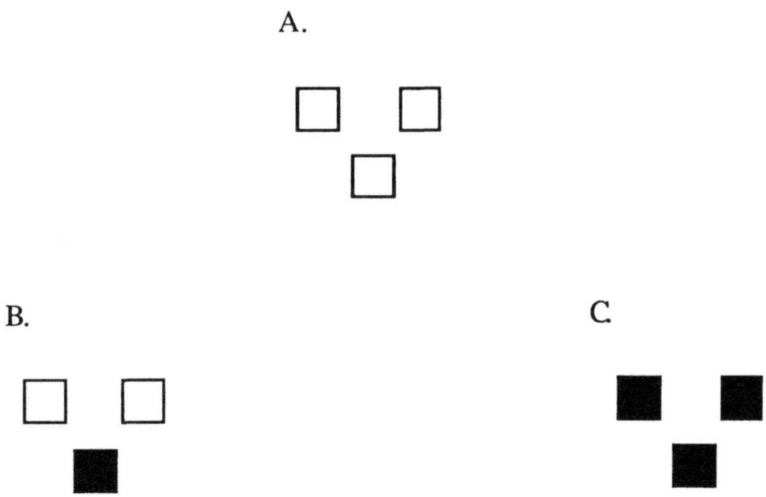

Figure 6.10: A stimulus set resembling (but not identical to) that used by Medin, Goldstone, and Gentner (1990) to demonstrate how attributes and relations have different effects on judgments of similarity and difference. Standard A seems more similar to Stimulus C than Stimulus B because A and C have a relational similarity; both are uniformly colored. Standard A also seems more different from Stimulus C than Stimulus B because A and C have high attribute dissimilarity; they share no attributes in common.

In other words, the same stimulus can be judged as both more similar to and more different from a standard, indicating that difference judgments are not the inverse of similarity judgments. Importantly, though, because the two kinds of "features" -- attributes and relations -- are at different levels of abstraction, the findings of Medin et al. are unlike those of Tversky and Gati (1978) in their investigations of similarity and difference among countries. In the latter work, certain countries, such as East Germany and West Germany, were found to be both very similar to *and* very different from each other when judged in the context of countries such as Nepal and Sri Lanka. The reason is that East Germany and West Germany enjoy more features -- *both* common and distinctive -- than Nepal and Sri Lanka. Subjects apparently stressed the common features when judging similarity and the distinctive features when judging difference. Stimuli tested in the Medin et al. study do not differ in number of features, however, and so the asymmetry cannot be explained by this version of contrast theory. Indeed, Medin and his colleagues claim that *no* weighting of common and distinctive features could reproduce the effects obtained in their study, and so no version of contrast theory provides an adequate account. The authors conclude that future theories of similarity need to acknowledge the different roles of attributes and relations in similarity judgments.

IX. Thurstone's Legacy: Multivariate Multidimensional Scaling

Although many cognitive psychologists working on higher-level cognitive uses of similarity have shied from geometric interpretations of similarity, many working with perceptual stimuli have continued to develop these models profitably. The traditional model of multidimensional scaling assumes that each perceptual stimulus is represented as a single point in some multidimensional space. Among recent developments is the rejection of this static conception of multidimensional space, replaced by a stochastic conception in which each stimulus at each moment is represented by a value sampled from a multivariate probability distribution. This change from static to stochastic mechanisms of similarity is directly analogous to the change wrought by Thurstone in response to Fechner's static conception of the jnd. It thus hallmarks the most recent advance in the tradition of metric similarity relations begun in psychophysics and carried over into cognitive psychology.

The approach described by Zinnes and MacKay (1983) is a good example of a multivariate model of similarity. They formalized the Hefner (1958) model, in which each stimulus is represented by a random vector having r dimensions, with each component of the vector distributed normally and independently. Thus, each stimulus is characterized by a location (mean) parameter, μ_{ik}, and a variability (uncertainty) parameter, σ_i^2. As noted by Zinnes and MacKay, the multidimensional Hefner model is, in one dimension, identical to Thurstone's paired comparison model. The variability parameter is permitted to change from stimulus to stimulus, but Zinnes and MacKay assume that, for a given stimulus, variance does not change from dimension to dimension, a rather severe assumption. This suggests a model similar to Thurstone's Case III unidimensional model.

In order to derive μ_{ik} and σ_i^2, Zinnes and MacKay define a random variable of distance, d_{ij}, determining its variance, σ_{ij}^2, and expected value, $E(d_{ij})$. In short, they compute the stimulus distributions from knowledge of the inter-stimulus distances. To calculate the location parameters, Zinnes and MacKay use the Young-Householder (1938) procedure described earlier. To estimate the variance parameters, the authors exploit an approximation based on the squared difference between dissimilarity judgments and Euclidean distances of means:

$$\sigma_i^2 + \sigma_j^2 = (D_{ij} - d_{ij})^2 \ , \tag{22}$$

where σ_i^2 is the approximated variability in Stimulus i, D_{ij} is the judged dissimilarity between Stimuli i and j, and d_{ij} is the Euclidean distance between the location values of Stimuli i and j estimated from the Young-Householder coordinates. The individual terms on the left side of Equation 22 are determined subsequently by standard least squares estimation techniques.

Zinnes and MacKay (1983) demonstrated how their model is superior to traditional models in recovering true stimulus configurations. In one test, they compared the scaling solutions of the Hefner model with those of a traditional static multidimensional model (Kruskal, 1964a, 1964b). The stimulus set comprised concentric hexagons as shown in Panel A of Figure 6.11. Zinnes and MacKay created similarity ratings for the stimuli in this set, making the variability in the inner hexagon more than twice that of the outer hexagon. As shown in Panel B, this manipulation caused the traditional scaling procedure to invert the hexagon. This is because greater variability is interpreted by such procedures as greater distance. Traditional models thus fail to recover the original map when stimulus distributions have different variances. As shown in Panel C, the Hefner model is suited to such changes in variability, recovering exactly the original configuration of stimuli.

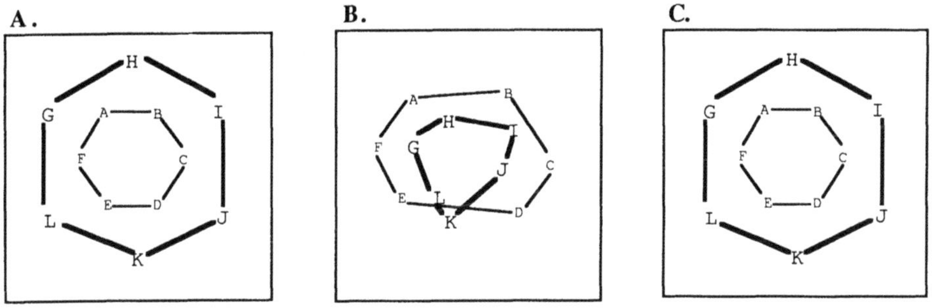

Figure 6.11: Panel A: Representation of the two-dimensional stimulus set tested by Zinnes and MacKay (1983). Simulated similarity judgments of this set were used as input to a traditional and stochastic multidimensional scaling procedure, with judgments of the inner hexagon given twice the variability as those of the outer hexagon. Panel B: Scaling solution from a traditional scaling procedure (KYST), which inverts the inner and outer hexagons. Panel C: Scaling solution from Zinnes and MacKay's stochastic scaling procedure, which accurately recovers the original stimulus set.

Ennis, Palen, and Mullen (1988) have recently developed a Hefner-style stochastic model and used it to transform distances into measures of similarity. They assume that each stimulus is represented by a normal, multivariate distribution, and that the distance between the means of these distributions is given by a generalized Minkowski equation:

$$\delta = \left[\sum_{k=1}^{n} \left| \mu_{xk} - \mu_{yk} \right|^{\beta} \right]^{\frac{1}{\beta}} \qquad r \geq 1 \ , \qquad (23)$$

where n is the number of dimensions, μ_{xk} is the mean of Stimulus x on dimension k, and β is the Minkowski exponent (i.e., $\beta = 1$ creates city-block space; $\beta = 2$ creates Euclidean space). Similarity is then based on an exponential transformation of the Minkowski distances:

$$g(s) = e^{\delta^{\alpha}} \quad , \qquad (24)$$

where g(s) is a similarity function that transforms distance, δ. Note that this function is identical to our earlier description of confusability (Equation 13). Thus, it would seem that the Ennis et al. model is better conceptualized as a multivariate model of confusability or generalization.

Multivariate models of psychological distance have the potential to account for observed violations of metric axioms. As noted by Ennis et al., it is relatively straightforward to reconsider Krumhansl's notions of spatial density in terms of a stochastic model. In this dress, dense regions of space are caused by stimulus distributions having high variance relative to other regions. Violations of symmetry and identity could thus be attributable to differences in variance among stimulus distributions. Such a conjecture has powerful implications if true, and certainly merits systematic investigation.

X. Thurstone's Legacy: Multivariate Signal Detection Theory

Thurstone's idea that physical stimulation creates a distribution of effects along a sensory continuum was developed further in the 1950's by engineers at the University of Michigan, MIT, and in the Soviet Union (see Macmillan & Creelman, 1991), although all were probably unaware of Thurstone's work. These engineers were concerned with the detection of radar and sonar signals amid the noise that is intrinsic to the signal itself. One can represent a signal within noise stochastically by a distribution of effects, as in Thurstone's conception. Noise in the absence of signal can also be represented by such a distribution, as shown in Fig. 12. Because the signal-with-noise distribution might overlap with the noise-alone distribution, the engineers were faced with describing how observers discriminate between a random value that conceivably may arise from either of the two distributions. This is a problem of decision making -- deciding whether, say, a radar display does (signal) or does not (noise) contain a blip; an answer to the problem was found in statistical decision theory. Decision theorists address the question of what decision rule an observer will adopt when achieving some specific goal. The observer's goal might be, for example, to maximize "hits" -- correctly identifying blips when they appear -- or to minimize "false alarms" -- incorrectly identifying blips when they do not appear. According to statistical decision theory, the optimal decision rule for a given goal can be determined mathematically. The decision rule needed to maximize hits *and* minimize false alarms, for example, can be represented by a vertical line β, called the criterion, which intersects the sensory axis, as shown in Figure 6.12. The observer identifies any effects falling in the region above the criterion as "signal" (e.g., blip), and any falling in the region below as "noise."

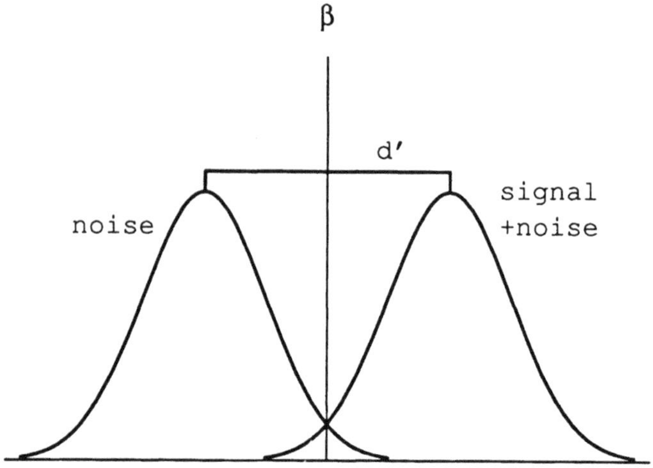

Figure 6.12: Signal detection representation of the perceptual effects of noise and a signal with noise for signals varying on a single dimension of perceptual experience. The two perceptual effects are distributed as univariate normal, the ordinate represents the probability of an effect and, in this example, the distributions are shown to overlap each other. A criterion is included that acts as a decision boundary for observers to maximize hits and minimize false alarms: Observers call signal those perceptual effects experienced above β, and noise those experienced below β.

These engineering ideas were borrowed by psychologists Tanner and Swets at the University of Michigan, and used to formalize what psychologists know as *signal detection theory* (see Green & Swets, 1966). According to signal detection theory, both the noise-alone distribution and the signal-with-noise distribution can correspond to the perceptual effects of physical stimulation, say, the effects of a 1000-Hz tone and a 1004-Hz tone, respectively. A hit occurs whenever the 1004-Hz tone is identified as high pitched; a false alarm occurs whenever the 1000-Hz tone is identified as high pitched. Assuming that the sensory distributions are normal and have equal variances, the sensory difference between the perceptual effects of these two stimuli can be described by a measure of sensitivity, specifically, the value d', which represents the difference between the means of the two distributions:

$$d' = \frac{\mu_{signal} - \mu_{noise}}{\sigma_{noise}} \quad . \tag{25}$$

The sensory effects of signals are independent of the decision rule. That is, the separation between distributions need not affect where the perceiver places the criterion β. The perceiver will make more hits (and more false alarms) the smaller the value of β, no matter how far apart the two distributions. Conversely, the less the distributions overlap, the easier it is to make a hit without committing a false alarm, no matter where the criterion is placed. Thus, signal detection theory separates the effect of sensory/perceptual experience from the rules perceivers use to make decisions (see also Luce, 1959, 1963).

When modelling similarity, one might describe perceptual differences using d' exclusively. d' is a distance measure, and so obeys all the metric axioms. d' is not limited to differences among stimuli varying unidimensionally: One can calculate d' for multidimensional stimuli with each stimulus represented, as in multivariate multidimensional scaling, by a multivariate distribution; d' is the difference between means of those distributions. Of course, the use of d' alone as a model of similarity is nothing more than Thurstone's paired comparison model, and so is merely a special case of a stochastic model of multidimensional scaling. Moreover, because d's are effectively bounded between 0 -- when hits equal false alarms -- and about 4.65 -- when hits equal .99 and false alarms equal .01 -- the perceptual differences indicated by this measure are quite restricted. What is needed is an approach that takes advantage of the unique features of signal detection theory, namely, sensory/perceptual effects independent of decision processes. Just such an analysis has been offered recently by Ashby and Perrin (1988).

Ashby and Perrin assert that distance-based models of similarity, like those of multidimensional scaling, are not adequate for similarity data that routinely violate the distance axioms. They believe that theorists should search for models of similarity not constrained by the metric assumptions. Signal detection theory offers partial freedom from metric assumptions because similarity is explained not solely by the distance-based measure, d', but also through the effects of decision rules. In their model, called General Recognition Theory, similarity co-varies with confusability: The more similar two stimuli, the more confusable they are. Multidimensional stimuli are each represented, in accord with signal detection theory, as multivariate distributions, like those shown in Figure 6.13. A decision rule, represented by the boundary line in Figure 6.13, determines the subjects'

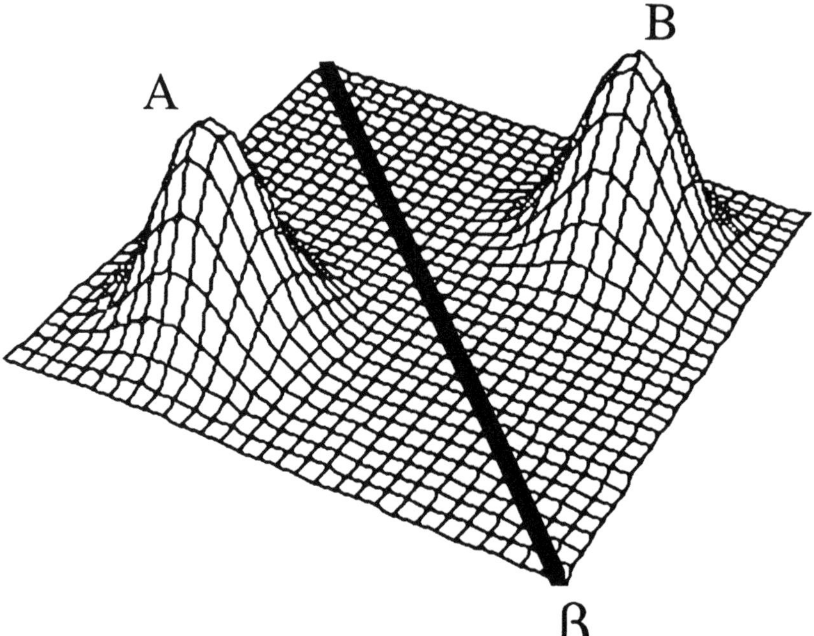

Figure 6.13: Signal detection representation of the perceptual effects of two stimuli, A and B, for signals varying on two dimensions of perceptual experience. The height of each multivariate distribution is the probability of a perceptual effect. The boundary line is a rule for deciding whether an experienced effect is Stimulus A or Stimulus B.

response to a particular perceptual effect (see also Ashby, 1989; Ashby & Gott, 1988; Ashby & Lee, 1991; Ashby & Townsend, 1986). In the example, all perceptual effects occurring in the region to the left of the line are called Stimulus A; all effects occurring in the region to the right of the line are called Stimulus B. According to the model, then, the perceived similarity of Stimulus A to Stimulus B is proportion of the Stimulus A perceptual distribution that crosses the decision boundary into the region associated with Stimulus B. Formally,

$$s(S_A, S_B) = k \iint_{R_B} f_A(x,y)\, dx\, dy \quad , \tag{26}$$

where $s(S_A,S_B)$ is the similarity of Stimulus A to Stimulus B, k is a positive constant, and R_B is the region in a two-dimensional (x,y) plane associated with Stimulus B.

Equation 26 is the full definition only in a two-stimulus absolute identification procedure, and in the absence of response biases. With more than two stimuli, the optimal decision boundary will change, and hence so will the similarity between two stimuli. Imagine adding a third multivariate distribution, Stimuli C, to the two appearing in Figure 6.13. Now imagine taking a horizontal slice from each of the three distributions at a constant vertical level of probability. If you then examine the three slices from above, you would see three circles or ellipses -- three contours of equal probability -- as shown in Figure 6.14. Notice that this figure contains three possible decision criteria: β_1, β_2, and β_3. In the Ashby-Perrin model, the optimal criterion depends on which set of stimuli observers experience. In Figure 6.14, for example, observers distinguishing Stimulus A from Stimulus C would respond optimally by using β_2 if Stimulus B was absent, by using β_3 if Stimulus B was present and assigned a response different from Stimulus C, and by using β_1 if Stimulus B was present and assigned the same response as Stimulus C. In this way, Ashby and Perrin distinguish cases in which two stimuli are compared in the presence of other stimuli, which they call the *context sensitive* similarity model, from cases in which two stimuli are compared in isolation, which they call the *context free* similarity model. The authors indicate that their context sensitive version is able to accommodate context effects of similarity, such as those demonstrated by Tversky, and so is superior to traditional spatial models of similarity that are not influenced by surrounding stimuli (but see Krumhansl, 1978).

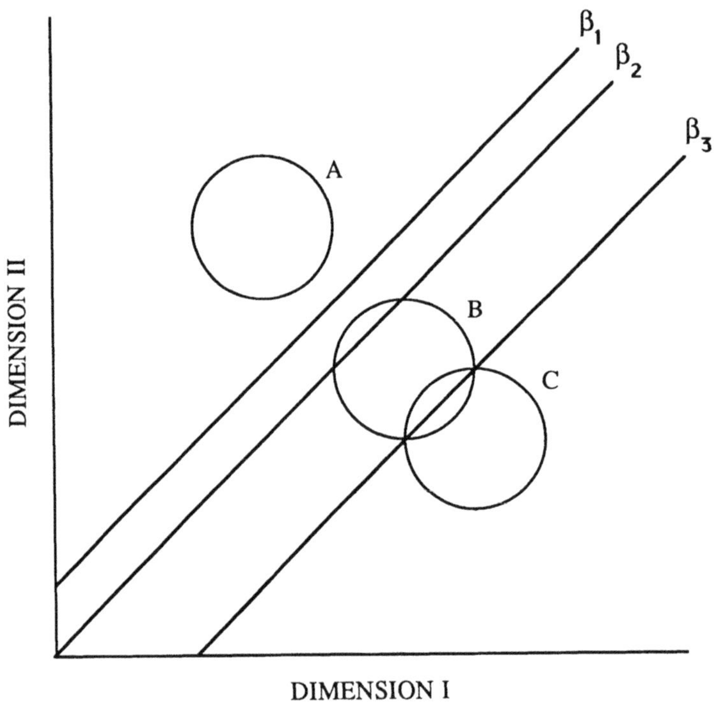

Figure 6.14: Three contours of equal probability, corresponding to the perceptual effects of three stimuli -- A, B, and C -- in a two-dimensional perceptual space. Also included are three different decision boundaries -- β_1, β_2, and β_3 -- used in Ashby and Perrin's (1988) context-sensitive and context-free similarity models as optimal decision rules (see text for details).

In comparing the General Recognition Theory with multidimensional scaling models, Ashby and Perrin stress that the former does not depend exclusively on the metric axioms. Moreover, unlike scaling models, similarity in General Recognition Theory is a "derived construct" dependent on determining the relations among perceptual distributions. "In fact, the General Recognition Theory predicts that the task of judging perceived similarity will be very difficult for subjects because it requires them to do something roughly analogous to multiple integration" (p.131). Nonetheless, the authors are able to show that a Euclidean scaling model is a special case of the context-free General Recognition Theory with a Gaussian distribution.

Evaluating General Recognition Theory is difficult because the hypothesized perceptual distributions, and hence their overlap, are not directly observable. In testing the model, Ashby and Perrin (1988) attempted to mimic perceptual distributions by building categories of stimuli that were either circular or elliptical in shape. The overlap between the category circles or ellipses was varied, and subjects were asked after learning to rate the similarity of the two categories to each other. Not surprisingly, the two categories having the greatest overlap (and hence the worst performance) were judged to be more similar than the two categories having the least overlap (and hence the best performance). Of course, this is hardly a definitive test of the model, as the perceptual effects specified by the model -- multivariate distributions in perceptual space -- may bear little psychological relation to contour-shaped categories used to perform the test. Moreover, subjects' ratings in this test were likely to be determined by their success in categorizing.

Apart from the limitations of their tests, the Ashby-Perrin model suffers from more general drawbacks. First, by linking similarity with confusability, the model is burdened by the problems of equating these two terms, as outlined earlier. Second, by describing similarity relations as "derived" and unnatural, the model seems to fly in the face of how fundamental these relations are in perceptual and cognitive acts. Finally, it is not clear what is meant by perceptual distributions in General Recognition Theory. If these distributions are like the sensory distributions of traditional signal detection theory, then the range of similarity relations that can be covered by the theory in practice is probably too limited, for the same reason that d' in signal detection theory is bounded in practice. An example will clarify the nature of the problem. Imagine that the perceptual effects of two stimuli, called Pair A, have little or no sensory overlap, and that the same is true for two stimuli in Pair B. It is still quite conceivable that similarity ratings to Pair A stimuli are very different from ratings to Pair B stimuli. This suggests that usual characterizations of sensory distributions, as defined by signal detection theory, are inadequate as a general framework for perceptual similarity. If a new characterization of psychological distributions is implied by the model, the authors fail to specify what it is.

Despite these problems, General Recognition Theory is an interesting development in the study of similarity for two reasons. First, it specifically incorporates the decision processes into mechanisms of forming similarity relations. Thus the model separates perceptual similarity per se from cognitive acts that may influence judgments of similarity. Second, it distinguishes between similarity relations that are context dependent from those that are context free. Thus, the model suggests that perceptual similarity can potentially be evaluated in the absence of context. As I discuss next, these issues must certainly be addressed by any complete account of similarity.

XI. Future Developments in the Study of Similarity: A Personal View

In this chapter, I have traced the idea of perceptual similarity from its beginnings in psychophysics through the modifications instigated by mathematically-oriented cognitive psychologists. I have argued that the Fechnerian notion of a psychological ruler still thrives in cognitive psychology, primarily in the guise of spatial models of stimulus similarity. Further, I have argued that, despite a history of criticism, these models have proved to be surprisingly resilient, and have been useful in characterizing many higher-order cognitive processes such as stimulus categorization.

What issues still need to be addressed? What direction should future study of similarity take? My personal answers to these questions emerge naturally from the lessons learned in the history of similarity relations, as reviewed in this chapter. My views are summarized simply: Theory should strive to elucidate how humans process the individual components of a multidimensional stimulus. Once elucidated, theory should be directed toward understanding how humans combine the components of experience into an overall judgment of stimulus similarity. In this section, I outline one possible model of stimulus similarity. This model uses the historical lessons to guide a set of constructs and principles. Admittedly, the model is now little more than a sketch requiring rigorous exploration in the future. Nevertheless, I think that the proposed approach captures many fundamental aspects of the experience of perceptual similarity.

Historical Lessons and New Constructs

Attneave argued persuasively that perceivers organize their experiences, either implicitly or explicitly, around psychologically real dimensions of change in the environment. I begin with this assumption. The evidence that my colleagues and I have collected (e.g., Melara & Marks, 1990; Melara, 1989b), using both speeded and unspeeded techniques, suggests that dimensions of experience are unique and not malleable. When presented with color stimuli in speeded classification, for example, perceivers give special status to the dimensions of hue, saturation, and brightness over other possible dimensions (i.e., orientations of axes) in the color space (see Melara, Marks, & Potts, 1991). Preference for these dimensions appears to be immediate and not the result of conscious effort. Moreover, such preferences exist whether the dimensions are interacting or separable. The evidence suggests, therefore, that, to the extent that the spatial metaphor holds, the structure of the psychological space cannot be Euclidean.

This *primacy of dimensions*, as I call it, indicates that similarity relations begin at the level of individual dimensions. Earlier, I advanced the construct of intradimensional similarity to characterize the psychological experience of difference along dimensions. Because the construct is hypothetical, one must decide how best to measure it. I argued earlier that the typical measure -- nonlinear transformations of distances that themselves reflect transformed confusabilities -- is probably incorrect because, psychologically speaking, its underlying rationale is faulty. Instead, it seems useful to begin with measures of similarity judged directly, thereby employing a more psychophysical approach to the problem of dimensional change. The idea is that perceivers *can* scale their experiences accurately, and that these direct measurements are related linearly to psychological distance. The difficulty with the approach, as I have alluded, is that subjects also are affected greatly by stimulus and task contexts: Subjects appear to stretch or shrink their rulers to the particular stimulus set or procedure to which they have been exposed. For example, a subject may span the same extent of rating scale for stimuli covering a relatively small range along a dimension as for stimuli covering a wide range (cf. Parducci, 1965). To date, it remains unclear whether (and which) contexts affect (a) the responses given by subjects (e.g., the particular way that subjects use numbers) or, more critically, (b) actual perceptual representations. Certainly, useful measures of intradimensional similarity must await a better understanding of how context affects judgments of similarity (cf. Ashby & Perrin, 1988).

But let us suppose that we *can* make unbiased, context-independent measures of intradimensional similarity using direct judgments. Now, we can raise the more fundamental cognitive question: What rules do subjects use to combine psychological discrepancies along each of several dimensions? Attneave (1950) found that his similarity data were described best when Minkowski's $r = 1$, the Householder-Landahl or city-block rule. In the years following Attneave, however, numerous studies using his approach have found that the city-block rule seems to work well only when dimensions do not interact perceptually; for interacting dimensions, the best-fitting rule is often the simple Euclidean distance rule, $r = 2$ (see Garner, 1974). The city-block model also appears inappropriate for reaction time data (e.g., Melara, 1989b) or any time subjects are under conditions of speed stress (e.g., Smith & Kemler-Nelson, 1984; Ward, 1983). Finally, the more complex the stimuli, that is, the more dimensions on which stimuli differ, the less likely that a city-block rule seems appropriate (e.g., Torgerson, 1965).

In contrast to evidence against the city-block metric, Melara, Marks, and Lesko (1991) showed recently that subjects *can* use an additive combination rule successfully, even with interacting dimensions. We tested three pairs of interacting dimensions, one visual, one auditory, and one cross-modal; in each case, we found that subjects could use a city-block rule when making similarity judgments with multidimensional stimuli. Thus, perceivers do appear to have clear access to this rule under certain circumstances. Moreover, the city-block rule, unlike the Euclidean rule, requires non-arbitrary axes in psychological space, a condition that I have argued is met by both interacting and separable dimensions.

What is the difference psychologically, then, between interacting and separable dimensions? In my view, these dimensions differ in their similarity relations. Specifically, interacting and separable dimensions differ in their degree of *cross-dimensional similarity*, a construct defined as the phenomenal similarity of one dimension of experience with another. I propose that interacting dimensions are higher in cross-dimensional similarity than separable dimensions. Consider, for example, two interacting dimensions of color, saturation and brightness. Students taught in a perception course about these dimensions will often show some initial confusion regarding the difference between a change in saturation and a change in brightness. For perceivers, changes in saturation are very similar to changes in brightness; these dimensions enjoy a high degree of cross-dimensional similarity. Thus, the degree of perceptual interaction between saturation and brightness, as measured by, say, Garner interference in speeded classification, can be attributed to the degree of cross-dimensional similarity. I submit that a pair of dimensions high in cross-dimensional similarity can always be expected to interact perceptually.

To measure the construct of cross-dimensional similarity, one might evaluate the speed to respond same or different to one dimension in the face of changes along other dimensions. Consider a subject deciding whether two patches of color are the same or different in brightness in the face of changes in saturation and in the shape of the patch. One might expect that cross-dimensional similarity between brightness and saturation is greater than that between brightness and shape. If so, then subjects should be slower to respond "same brightness" if the standard and test stimuli differ in saturation than if they differ in shape. Similarly, subjects might be faster to respond "different brightness" if the standard and test differ in saturation than if they differ in shape. One can then use these estimates to predict Garner interference in speeded classification. In this example, one would predict more Garner interference between the pair brightness-saturation than between the pair brightness-shape. Preliminary evidence from my laboratory suggests that this is exactly what happens: Cross-dimensional similarity among brightness, saturation, hue, size, and shape, as measured by same-different reaction times, explained 98% of the Garner interference in speeded classification.

A Model of Multidimensional Perceptual Similarity

Once delimiting the constructs of intradimensional similarity, measured by direct judgments, and cross-dimensional similarity, measured by reaction times, we are now in a position to identify how perceivers combine dimensional differences. The model that I propose in this chapter takes a strong stance with respect to rules of combination: I believe that perceivers always base their judgments on an *additive combination of intradimensional dissimilarities*. In other words, I claim that (1) multidimensional similarity is decomposable into a set of intradimensional similarities and (2) for any given pair of perceptual dimensions, one can almost always find evidence for a city-block distance function. Theoretically, these ideas follow from the framework developed throughout this chapter: Perceivers have access to unique, primary dimensions, and they build up the experiential differences along these dimensions to compute similarity relations.

Despite the strong stance, I also believe that similarity data are more likely to *appear* additive when (1) the number of dimensions of difference between stimuli being compared is small, (2) the processing time permitted to attend to (i.e., learn) each dimension of difference is ample, and (3) the degree of cross-dimensional similarity is minimal. In general, I hypothesize that the higher the degree of cross-dimensional similarity, or the less a task permits subjects to attend to the individual dimensions, the less likely that the combination rule will appear strictly city-block, all things being equal. I believe that these factors are what make additive models appear incorrect for similarity data. For example, interacting dimensions are probably higher in cross-dimensional similarity than separable dimensions. Thus, similarity judgments of stimuli created from interacting dimensions are more likely to appear non-additive.

By non-additive, I have in mind something specific, namely that the combination rule will approximate a Euclidean function. The Euclidean metric is approximated, I think, because when making multidimensional judgments (i.e., judgments of stimuli differing along, say, two dimensions) perceivers often *underestimate* intradimensional dissimilarity relative to unidimensional judgments (i.e., judgments of stimuli that differ on a single dimension). Consider Stimuli A, B, and C represented in Panel A of Figure 6.15 as three points in bidimensional space. The hypothesis is that the Euclidean metric is approximated when perceivers underestimate the length of the AB leg (i.e., intradimensional similarity) in comparing Stimulus A with C (a multidimensional judgment) versus comparing Stimulus A with B (a unidimensional judgment). There exists a unique relation between city block and Euclidean metrics such that

$$CB = \sqrt{E^2 + 2 \left[\prod_{k=1}^{N} | x_{ik} - x_{jk} | \right]} \; , \qquad (27)$$

where CB is city-block distance, E is Euclidean distance, x_{ik} is the value of Stimulus i and Dimension k, and N is the number of dimensions of difference. This relation is significant psychologically because, as shown in Panel B of Figure

6.15, it implies that bidimensional Euclidean distance is always less than bidimensional city-block distance. Moreover, the former approximates the latter when intradimensional dissimilarity on one dimension is much greater than that on the other dimension: that is, when the bidimensional judgment approximates a unidimensional judgment.

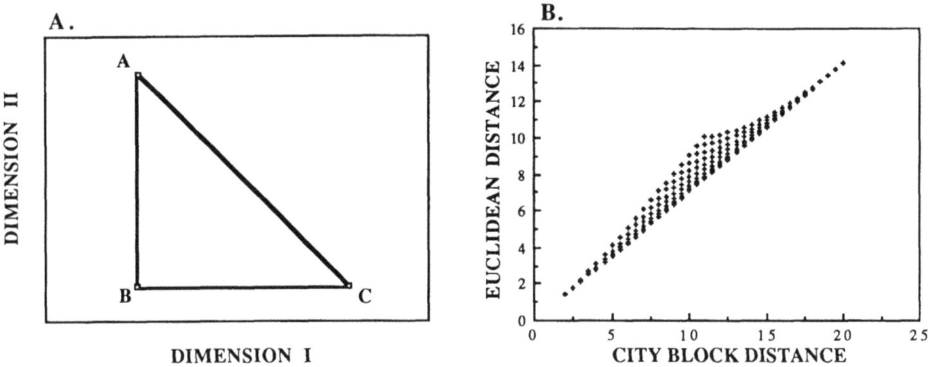

Figure 6.15: Panel A: Representation of three stimuli -- A, B, and C -- in a two-dimensional perceptual space. A versus B is a unidimensional similarity judgement, A versus C a multidimensional judgment. Panel B: The relationship between city-block and Euclidean distances in two-dimensional space, with values along each dimension from 1 to 10 in steps of 0.5.

This quantitative account can be readily conceptualized psychologically: Perceivers combine intradimensional differences additively; however, under certain conditions, intradimensional dissimilarity is underestimated, causing the combination rule to appear Euclidean. I argue, therefore, that what was regarded previously to be evidence that, when dimensions interact, subjects make

Pythagorean calculations in a space having arbitrary reference axes, is explained better by assuming that high cross-dimensional similarity increases the like.'hood that dimensions with unique reference axes will be combined under-additively. Importantly, however, I believe that, under the proper conditions, additivity will be achieved in similarity data even with dimensions high in cross-dimensional similarity, as long as these dimensions are psychologically primary. Based on previous research, I suggest that three main factors underlie the tendency to underestimate: (1) cross-dimensional similarity, (2) number of dimensions of difference, and (3) inadequate processing time. Hence, these factors work to undermine additivity. Critically, though, because the Euclidean rule is only approximated, the implication is that this rule is never an adequate model of perceptual similarity.

The foregoing analysis leads us, finally, to a formal model of perceptual similarity:

$$D_{ij} = \sum_{k=1}^{N} \frac{|x_{ik} - x_{jk}|}{CS_k N/t_k} , \qquad (28)$$

where $CS_k \geq 1$, $N \geq 1$, $t_k > 0$, D_{ij} is the judged dissimilarity of Stimulus i with Stimulus j, $|x_{ik}-x_{jk}|$ is intradimensional dissimilarity, N is the number of primary perceptual dimensions on which the stimuli differ, t_k is the functional processing time devoted by the perceiver to Dimension k, and CS_k is the cross-dimensional similarity between Dimension k and the remaining N-1 dimensions. I will assume multiplicative growth in cross-dimensional similarity:

$$CS_k = \prod_{m=1}^{N-1} CS_{km} \qquad m \neq k \ , \tag{29}$$

where CS_{km} is the cross-dimensional similarity of dimension k with dimension m. I also assume a concave downward relationship between functional time and real time. That is, as real time increases, functional time grows at a progressively smaller rate until it asymptotes:

$$t_k = c\ [1 - e^{-(T^{\alpha})}\ ] \qquad 0 < \alpha \leq 1 \ , \tag{30}$$

where T is real time, c is a scaling constant, and the exponent α is matched to data. In many respects, t_k is analogous to the weight that subjects attach to each dimension because, the more functional time subjects are given, the better able they are to weight a particular dimension. Thus, t_k can be seen to have its historical roots in the work of Attneave, Shepard, and Nosofsky. Outside the domain of perception, it may prove heuristic to regard functional time as a surrogate measure either of learning, on the one hand, or of memory, on the other. If so, then one would predict relatively small values of t_k when the stimuli to be judged are either poorly learned (e.g., tactile stimuli to a novice of the Optacon) or poorly remembered (e.g., stimuli separated in time from the judgments of similarity). This extrapolation dramatizes one possible way in which a model of perceptual similarity can form the foundation for a more general model of similarity.

In words, the model states that perceivers will tend to underestimate unidimensional distances in multidimensional over unidimensional judgments (1) as the number of dimensions of difference increases, (2) whenever cross-dimensional similarity is large, and (3) whenever functional time is short. Conversely, functional time acts to moderate the effects of number and cross-dimensional similarity; thus, greater time implies more accurate distance estimation. To the extent that distance underestimation is minimized, judged similarity will be fit better by a city-block metric.

This model is now only a framework for thinking about similarity relations among perceptual stimuli. Nonetheless, it is a fairly straightforward matter to subject the model to empirical test, and future reports will contain these tests. But even in its current state of development, the model has several attractive features. First, it captures and extends the psychophysical approach to similarity relations that has been a theme of study since Fechner. In this way, it marks a new stage in the intellectual development of a set of ideas, development itself being a quality that is difficult to identify in many fields of psychology. Second, the model incorporates many characteristics of similarity relations that have been discovered over the past century. For example, the phenomenon of dimensional interaction, long a source of concern for those modeling similarity, is here re-conceptualized as a special form of similarity. The model can account for a variety of effects noticed frequently in the past, doing so with a minimal number of free parameters. Thus, in this model we can identify an evolution of ideas, much as I have done in reviewing the history of similarity. These ideas lead, through the model, to possible answers to some notoriously difficult and nagging questions. Still, only the future can evaluate the merit of this approach.

References

Anderson, N.H. (1975). On the role of context effects in psychophysical judgment. *Psychological Review*, **82**, 462-482.

Ashby, F.G., & Townsend, J.T. (1986). Varieties of perceptual independence. *Psychological Review,* **93**, 154-179.

Ashby, F.G. (1989). Stochastic general recognition theory. In D. Vickers and P.L. Smith (Eds.), *Human Information Processing: Mechanisms and Models* (pp.435-457). Amsterdam: Elsevier Science.

Ashby, F.G., Gott R.E. (1988). Decision rules in the perception and categorization of multidimensional stimuli. *Journal of Experimental Psychology*, **14**, 33-53.

Ashby, F.G., & Lee, W.W. (1991). Predicting similarity and categorization from identification. *Journal of Experimental Psychology: General* **120**, 150-172.

Ashby, F.G., & Perrin, N.A. (1988). Toward a unified theory of similarity and recognition. *Psychological Review*, **95**, 124-150.

Attneave, F. (1950). Dimensions of similarity. *American Journal of Psychology*, **63**, 516-556.

Barsalou, L.W. (1983). Ad hoc categories. *Memory & Cognition*, **10**, 82-93.

Beals, R., Krantz, D.H., & Tversky, A. (1968). Foundation of multidimensional scaling. *Psychological Review*, **75**, 127-142.

Birnbaum, M.H. (1974). Using contextual effects to derive psychophysical scales. *Perception & Psychophysics*, **15**, 89-96.

Birnbaum, M.H., Parducci, A., & Gifford, R.K. (1971). Contextual effects in information integration. *Journal of Experimental Psychology*, **88**, 158-170.

Boring, E.G. (1933). *The physical dimensions of consciousness*. New York: Appleton-Century-Crofts.

Bower, G.H. (1971). Adaptation-level coding of stimuli and serial position effects. In M. Appley (Ed.), *Adaptation-level theory* (pp. 175-201). New York: Academic Press.

Carroll, J.D., & Chang, J.J. (1970). Analysis of individual differences in multidimensional scaling via an N-way generalization of Eckart-Young decomposition. *Psychometrika*, **35**, 283-319.

Carroll, J.D., & Wish, M. (1974). Models and methods for three-way multidimensional scaling. In D.H. Krantz, R.C. Atkinson, R.D. Luce, & P. Suppes (Eds.), *Contemporary developments in mathematical psychology* (Vol. 2). San Francisco: W.H. Freeman.

Coombs, C.A. (1964). *A theory of data*. New York: Wiley.

Ennis, D.M. (1988). Technical comment: Toward a universal law of generalization. *Science*, **242**, 944.

Ennis, D.M., Palen, J.J., & Mullen, K. (1988). A multidimensional stochastic theory of similarity. *Journal of Mathematical Psychology*, **32**, 449-465.

Fechner, G.T. (1860). *Elemente der Psychophysik*. Leipzig: Breitkopf and Härterl. English translation of Vol. 1 by H.E. Adler (1966; D.H. Howes and E.G. Boring, Eds.). New York: Holt, Rinehart, and Winston.

Garner, W.R. (1974). *The processing of information and structure*. Potomac, MD: Erlbaum.

Garner, W.R., & Felfoldy, G.L. (1970). Integrality of stimulus dimensions in various types of information processing. *Cognitive Psychology*, **1**, 225-241.

Garner, W.R., Hake, H.W., & Eriksen, C.W. (1956). Operationism and the concept of perception. *Psychological Review,* **63**, 49-159.

Getty, D.J., Swets, J.B., Swets, J.A. (1980). The observer's use of perceptual dimensions in signal identification. In R.S. Nickerson (Ed.), *Attention and Performance VIII* (pp. 361-381). Hillsdale, New Jersey: Lawrence Erlbaum Associates.

Getty, D.J., Swets, J.B., Swets, J.A., & Green, D.M. (1979). On the prediction of confusion matrices from similarity judgments. *Perception & Psychophysics,* **26**, 1-19.

Grau, J.W., & Kemler Nelson, D.G. (1988). The distinction between integral and separable dimensions: Evidence for the integrality of pitch and loudness. *Journal of Experimental Psychology: General*, **117**, 347-370.

Gravetter, F., & Lockhead, G. (1973). Critical range as a frame of reference for stimulus judgment. *Psychological Review*, **80**, 203-216.

Green, D.M., & Swets, J.A. (1966). *Signal detection theory and psychophysics*. New York: Wiley.

Gregson, Robert A.M. (1975). *Psychometrics of Similarity*. New York: Academic Press.

Handel, S., & Imai, S. (1972). The free classification of analyzable and unanalyzable stimuli. *Perception & Psychophysics*, **12**, 108-116.

Hefner, R.A. (1958). *Extensions of the law of comparative judgment to discriminable and multidimensional stimuli.* Unpublished doctoral dissertation, University of Michigan.

Hovland, C.I. (1937a). The generalization of conditioned responses: I. The sensory generalization of conditioned responses with varying frequencies of tone. *Journal of General Psychology*, **17**, 125-148.

Hovland, C.I. (1937b). The generalization of conditioned responses: II. The sensory generalization of conditioned responses with varying intensities of tone. *Journal of Genetic Psychology*, **51**, 279-291.

Hull, C.L. (1943). *Principles of behavior.* New York: Appleton-Century.

Hyman, R., & Well, A. (1967). Judgments of similarity and spatial models. *Perception & Psychophysics*, **2**, 233-248.

Hyman R., & Well, A. (1968). Perceptual separability and spatial models. *Perception & Psychophysics*, **3**, 161-165.

Indow, T. (1988). Multidimensional studies of Munsell color solid. *Psychological Review*, **95**, 456-470.

Indow, T., & Kanazawa, K. (1960). Multidimensional mapping of Munsell colors varying in hue, chroma, and value. *Journal of Experimental Psychology*, **59**, 330-336.

James, W. (1890). *The principles of psychology*. New York: Dover.

Johnson, G.J. (1975). Positional mediation of intraserial associations. *American Journal of Psychology,* **88**, 49-63.

Johnson, G.J. (1991). A distinctiveness model of serial learning. *Psychological Review*, **98**, 204-217.

Krantz, D.H. (1967). Rational distance functions for multidimensional scaling. *Journal of Mathematical Psychology*, **4**, 226-245.

Krantz, D.H., Luce, R.D., Suppes, P., & Tversky, A. (Eds.) (1971). *Foundations of measurement: Vol. 1. Additive polynomial representations*. San Diego: Academic Press.

Krueger, L. (1989). Reconciling Fechner and Stevens: Toward a unified psychophysical law. *Behavioral and Brain Sciences*, **12**, 251-320.

Krumhansl, C.L. (1978). Concerning the applicability of geometric models to similarity data: The interrelationship between similarity and spatial density. *Psychological Review*, **85**, 445-463.

Kruskal, J.B. (1964a). Multidimensional scaling by optimizing goodness of fit to a nonmetric hypothesis. *Psychometrika*, **29**, 1-27.

Kruskal, J.B. (1964b). Nonmetric multidimensional scaling: A numerical method. *Psychometrika*, **29**, 115-129.

Lockhead, G.R. (1972). Processing dimensional stimuli: A note. *Psychological Review*, **79**, 410-419.

Lockhead, G.R. (1979). Holistic versus analytic process models: A reply. *Journal of Experimental Psychology: Human Perception and Performance*, **5**, 746-755.

Luce, R.D. (1959). *Individual choice behavior*. New York: Wiley.

Luce, R.D. (1963) Detection and recognition. In R.D. Luce, R.R. Bush, & E. Galanter (Eds.), *Handbook of Mathematical Psychology*. (Vol. 1, pp.103-189). New York: Wiley.

Macmillan, N.A., & Creelman, C.D. (1991). *Detection theory: A user's guide*. Cambridge: Cambridge University Press.

Marks, L.E. (1974). On scales of sensation: Prolegomena to any future psychophysics that will be able to come forth as a science. *Perception & Psychophysics,* **16**, 358-376.

Medin, D.L. (1989). Concepts and conceptual structure. *American Psychologist,* **44**, 1469-1481.

Medin, D.L., Goldstone, R.L., & Gentner, D. (1990). Similarity involving attributes and relations: Judgments of similarity and differences are not inverse. *American Psychological Society*, **1**, 64-68.

Medin, D.L., & Schaffer, M.M. (1978). Context theory of classification learning. *Psychological Review*, **85**, 207-238.

Melara, R.D. (1989a). Dimensional interaction between color and pitch. *Journal of Experimental Psychology: Human Perception and Performance*, **15**, 69-79.

Melara, R.D. (1989b). Similarity relations among synesthetic stimuli and their attributes. *Journal of Experimental Psychology: Human Perception and Performance*, **115**, 212-231.

Melara, R.D., & Marks, L.E. (1990). Perceptual primacy of dimensions: Support for a model of dimensional interaction. *Journal of Experimental Psychology: Human Perception and Performance*, **16**, 398-414.

Melara, R.D., Marks, L.E., & Lesko, K.E. (1991). *Optimal processes in similarity judgments*. Manuscript submitted for publication.

Melara, R.D., Marks, L.E., & Potts, B. (1991). *The primacy of dimensions in color perception*. Manuscript submitted for publication.

Murphy, G.L., & Medin, D.L. (1985). The role of theories in conceptual coherence. *Psychological Review*, **92**, 289-316.

Nosofsky, R.M. (1984). Choice, similarity, and the context theory of classification. *Journal of Experimental Psychology: Learning, Memory, and Cognition*, **10**, 104-114.

Nosofsky, R.M. (1986). Attention, similarity, and the identification-categorization relationship. *Journal of Experimental Psychology: General*, **115**, 39-57.

Nosofsky, R.M. (1987). Attention and learning processes in the identification and categorization of integral stimuli. *Journal of Experimental Psychology: Learning, Memory, and Cognition*, **13**, 87-109.

Nosofsky, R.M. (1991). Tests of an exemplar model for relating perceptual classification and recognition memory. *Journal of Experimental Psychology*, **17**, 3-27.

Parducci, A. (1965). Category judgments: A range-frequency model. *Psychological Review*, **72**, 407-418.

Pavlov, I. (1927). *Conditioned reflexes*. Oxford: Oxford University Press.

Podgorny, P., & Garner, W.R. (1979). Reaction time as a measure of inter- and intraobject visual similarity: Letters of the alphabet. *Perception & Psychophysics*, **26**, 37-52.

Pomerantz, J.R. (1983). Global and local precedence: Selective attention in form and motion perception. *Journal of Experimental Psychology: General*, **112**, 515-540.

Pomerantz, J.R. (1986). Visual form perception: An overview. In E.C. Schwab & H.C. Nusbaum (Eds.), *Pattern recognition by humans and machines: Visual perception* (pp. 1-30). New York: Academic Press.

Restle, F. (1961). *Psychology of judgment and choice*. New York: Wiley.

Richardson, M.W. (1938). Multidimensional psychophysics. *Psychological Bulletin*, **35**, 659-660.

Rips, L.J. (1989). Similarity, typicality, and categorization. In S. Vosniadou & A. Ortony (Eds.), *Similarity and analogical reasoning* (pp. 21-59). Cambridge: Cambridge University Press.

Schönemann, P.H. (1990). Psychophysical maps for rectangles. In H.-G. Geissler (Ed.) *Psychophysical explorations of mental structures* (pp. 149-164). Toronto, Canada: Hogrefe & Huber.

Schönemann, P.H., Dorcey, T., & Kienapple, K. (1985). Subadditive concatenation in dissimilarity judgments. *Perception & Psychophysics*, **38**, 1-17.

Schönemann, P.H., & Lazare, A. (1987). Psychophysical maps for subadditive dissimilarity ratings. *Perception & Psychophysics*, **42**, 342-354.

Shepard, R.N. (1957). Stimulus and response generalization: A stochastic model relating generalization to distance in psychological space. *Psychometrika*, **22**, 325-345.

Shepard, R.N. (1958a). Stimulus and response generalization: Deduction of the generalization gradient from a trance model. *Psychological Review*, **65**, 242-256.

Shepard, R.N. (1958b). Stimulus and response generalization: Tests of a model relating generalization to distance in psychological space. *Journal of Experimental Psychology*, **65**, 509-523.

Shepard, R.N. (1962a). The analysis of proximities: Multidimensional scaling with an unknown distance function. I. *Psychometrika*, **27**, 125-140.

Shepard, R.N. (1962b). The analysis of proximities: Multidimensional scaling with an unknown distance function. II. *Psychometrika*, **27**, 219-246.

Shepard, R.N. (1964). Attention and the metric structure of the stimulus space. *Journal of Mathematical Psychology*, **1**, 54-87.

Shepard, R.N. (1974). Representation of structures in similarity data: Problems and prospects. *Psychometrika*, **39**, 373-421.

Shepard, R.N. (1986). Discrimination and generalization in identification and classification. *Journal of Experimental Psychology: General*, **115**, 58-61.

Shepard, R.N. (1987). Toward a universal law of generalization for psychological science. *Science*, **237**, 1317-1323.

Smith, J.D., & Kemler Nelson, D.G. (1984). Overall similarity in adults' classification: The child in all of us. *Journal of Experimental Psychology: General*, **113**, 137-159.

Smith, L.B. (1989). A model of perceptual classification in children and adults. *Psychological Review*, **96**, 125-144.

Stevens, S.S. (1975). *Psychophysics: Introduction to its perceptual, neural, and social prospects*. New York: Wiley.

Suppes, P., Krantz, D.H., Luce, R.D., & Tversky, A. (Eds.). (1989). *Foundations of measurement: Vol. 2. Geometrical, threshold, and probabilistic representations*. San Diego: Academic Press.

Thurstone, L.L. (1927). A law of comparative judgment. *Psychological Review*, **34**, 273-286.

Torgerson, W.S. (1958). *Theory and methods of scaling*. New York: Wiley.

Torgerson, W.S. (1965). Multidimensional scaling of similarity. *Psychometrika*, **30**, 379-393.

Tversky, A. (1977). Features of similarity. *Psychological Review*, **84**, 327-352.

Tversky, A., & Gati, I. (1978). Studies of similarity. In E. Rosch & B.B. Lloyd (Eds.), *Cognition and Categorization* (pp. 79-99). Hillsdale, New Jersey: Lawrence Erlbaum Associates.

Tversky, A., & Gati, I. (1982). Similarity, separability and the triangle inequality. *Psychological Review*, **89**, 123-154.

Tversky, A., & Krantz, D.H. (1970). The dimensional representation and the metric structure of similarity data. *Journal of Mathematical Psychology*, **7**, 572-596.

Ward, T.B. (1983). Response tempo and separable-integral responding: Evidence for an integral-to-separable processing sequence in visual perception. *Journal of Experimental Psychology: Human Perception and Performance*, **9**, 103-112.

Young, G., & Householder, A.S. (1938). Discussion of a set of points in terms of their mutual distances. *Psychometrika*, **3**, 19-21.

Zinnes, J.L., & MacKay, D.B. (1983). Probabilistic multidimensional scaling: Complete and incomplete data. *Psychometrika*, **48**, 27-48.

Psychophysical Approaches to Cognition
D. Algom (Editor)

7

PSYCHOPHYSICS OF VISUAL IMAGERY

John C. Baird

Dartmouth College

and

Timothy L. Hubbard

Eastern Oregon State College

Table of Contents

I. Visual Imagery

I see my mother's face. I remember my mother's face. I image my mother's face. One difference in these experiences is that my mother's face needs to be physically present for perception to occur, but my mother's face need not be physically present for memory or imagery to occur. Despite this difference, the experience of the specific shape, size, coloring and features of my mother's face is highly similar, regardless of whether the face is perceived, remembered, or imaged. In the past decade a considerable amount of research has documented such similarities among perception, memory, and imagery; quite often, the methods used to compare these types of experiences have been borrowed from psychophysics. Regardless of which theories of perception and cognition we care to entertain, the objective methods of psychophysics allow us to compare results obtained when subjects are assumed to be utilizing skills associated with perception, memory and imagery. This chapter reviews our own research program in this area, and in particular, the functional relationships we have discovered between the recalled and imaged sizes and distances of familiar and unfamiliar objects.

According to Kosslyn (1990), there are two major purposes of imagery: a means to retrieve information from memory and a means to anticipate future events. In both instances, it is assumed that a visual image is formed as a unitary depiction, available to the person as an analogue representation, rather than as a propositional form involving the listing of object properties and their relations. When we say that we see a train approaching us in the distance, we do not mean that we are mentally sorting through a verbal list of the train's size, shape, speed, weight, etc. Similarly, when we consider an image of a train moving down the track, we experience a wholistic depiction of the scene, and do not find ourselves checking off a list of declarative statements about the train's characteristics.

Ever since the original experiments by Shepard and his colleagues on people's ability to mentally rotate images of perceived objects (Shepard & Cooper, 1982) and by Kosslyn and his colleagues on people's ability to scan or transform images of described or perceived objects (Kosslyn, 1980), a debate has raged concerning whether mental imagery should be considered a closer relative of perception and hence more depictive (Kosslyn, 1980, 1981; Kosslyn & Pomerantz, 1977) or of language and hence more descriptive (Pylyshyn, 1973, 1981, 1984). Some theorists (Anderson, 1978) have disparaged of ever finding data capable of deciding this issue, while others (Marschark, Richman, Yuille, & Hunt, 1987) feel that data on how imagery is used (e.g., processes and functions) cannot address questions of how imagery is constructed (e.g., structure).

Some theorists have suggested that aspects of imagery which are attributed to the depictive nature of imagery are in fact not due to properties of imagery per se, but are due to non-imagistic factors such as cognitive penetrability or tacit knowledge (Pylyshyn, 1981), demand characteristics (Mitchell & Richman, 1980), and experimenter bias (Intons-Peterson, 1983; Intons-Peterson & White, 1981; see also Goldston, Hinrichs, & Richman, 1985). Although these criticisms certainly involve valid methodological issues, numerous studies have also suggested that imagery can nonetheless function as a depictive representation in its own right (Finke & Pinker, 1982, 1983; Hubbard & Stoeckig, 1988; Jolicoeur & Kosslyn, 1983, 1985; Pinker, Choate, & Finke, 1984).

Hubbard (1991) has argued that abstract, propositional, and descriptive representations do not account for what is central about images -- the qualia, the depictive sensory-like aspects. Thus, imagistic depiction goes beyond the mere propositional description. These depictive elements of imagery can and do play a functional role in human cognition (for reviews, see Finke, 1989; Kosslyn, 1990; Paivio, 1971, 1986) and imagery is thus more than just an epiphenomenon of linguistic or propositional representation. From a psychophysical standpoint this is fortunate, because psychophysical methods and theory seem much more relevant to the study of the imagery experience if imagery is considered a depictive quasi-perceptual form of representation and not a part of linguistic structure. Regardless of the ultimate representational basis of imagery and perception, however, the experience of imagery seems highly similar to the experience of perception, and we discuss some ways in which researchers can exploit that similarity by using psychophysical methods and theory.

II. Functional Equivalence

The phenomenal similarity of perception and imagery and the successful use of psychophysical techniques to investigate properties of images suggest that there may be similarities in the cognitive structures, mechanisms or processes that are invoked by subjects when engaged in either perceptual or cognitive tasks (Shepard & Podgorny, 1978). The idea that images may use some of the same cognitive processes or structures used in perception has been referred to as "functional equivalence" and is supported by psychophysical (e.g., Farah, 1985), chronometric (Brooks, 1968; Hubbard & Stoeckig, 1988; Kosslyn, 1980; Shepard & Cooper, 1982) and neurophysiological (Farah, 1988) evidence. Alternative hypotheses to each functional equivalent result can be given, but the hypothesis of a functional equivalence between imagery and perception is the single best overall explanation for results across a wide range of tasks (Finke & Shepard, 1986). Even in a strong form, however, the notion of functional equivalence need not completely equate images and percepts. In most nonpathological cases we are able to distinguish between perceived reality and imaged fantasy (though see Johnson, 1988; Johnson & Raye, 1981). Although many researchers accept the hypothesis that images are processed by mechanisms similar to or even identical with those used in the processing of percepts (Farah, 1985, 1988; Finke, 1985;

Finke & Shepard, 1986; Kosslyn, 1980, 1987), such a position is not universally accepted (Pylyshyn, 1984; Reisberg & Chambers, 1985).

To date, there have been two main strategies for testing the functional equivalence hypothesis. One strategy is to show that imagery in one modality interferes with perception in that modality but not with perception in other modalities (Brooks, 1968; Segal & Fusella, 1970) and that subjects instructed to image a given stimulus produce response patterns similar to subjects who perceive that stimulus (Finke & Kurtzman, 1981; Hubbard & Stoeckig, 1988; Podgorny & Shepard, 1978). A second strategy is to test patients in whom brain activity can be noninvasively tracked or who have suffered strokes or other cortical damage (for review, see Farah, 1984, 1988). Patients who have suffered strokes that disrupt perception in selected parts of their visual fields also experience similar difficulties in imaging objects that would be "seen" in that part of the visual field. For example, Bisiach and Luzzatti (1978) asked patients to assume they were standing in a familiar outdoor setting and to report the buildings that they "saw." The patients reported only buildings whose images would have fallen in that part of the visual field that was unaffected by the stroke. It was not a matter of simply not remembering those particular buildings, because if the subjects later visualized the same scene from a different vantage point, they were then able to image the buildings that had previously fallen within the damaged part of their visual field, but were unable to visualize buildings which they had previously "seen" but which now fell within the damaged portion of their visual field (see also Sacks, 1990). Levine, Warach, and Farah (1985) report that patients who are unable to recognize faces are also unable to image faces, and that patients who are unable to perceive object locations are also unable to image those object locations.

The clearest example of a strong form of functional equivalence in a theory of imagery is found in Kosslyn (1980, 1981) who treats a percept or image as though it were constructed in a "visual buffer." The visual buffer is a "functional space," with its functionality defined by the way various cognitive processes access locations in the buffer. For example, the finding that subjects take longer to scan across a greater imaged distance, just as they would take longer to visually scan across a greater perceived distance, shows that functional space is preserved within an image (Kosslyn, Ball & Reiser, 1978). Once a visual image is created, there are a number of processes that operate on it, including procedures that generate, inspect, and transform. A functional equivalence suggests that these processes operate in a similar fashion regardless of whether the stimulus portrayed in the buffer arises from long-term memory (imagery) or impinges through the sense channels (perception). Jackendoff (1987) has specified this equivalency in even greater detail, suggesting that the "visual buffer" in Kosslyn's theory is equivalent to the "2½ D" sketch in Marr's (1982) theory of vision.

A strong form of functional equivalence is also found in Shepard's research on internal representation. Shepard and Chipman (1970) had subjects rank-order states of the US according to the similarity of their shapes. In one condition, subjects sorted cards containing actual outline drawings of each state, while in another condition, cards contained only the printed names of each state. The average rank number for each pair of states was highly similar across the two conditions, leading the authors to conclude that a "second-order isomorphism" existed between the external objects and their internal representations. Shepard, Kilpatric, and Cunninghum (1975) had subjects rate the similarities of pairs of numbers in a variety of formats (sound of spoken English names, Arabic numerals, rows of dots). Similarity judgments depended on the form in which the numbers were judged and not on the form in which they were presented, an outcome consistent with the notion that functional similarities of the external referent objects to which the representations corresponded.

Shepard's well-known studies on mental rotation (reviewed in Shepard & Cooper, 1982) demonstrate that subjects require greater amounts of time to compare targets if the targets differ by greater degrees of angular disparity, and these results also support the idea that the internal representation of an object is isomorphic to the external object (since external objects also require greater amounts of time to move through greater degrees of angular disparity). Shepard (1981) also hypothesizes that in establishing the equivalency of physical objects A and C, the mental representation of object A is transformed and compared to the mental representation of object C. If object A is transformed (i.e., rotated or translated) to object C, object A has to pass through an intermediate form B. Shepard proposes that the mental representation of A, say A*, must pass through an intermediate form B* on its way to C*. Thus, the intermediate states of the mental representation are in one-to-one correspondence (isomorphism) with the intermediate states of the physical and proximal stimuli, even when the physical or proximal stimuli are not seen in the intermediate state (see also Cooper, 1976). For example, in rotating a physical object from the upright to 90 degrees, the physical object has to pass through all the orientations intermediate to the upright and 90 degrees; Shepard's idea is that the mental representation of an object undergoing the same transformation must also pass through all the same intermediate orientations.

A weaker form of functional equivalence is given by Finke (1980), who restricts the level of equivalence somewhat by linking it to the level of processing. Higher-level visual processing (perceiving/imaging size, shape or orientation) results in more overlap, that is, more equivalence, than lower-level processing (perceiving/imaging brightness and relative contrast). A comparable form of functional equivalence in a nonvisual domain is reported in Hubbard and Stoeckig (in press) who propose that many aspects of musical imagery can be accounted for within a modular processing system consisting of a "surface" representation module whose outputs correspond to the experienced qualia of music (e.g., pitch, timbre). In perception, the input to such a module would come through the sense organs, while in imagery, the input would come from a memory store. By utilizing the same structural or processing modules, similar outputs for perception and imagery are obtained, thus accounting for the similarities in perceived and imaged musical stimuli. Algom, Wolf, and Bergman (1985) address functional equivalence from a different direction. They note that judgments of perceived and remembered quantities are computed in the same fashion. In this case, use of the same "cognitive algebra" (see the chapter by Anderson)[1] for both perception and imagery would be tantamount to a functional equivalence.

III. Visual Memory

Among the many distinctions made between different types of memory systems, perhaps the most useful from the standpoint of imagery and psychophysical research is between "semantic" and "episodic" memory (Tulving, 1983). As long ago as 1951, Furlong noted this distinction by pointing out the differences between a situation where a person remembers seeing someone at the grocery store and when a person remembers the square root of nine: "In the former case the mind looks back to a past event: we recollect, reminisce, retrospect; there is imagery. In the latter case this looking-back is absent, and there is little or no imagery." (Furlong, 1951, p.6). According to Tulving, specification of the time and place of the remembered event is a necessary component of episodic memory, but not of semantic memory. Tulving further states that "the registration of information into the episodic system is more direct than that into the semantic system. The episodic system is capable of recording and retaining information about perceptible properties of stimuli that can be apprehended immediately by the senses." (1983, p.41).

---

[1] Editor's note.

Whereas the distinction between these two memory systems is admittedly more blurred than Tulving suggests, there are real advantages to maintaining this distinction when discussing the psychophysics of memory and imagery. In particular, the theoretical story linking perception, memory and imagery hangs together in a coherent fashion only if one considers events that fall under the rubric of episodic, rather than semantic, memory. Perception is the apprehension of actual events unfolding over time and existing in real space. Memory for these events at a later point in time involves memory for the contextual situation surrounding the original event perceived; and if one is asked to image this same event from the past, the contextual information provided by time and space is once again an inextricable part of the total image containing the event in question. Although people may not be able to remember exact details surrounding perceptual episodes from the past, they do appear to recall, and are adept at imaging, an incredible amount of information concerning events occurring in their everyday environment. If it were otherwise, people would not be able to navigate safely through a single day, and would be unable to plan for the next.

IV. Psychophysics

The similarities among perception, memory, and imagery can be profitably explored by psychophysical methods, and in fact, the so-called "cognitive" psychologists working on such problems typically employ methods from scaling and psychophysics, or offshoots of these methods, sometimes without even being aware of the link between their research and traditional psychophysics. It is a great advantage from a theoretical standpoint if exactly the same methods can be applied in all three domains (perception, memory, imagery), because this allows us to attribute differences in results to differences in the phenomena of interest, rather than to differences in the methods used in their investigation.

Two types of psychophysical responses seem most relevant to research on memory and imagery: (a) reaction time and (b) scaling of response magnitudes. Within traditional psychophysics the use of reaction time is discussed extensively by Luce (1986) and scaling of response magnitudes is discussed by Baird and Noma (1978), Gescheider (1985), and Stevens (1975). Within visual imagery, these two types of responses can help define the functional relationships between quantities such as the size and distance of an imaged object. For reaction time, an investigator may look at the speed with which a subject changes focus on different parts of an imaged object as a function of their separation in space. For scaling of response magnitudes, an investigator may look at the response magnitude as a function of the physical separations (distances) among the stimuli, and compare the response magnitude of an imaged stimulus to the intensity of the physical stimulus or another imaged stimulus. For both reaction time and scaling functions, the question of interest is whether relationships between imaged and perceived magnitudes, or imaged magnitudes and physical intensities are the same as the relationships between perceived magnitudes and physical intensities. If they are the same, then similar lines of theoretical arguments might apply to both the domains of imagery and perception. In our discussion, we focus primarily on the scaling of response magnitudes.

V. Perceptual Memory

A literature has emerged on what is referred to as "memory psychophysics". Here subjects are asked to give magnitude estimates of the intensities (sizes, distances) of familiar objects; familiar either through the commerce with them in the everyday environment, or by dint of the fact that they have been previously observed in the laboratory under controlled conditions. The results of such studies may yield important clues as to the relationship between memory and perception, and what it is that actually is stored in memory concerning the physical characteristics of objects (Moyer, Bradley, Sorenson, Whiting, & Mansfield, 1978). However, because this topic is treated in detail by Algom in this volume (see also, Weist & Bell, 1985; Da Silva, 1985), it will not be reviewed here, except to note that such results must someday be tied in with results arising from much earlier experiments on the role played in perception by the subject's assumptions about the metric characteristics of objects about which he or she is asked to render a judgment. We now turn to this topic.

Familiar Size

For over a century the link between the perceived size and distance of objects has been a prime focus for research in visual space perception (see Sedgwick, 1986). One aspect of this problem that has received considerable attention concerns the role of familiarity in perception, and whether familiarity with one or two dimensions of an object (such as size and subtended visual angle) can uniquely determine the value of a third dimension (such as distance). The data generally support the contention that familiar size can influence perceived distance, although there is substantial variability among subjects (Baird, 1963; Baird, 1970; Epstein, 1967). For example, if a line of light is presented to a subject in an otherwise dark room, then there is no significant correlation between judgments of size and distance; however, if the experimenter states that the line has a certain metric length (e.g., 12 inches), then this information combines with the subtended visual angle to determine a unique perceived distance, and this distance is in accord with what it would be in the real world for an object of that length and subtended visual angle (Baird, 1964).

If we examine what occurs in experiments such as this, we see that the subjects' task involves, in addition to perception, elements of long-term memory and imagery. The subject must recall, or image, an object from the past that had the same stated length and subtended visual angle as the experimental stimulus. For example, the subject might imagine positioning himself so that a hiking boot standing one foot high in the hallway appears to subtend the same visual angle as the line of light now being exposed for judgment in the dark room. The subject's stated estimate of target distance in the image depends on how far away the particular subject images himself to be when the familiar boot would subtend that particular visual angle. Familiar size, when combined with a visual angle, can thus influence perceived distance; similarly, familiar distance, when combined with a visual angle, can also influence perceived size (Coltheart, 1970). We can account for the effect of familiar distance by similar reasoning -- the subject must recall (image) an object from the past that satisfies the constraints set by the distance stated by the experimenter and visual angle subtended at the eye by the target stimulus.

Although this research tradition on the effects of familiar size and distance on perception was not the primary impetus for the much later experiments conducted by Kosslyn (1980) and others on imaged distance as a function of stated object size, the similarities in the two research traditions are striking. The only real difference is that in an imagery experiment, a particular visual angle is not presented, but must be supplied by a subject-generated image. However, such a standardized visual angle is often provided by asking subjects to position themselves in such a way that the familiar object appears to fill a specified portion of the visual field (in the case of Kosslyn's studies, subjects were instructed to image the named object such that the image completely filled the imaginal visual field) -- which is in fact a fixed visual angle. This topic will be addressed more fully below.

Cognitive Mapping

The ability to anticipate events and move about successfully in the environment seems to require that we maintain some cognitive representation of the environment, which is used in conjunction with the stimulus information available to the sense organs. This assumption has been a keystone for most empirical theories of perception (see Ames, 1946-1947; Epstein, 1967; Neisser, 1967; Pastore, 1971; Rock, 1983).

Over the past few decades interest has grown about how well people are able to cognitively represent their familiar environments, and research on memory for spatial environments has increased. Studies that focus on a person's awareness of large-scale environments such as countries, cities, and neighborhoods are generally referred to as investigations of "cognitive maps" (Saarinen, 1976). One approach to determine the accuracy of cognitive maps is to have subjects estimate the relative distances between items in their familiar environment by the use of magnitude estimation. For example, all possible pairs of buildings on a campus can be presented to a subject who estimates the distance between the two members of each pair. Since the physical distances can be obtained by direct measurement, it is possible to plot a Stevens function (Baird & Noma, 1978; chap. 5) relating judged and physical distances (Baird, Merrill, & Tannenbaum, 1979). It is generally reported that the power law holds well for these conditions:

$$J = \lambda D^{\gamma} \tag{1}$$

Here, J is judged distance, D is physical distance between a pair of buildings, γ is the exponent, and λ is the multiplicative constant. In our studies of the cognitive mapping of a campus (Baird et al., 1979), we found that the exponent of Equation 1 was slightly less than 1 (approximately .9), indicating that people were quite accurate in recalling and representing the distances between buildings in their familiar environment.

When subjects are queried as to their judgment strategies in this task, they typically report that they imagined themselves standing at some particular location in the environment from which they could gain a clear view of the buildings in question. The estimate of distance between the buildings was then based upon the nature of the information in this image. Similarly, if you ask students to draw a map of their campus, they typically map buildings in a systematic order that suggests they are imagining themselves seeing the buildings from a specific vantage point. For example, they may imagine themselves in the center of campus, and consequently, the symbols of the buildings are placed on the map as if they were moving their eyes around a 360 degree arc and reading off the successive images that represent the buildings (comparable findings supporting the impressive veridicality of cognitive maps are reported by Sherman, Croxton, & Giovanatto, 1979).

Images of Aesthetic Quality

Memories of more complex and subtle aspects of the natural environment have also been investigated by judgment methods taken directly from psychophysics. The field of experimental aesthetics was in fact established by Fechner (1876), and rested upon the methods he had developed earlier for studies of sensory systems. In our research (Merrill & Baird, 1980), magnitude estimates were obtained of the aesthetic quality of outdoor locations on a familiar campus and these estimates were compared to those obtained indoors where subjects were asked to imagine themselves in the same outdoor locations, and to base their judgments on visual impression, auditory impression, and overall, composite sensory quality.

One group of students toured the Dartmouth College campus and nearby commercial district and gave magnitude estimates of aesthetic quality at each of 32 locations. A second group made the same judgments based on their memory of the aesthetic quality at each of the same locations -- identified briefly by the experimenter (e.g., "imagine you are in front of the hardware store," or "you are standing in front of the computer center").

The relationships between on-site judgments (Exp. I) and judgments based on imagery (Exp. II) are given in Figure 7.1. Results based on memory/imagery and actual perception of the environment are highly correlated, suggesting that students carried with them a fairly detailed mental representation of their aesthetic outdoor environment. In addition, the relative ratings given for the different locations stayed roughly constant across seasons of the year. The highest correlations occurred for the composite quality ratings and the ratings based on vision alone, indicating that overall aesthetic quality is strongly influenced by visual impressions.

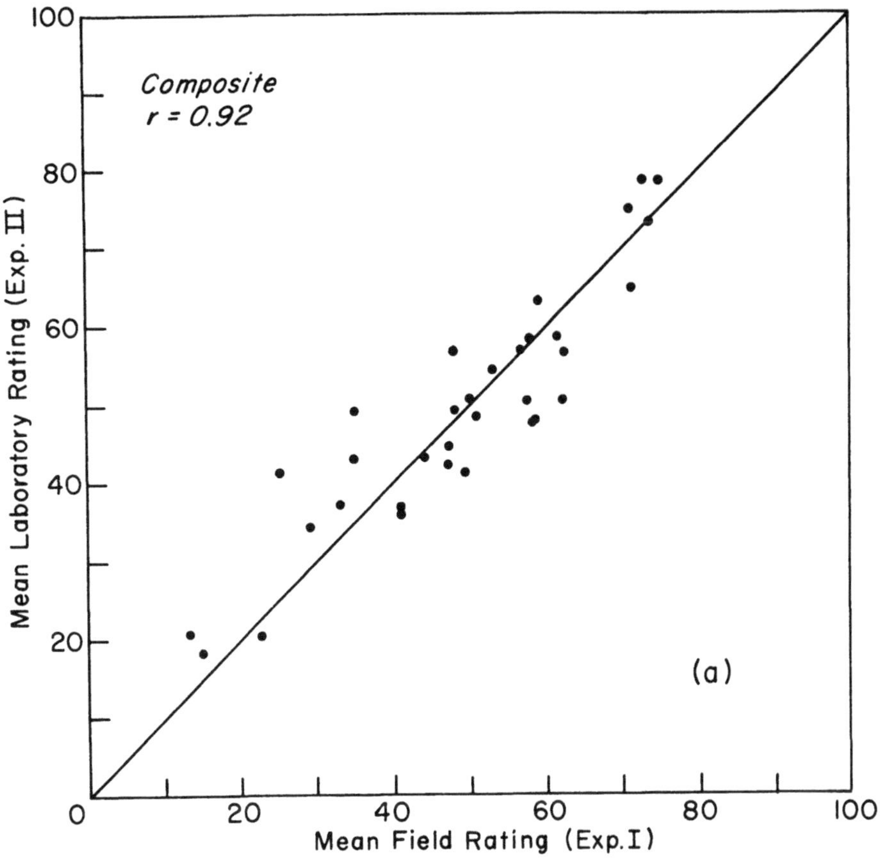

Figure 7.1: The relationship between ratings based on direct observation in the field (Exp. I) and ratings based on imaging the environment from the same familiar locations (Exp. II). Aesthetic judgments based on composite stimuli. After Merrill & Baird (1980).

Imaging Social Activities

In addition to their awareness of object properties in the environment, people also are able to image familiar social settings and accurately report on the specific activities taking place in them. In a study of predicted and observed activity patterns in a campus setting we observed the activity patterns of students in 12 different locations associated with two well-known campus buildings, and then had a group of students enter their predictions of such activities by typing numerical estimates into a computer. Although the absolute estimates of the frequencies of all activities greatly exceeded the actual numbers of people engaged in such activities, students did render accurate relative estimates; for instance, the percentage of individuals engaged in *reading* and *conversing* matched quite well the actual percentage of people performing that activity at specified periods of the day (Baird, Noma, Nagy, & Quinn, 1976).

Figure 7.2 shows the mean percent of people for activities in two campus buildings (center and library) at each of three times of day and for all times combined (top graphs). Data are presented for direct, on site, observations and for student predictions, where N is the number of occasions on which the means are based. Our interpretation of these results is that students are able to image a familiar scene of a location and then simply count (or estimate) the number of individuals in that scene engaged in the various activities. Discussion with subjects after the experiment suggests that imagery of this sort was often used, and that estimates were based on a pictorial representation rather than on some logical derivation from knowledge of the type of function one might expect to see in each location. As with the case of cognitive mapping and estimates of aesthetic quality, it appears that subjects are retrieving episodes from memory and relying on such images in making their estimates about various characteristics of the familiar environment.

Abstract Images

There is evidence that on occasion people who are asked to judge non-perceptual features of their environment, based only on memory/imagery, in fact rely on some perceptual feature instead. In order to explain this we postulate that

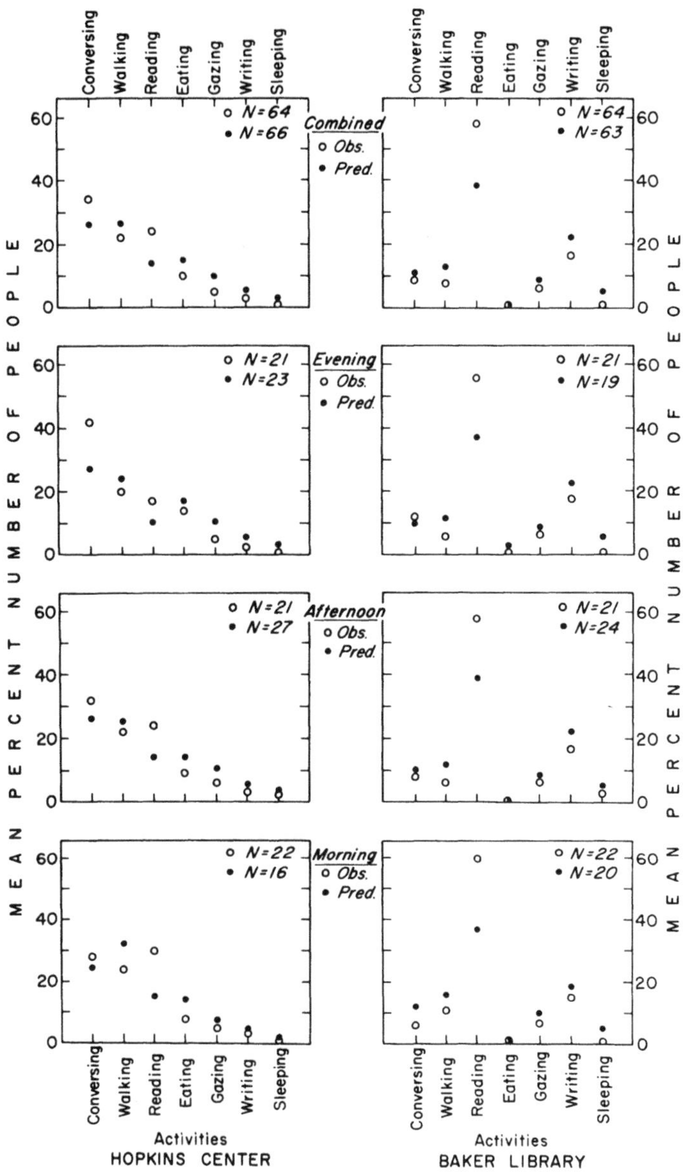

Figure 7.2: Mean percent number of people for activities in two campus buildings (center and library) at each of three times of day and for all times combined (top graphs). Data are presented for observations and student predictions, presumably based on imagery, where N is the number of occasions on which the means are based. After Baird et al. (1976).

subjects retrieve episodes from memory and form an image of the object in question. It is this visual image that constitutes the immediate basis for judgment. For instance, we conducted experiments to assess students' awareness of the energy requirements of familiar household appliances, such as *electric toothbrush, shaver, desk lamp, stereo, blanket, dishwasher, toaster,* and *range* (Baird & Brier, 1981). Subjects were told to assume that the average *clothes washer* uses 100 units of energy per hour and that other appliances presented (verbally) for judgment should be assigned a number such that it represents a relative value in respect to the washer. The median estimate of electrical expenditure ranged from 7.5 for an *electric toothbrush* to 200 for a *water heater*.

When we regressed the logarithm of the magnitude estimates against the logarithm of the actual wattage required by an appliance, as determined by direct inspection of the wattage labels on products in local stores, the slope (exponent) was .3, indicating a compression of the awareness of energy in respect to the actual values. On the other hand, when college students judged the physical volume occupied by these same appliances and we regressed judged energy against judged volume (in log-log coordinates) the exponent was approximately .7 (see Fig. 7.3). Such a result implies that people are relying heavily on their memory of the appearance of an actual appliance, and in particular, its size, when making judgments of its energy requirements. Such a finding is at least consistent with the view that subjects asked to judge energy requirements form a mental image of the appliance in question, and then utilize the relative size of the object in their image (compared to the standard) when deciding upon a numerical estimate. Unless they happen to have direct semantic knowledge about the physics of how these various appliances work, it is simply more expedient to base judgments on specific memories of past episodes in which they have observed such appliances. It seems that size is not the only variable of importance here, however, since if it were, then the exponent of the power function relating judged energy and judged volume (size) should be 1.

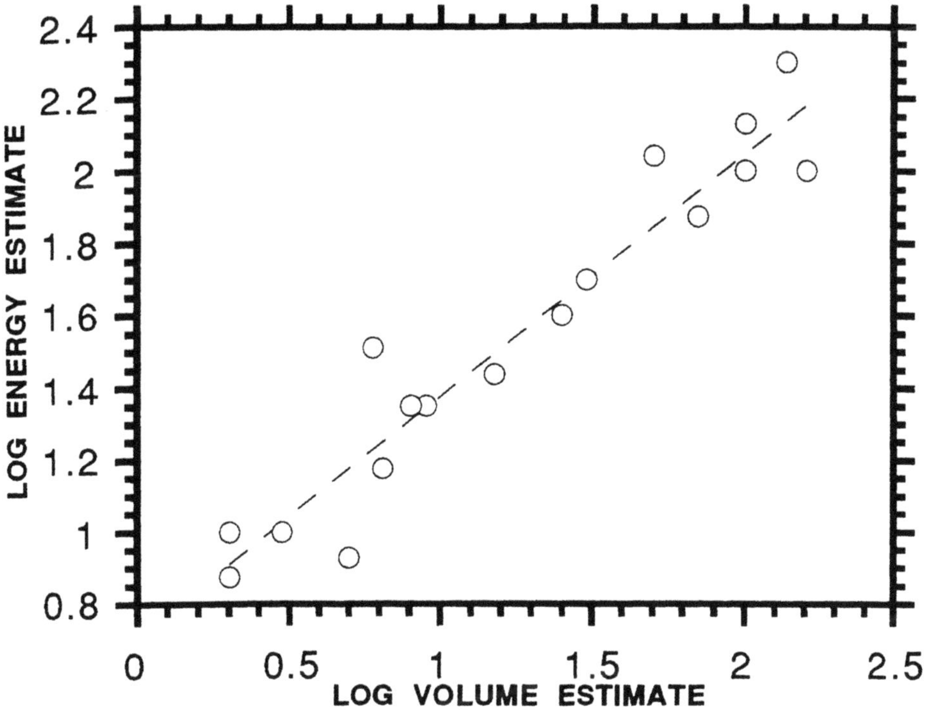

Figure 7.3: Median energy consumption estimates as a function of median volume estimates for 18 different electrical appliances. Logarithmic coordinates, where the linear function through the points has a slope of .7. After Baird & Brier (1981).

VI. Psychophysics of the Structure of Images

Structural properties of visual images have been a topic of interest for several years (for review, see Finke, 1989; Kosslyn, 1980; Shepard & Cooper, 1982), and we now consider how the use of magnitude estimation sheds light on this issue. The structural property we focus on involves distance, specifically, the way that distance is portrayed in a visual image.

Overflow Distance

One of the earliest systematic studies of the portrayal of distance in images was carried out by Kosslyn (1978, 1980) in his investigations of the "visual angle of the mind's eye." Kosslyn described some object (e.g., an animal, a featureless rectangle of a specific size) and asked subjects to visualize an object of the described type and size. Subjects then imagined "mentally walking," that is, imagined they were approaching the object in their image. When asked if the object appeared to loom larger, all subjects agreed that it did. Eventually, subjects reached a point where they had approached so close to the imaged object that it filled their entire visual imaginal field, where they could see all of the object at once, but if it were any closer, they could not see it all at once (i.e., it would overflow the edges of their image). When subjects reached this point, they estimated the distance to the imaged object that was portrayed in their image. Kosslyn named this distance the "overflow distance." The procedure was repeated for objects of different sizes, thus allowing examining of how imaged overflow distance varies as a function of the physical size of the referent object.

Kosslyn found a linear relationship between the stated size of the referent object and the distance at which an image of that object overflowed the edges of the mind's eye. Such a linear relationship suggests that the relationship between imaged distance at overflow, size of the referent object, and visual angle agreed with the size-distance invariance hypothesis (SDIH): for a fixed visual angle (θ), the ratio of perceived size (S) to perceived distance (D) of an object is constant (Epstein, Park & Casey, 1961):

$$\tan \theta = S/D \quad or \quad D = (1/\tan\theta)\ S \tag{2}$$

Somewhat surprisingly, Kosslyn found that although the SDIH held for many types of imaged objects, different objects had overflow angles of different sizes (different maximum "visual angle of the mind's eye"). Nonetheless, the portrayal of overflow distance in visual imagery appeared to be governed by (or is at least consistent with) the SDIH.

One aspect of these results should now be made more explicit. In typical perception experiments, a stimulus is presented and subjects estimate the value of some feature of that stimulus, often by exploiting other cues that are present. For example, subjects estimating distance may use the cues of familiar size and familiar visual angle as aids in estimating distance (see discussion of familiar size above). Thus, subjects have information about two of the terms in the SDIH (size, visual angle) and are able to use this information to estimate the value of the third term (distance). In an imagery experiment such as Kosslyn's, however, subjects are given explicit information about only one of the terms (size), and have to use a created image to "fill in" at least one of the missing values.

If only one of the three values is known, subjects should be unable to arrive at a unique solution. Specifically, if subjects are unable to retrieve either familiar visual angle or familiar size from imagery or memory, then they should not be able to specify a unique distance for any given object size. What subjects actually seem to do, however, is to create a visual image of the referent object and read the resultant values of at least one of the other parameters off the image. For example, if subjects are given only the stated size of the referent object (e.g., refrigerator, 6 feet tall), the distance and the visual angle could take any of a number of values (from a short distance and large visual angle ranging to a large distance and small visual angle). If subjects are able to retrieve information concerning a second parameter, in this case visual angle, then the combination of stated size and retrieved visual angle uniquely specify a single distance.

In the case of the overflow condition, subjects manipulated their images until a specified visual angle (the overflow angle) was obtained, thus they had access to two of the three terms in the SDIH. It then becomes a trivial exercise to specify the final term. For overflow data, the imaged distance was a linear function of stated size (for any given class of objects), thus implying that the visual angle was constant. Kosslyn felt that this constant visual angle defined the size of the imagery buffer, the "maximum visual angle of the mind's eye." This example used a psychophysical technique, magnitude estimation, and discovered a previously unknown property of visual images, namely, that the medium or structure within which images (perhaps the visual buffer) are created has a maximum, constant size for a given type of object.

First-sight Distance

An alternative interpretation of the overflow data is possible, however. It may be that the linear overflow function resulted not from properties of the imagery buffer, but from metric information contained within the image itself. More specifically, perhaps subjects imaged or remembered familiar objects at familiar distances that just happened to satisfy the SDIH because they were accustomed to seeing larger objects at larger distances and smaller objects at smaller distances. These familiar distances would be stored as specific episodes in memory and would be part of the metric information retrieved at the creation of an image. If a person imaged a house, the distance portrayed in the image of the house would probably be larger than the distance portrayed in an image of a flea, just because houses are generally seen at greater distances than are fleas. If sizes and distances were systematically related simply because familiar objects were imaged in their familiar settings, then the SDIH might be satisfied by default and not because the subject manipulated the image to achieve a constant point of overflow in the mind's eye or because of any structural property of the visual buffer.

To examine this, we asked subjects to visualize images of familiar objects and to report the distance at which the object was initially imaged in an untransformed image. We named this the "first-sight distance." If the SDIH held for the function relating first-sight distance to stated object size, then the results of Kosslyn's overflow experiments need not be due to any properties of the imagery buffer, but could be due to the more general metric information within the image (and the memory material from which the image was created). In fact, we obtained a nonlinear relationship between the stated size of the object and the distance at which that object was initially imaged, a relationship best described by a power function with an exponent less than 1 (Hubbard, Kall, & Baird, 1989; Hubbard & Baird, 1988). First-sight distance, while determined partly by metric size, was also affected by the type of object. In general, small objects were imaged at closer distances than large objects, but small objects which were typically experienced at further distances (e.g., a bird's nest) were imaged at relatively far distances while large objects typically experienced at near distances (e.g., refrigerator) were imaged at relatively close distances. As a result, the first-sight functions were considerably more variable than Kosslyn's overflow functions. There clearly was some metric information in the untransformed image before subjects began their imaginary walk toward overflow, but because the first-sight functions differed from the overflow function, we were able to rule out the possibility that the overflow functions Kosslyn reported were due solely to the metric information within the image itself.

Remembered Distance

The results of the first-sight imagery functions can also be compared with a condition in which subjects were asked to remember when they saw an object of a certain type, and to estimate how far away from their head the object was at that time (no mention of imagery being made). As shown in Figure 7.4, when remembered distance is plotted as a function of object size, and the function for remembered distance is compared with the function for imaged first-sight, the two functions are practically identical. Such similarity also supports the notions discussed earlier concerning visual memory and episodic memory: the percept and the image may both be encoded within a common episodic memory framework; thus, the basic functions are similar, even though (as discussed in more detail below) parameter values of the specific functions may vary. The similarity of functions is consistent with the notion of functional equivalence discussed earlier and implies a common underlying cognitive process. This conclusion is strengthened by the finding that during debriefing, practically all subjects claimed to have visualized the object, regardless of whether they were instructed to remember or image.

Additionally, subjects in both first-sight imagery and remembered distance conditions were asked to write down the physical contexts in which the imaged object appeared to be embedded. These contexts were written on individual cards and presented for free sorting to a separate group of naive subjects. The contexts in which remembered and imaged objects were embedded were

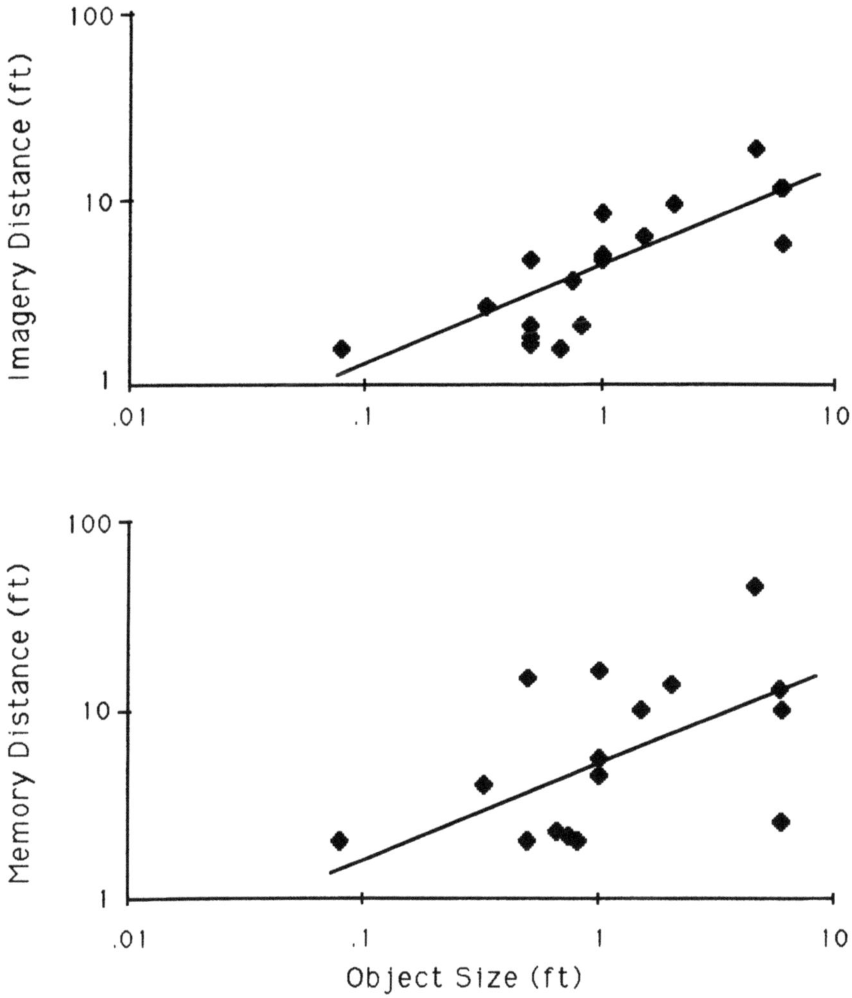

Figure 7.4: Median distance of imaged and remembered objects as a function of object size. The top panel shows the distance of imaged objects; the bottom panel shows the distance of remembered objects. After Figure 2 in Hubbard, Kall, & Baird (1989).

indistinguishable. Subjects could not reliably sort the contexts into those generated by the imagery group and those generated by the recall group.

We then asked subjects to report both a first-sight distance and an overflow distance (Hubbard & Baird, 1988). As shown in Figure 7.5, the first-sight functions were again best described by a power function with an exponent less than 1, while the overflow functions were strikingly linear (power function exponent = 1). Even though distances between first-sight and overflow points increased as object size increased, the relationship between overflow and first-sight was not simply a scalar multiplier, thus suggesting that the process underlying transformation to overflow distance is different from the process that yields first-sight distance. Another way to consider these results is to say that the transformation of a first-sight distance into an overflow distance is nonlinear.

In summary, when asked to recall or image a familiar object, subjects do indeed seem to form an image. That image, once formed, contains metric information such as size and distance, and subjects are able to report on these properties prior to any manipulations of the image. Specification of one variable (size) leads to constraints on other variables (distance) even in untransformed (first-sight) images. If subjects are given instructions to mentally approach the object, they can manipulate size, distance, and visual angle information in such a way as to bring about the desired relationship between themselves and the object; this manipulation will lead to further changes in the portrayed metric values of the other dimensions (e.g., approach means increasing visual angle and decreasing distance).

Image Grain

The experiments on first-sight and overflow distance functions suggest that metric information concerning size, distance, and visual angle is contained within the image. One aspect of metric space not addressed by either first-sight or overflow tasks, however, involves whether images possess a "minimum resolution."

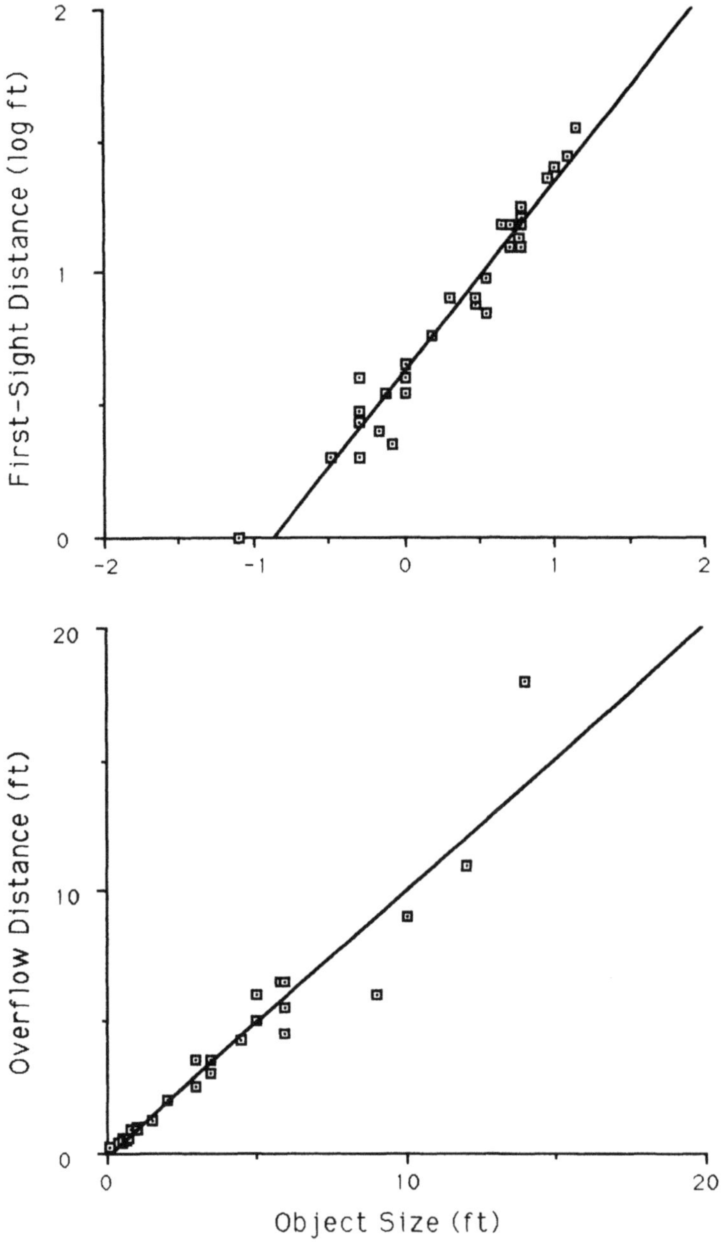

Figure 7.5: Median distance of imaged objects as a function of object size. The top panel shows imaged first-sight distance; the bottom panel shows imaged overflow distance. After Figures 1 and 2 in Hubbard and Baird (1988).

This issue is often discussed in terms of the "grain" of the image, where grain is similar to minimum resolution in a photograph or the size of pixels on a CRT screen. In a photograph, there is a minimum resolution, and objects smaller than this resolution, smaller than this grain size, cannot be portrayed in the photograph. Similarly, while many wonderful, complicated, and detailed pictures can be drawn on a computer graphics terminal, an object smaller than the size of an individual pixel (grain element) cannot be drawn. Some theorists have proposed that the grain of a visual image may change across the surface of the image (paralleling the lessening of acuity from fovea to periphery on the retina, Finke & Kosslyn, 1980; Finke & Kurtzman, 1981; but see also Intons-Peterson & White, 1981). Implicit in this idea, though, is that the grain at any given point in the visual image is constant, just as grain at any given point in the visual field is constant.

The initial evidence for the concept of grain in imagery comes from studies in which subjects imaged pairs of differently-sized objects together and then reported on their features. For example, a rabbit would be imaged next to either a fly or next to an elephant (Kosslyn, 1975). When the rabbit was imaged next to a fly, it would be portrayed as relatively large in the imaginal visual field, but when the rabbit was imaged next to an elephant, that same rabbit would subsume a relatively small portion of the visual field. When subjects were asked questions about the rabbit, and the rabbit was imaged next to the elephant (i.e., the rabbit was subjectively small), they took longer to answer than when the rabbit had been imaged next to the fly (i.e., the rabbit was subjectively large). Furthermore, many subjects reported having to "zoom in" and magnify parts on the smaller image before those parts could be "seen." The point of note is that some parts on the subjectively small rabbit would have been below the minimum resolution of the image, and so the entire animal (or at least a portion of the animal) would have to be increased in subjective size (i.e., "zoomed in" on) before the queried part was large enough to be successfully resolved.

Finke and his colleagues have examined acuity in visual images more closely. Finke and Kosslyn (1980) had subjects visualize two dots that were either vertically or horizontally some distance away from the point of fixation, and they reported that the visual fields within which the pairs of imaged dots could be resolved decreased in size as the distance separating the dots decreased and that the rate of decreasing size was approximately the same in imagery as in perception. Finke and Kurtzman (1981) presented subjects with sine wave gratings of various spatial frequencies. The gratings were presented within a small circular area; the upper half of the circle had gratings oriented vertically, while the bottom half had gratings oriented horizontally. Eight equally-spaced radii extended outward from the circle containing the gratings, and along each radii was a red dot which subjects could move and also use as a fixation point. In the perception condition, subjects would fixate on the dot and then move it outward from the gratings until they could no longer resolve that the circle consisted of gratings in two different orientations. Subjects would then place the dot at the far end of the rod and move it inward until they could just barely begin to see that the stimulus field consisted of two distinct halves. The imagery condition was similar to the perception condition except the subject imaged the sine wave grating in the center of the radii. The resulting visual field sizes and shapes were the same for both imagery and perception.

Vanishing-point Distance

We have further explored the notion of grain in visual images by explicit use of psychophysical techniques (Hubbard & Baird, 1988; 1991). If, in fact, the grain size at a given point in the image is constant, then a constant minimum resolution (a minimum "visual angle of the mind's eye") should be obtained. Additionally, since grain size corresponds to the minimum subjective size of the object (an object cannot be drawn at a smaller resolution), then imaged vanishing-point distance should be linearly related to the stated referent object size. However, as shown in Figure 7.6, we discovered that the function relating stated size to imaged vanishing-point distance is not linear, but is instead a power function with an exponent (γ) of approximately .7 (Hubbard & Baird, 1988). Similar power functions were found when descriptions of both familiar objects and featureless rods were used as stimuli, suggesting that the form of this function was due to properties of the imagery system and not to the properties of the particular stimuli.

Vanishing-point distance in imagery can be thought of as a type of threshold in that stimuli beyond the vanishing point cannot be imaged, while stimuli closer than vanishing point can be imaged. Difficulties with threshold measurement, however, have been well documented. For example, in the Method of Limits in classical psychophysics, a subject is presented with a sequence of stimuli in which the intensity is gradually increased or gradually decreased, and after each stimulus presentation, the subject reports if a stimulus was perceived. If the stimulus intensity begins at a subthreshold level and gradually increases, the subject may nonetheless continue to report "NO" after the stimulus intensity has reached suprathreshold levels, thus making the threshold appear to be higher than it really is (an error of habituation). Conversely, the subject may anticipate the arrival of the stimulus at threshold and prematurely report perception of the stimulus (an error or anticipation).

In our initial experiments on vanishing point, subjects gave a first-sight judgment before making their vanishing-point judgment; therefore, they always gave the shorter first-sight distance before giving the longer vanishing-point distance. This methodology may have inadvertently biased their judgments of vanishing point because estimation of the vanishing-point threshold was always approached from the same direction, that is, by increasing the distance. Therefore, errors of anticipation or habituation may have biased the distance

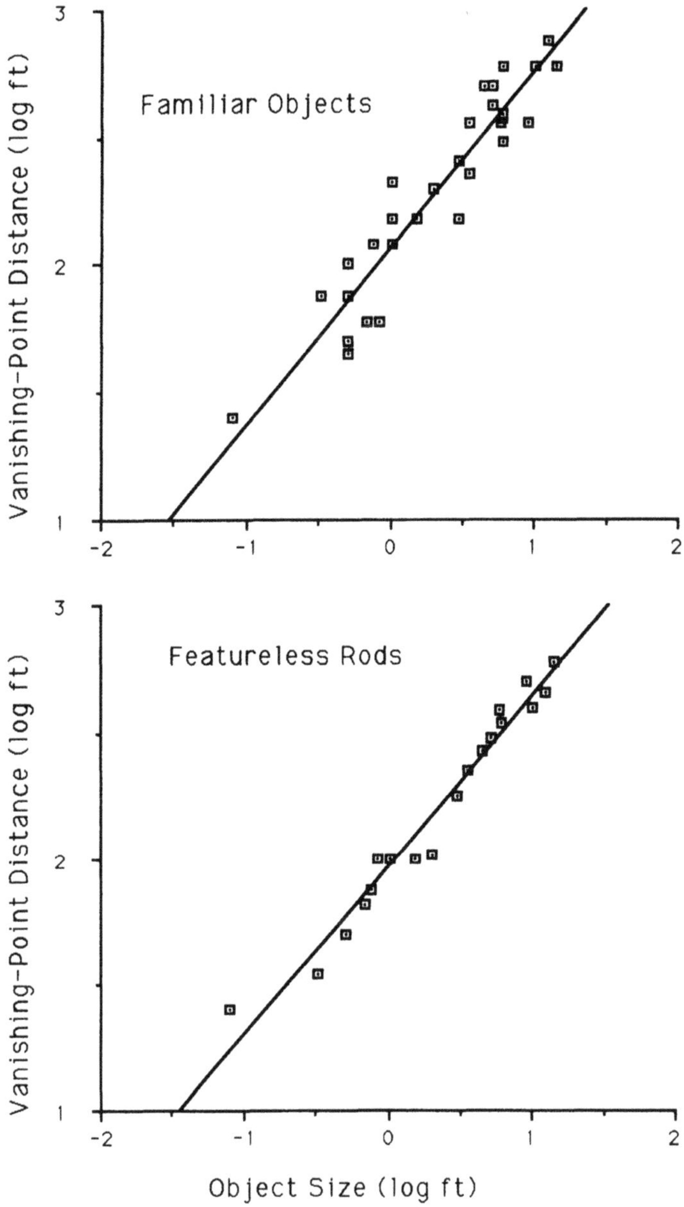

Figure 7.6: Median imaged vanishing-point distance as a function of object size. The top panel shows vanishing-point distance for familiar objects; the bottom panel shows vanishing-point distance for featureless rods. After Figures 8 and 9 in Hubbard and Baird (1988).

estimates. One standard way to limit such errors is to vary the starting point of stimulus intensity, and in a more recent study (Hubbard & Baird, 1991), one group began from a starting point closer than the vanishing point, while the second group began from a starting point beyond the vanishing point. The vanishing-point slopes and y-intercepts (logarithmic coordinates) obtained for the two groups were nearly identical, suggesting that errors of anticipation or habituation do not systematically effect either the exponent or the multiplicative constant of the power function.

Surface Detail

For overflow, surface detail is thought to be less important than length along the longest axis (Kosslyn, 1978), but it is not clear that a similar relationship must hold for vanishing-point. For example, considerations of acuity suggest that less detailed objects might be recognizable at greater distances than more detailed objects of the same size. We had subjects give estimates of both first-sight and vanishing-point imaged distances for 30 objects of various stated sizes and levels of surface complexity (Hubbard & Baird, 1991). As shown in Figure 7.7, for first-sight distances, there was no clear tendency for either the slope or the y-intercept to change with changes in complexity. For vanishing point distances, however, the slope increased slightly and the y-intercept decreased slightly as complexity increased. This pattern is a reasonable one: For first-sight images, there is no reason to suppose that more complex objects need be imaged at closer distances, but for vanishing-point images, acuity may demand that a more complex object (i.e., a surface with fine details) becomes indiscernible at a much closer distance than an object of the same size that is relatively featureless.

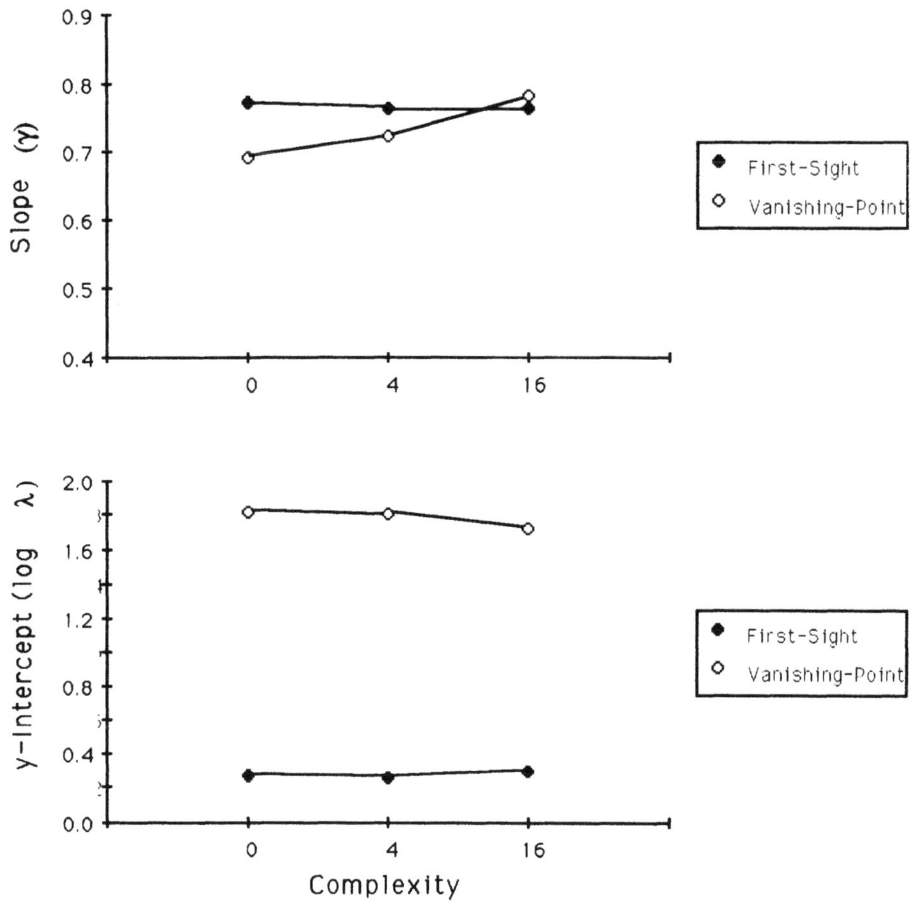

Figure 7.7: Imaged first-sight and vanishing-point distance exponents and multiplicative constants as a function of object complexity (level of surface detail). Exponents are in the top panel and multiplicative constants are in the bottom panel. After Figure 1 in Hubbard and Baird (1991).

Visual Clutter

We have also examined how the context in which an imaged object is embedded influences the vanishing-point distance. It is possible that context may influence distance estimates; for example, a "filled" space is often judged to be longer or larger than an "unfilled" space of the same objective dimensions (Coren & Ward, 1979; Luria, Kinney, & Weisman, 1967; Pressey, 1974). One related finding in the cognitive mapping literature is that when there is a greater amount of "clutter" between two locations, the estimates of distance are larger than when there is no clutter (Thorndyke, 1981).

Since clutter obviously cannot be interposed directly between the observer and the imaged vanishing point (as that would obscure the vanishing point), subjects filled the imaginal visual field on either side of imaged squares with imaged clutter. Subjects in a clutter group were instructed to image that they were standing between the rails of a railroad track and that a square of specified size and level of surface detail was placed atop a railroad flatcar directly in front of them. The square was placed on the flatcar such that its surface was perpendicular to the line of sight. The sides of the railroad track, stretching from where the subject stood out to the horizon, were to be lined with buildings, loading docks, warehouses, and other structures (for large squares, these structures might be hidden behind the square initially but would be revealed as the square receded into the distance). Subjects then imaged that the square and the flatcar upon which it was riding moved down the track away from where they were standing. Eventually the square reached a point where it was just barely identifiable (subjects were asked to ignore whether or not the flatcar itself was visible), and subjects then estimated the vanishing-point distance. The instructions for subjects in a "clear" group were identical to those in the "clutter" group except that instead of imaging loading docks, warehouses and other structures beside the tracks, the clear group imaged a wide open plain on both sides of the tracks (see results in Figure 7.8).

As shown in Figure 7.8, there was a trend (albeit nonsignificant) for exponents in the clutter condition to be slightly higher than exponents in the clear condition. The surprising result might be accounted for by considering the spacing of the clutter. In many previous experiments (e.g., Thorndyke, 1981), clutter was not distributed uniformly, that is, clutter consisted of at most three intervening points which were themselves separated by large clutter-free areas. In the imaged vanishing-point experiments, however, clutter was distributed much more uniformly. Rather than just having one, two, or three points, each of which was surrounded by relatively large uncluttered space, the clutter instructions of the previous experiments specified a more uniform distribution of clutter, as the flatcar and railroad track were lined by numerous buildings, warehouses, docks, and so forth, along the entire length of the railroad track from the observer to the vanishing point. If a point of clutter adds the same absolute amount to a distance estimate, and the uniform distribution of clutter produces an approximate one-to-one correspondence between a unit of distance and a unit of clutter, then we would expect the imaged distance to be larger in the clutter condition than in the clear condition because every "unit of distance" in the clutter condition is slightly larger than the equivalent "unit of distance" in the clear condition.

Partial Clutter

Estimates of vanishing-point distance were then collected in two conditions of "partial clutter." In an "asymmetric" partial-clutter condition, subjects were instructed to form images in which a small river flowed underneath the railroad track, and a small railroad station stood beside the track. Subjects in the "symmetric" partial-clutter condition formed images which contained a small cluster

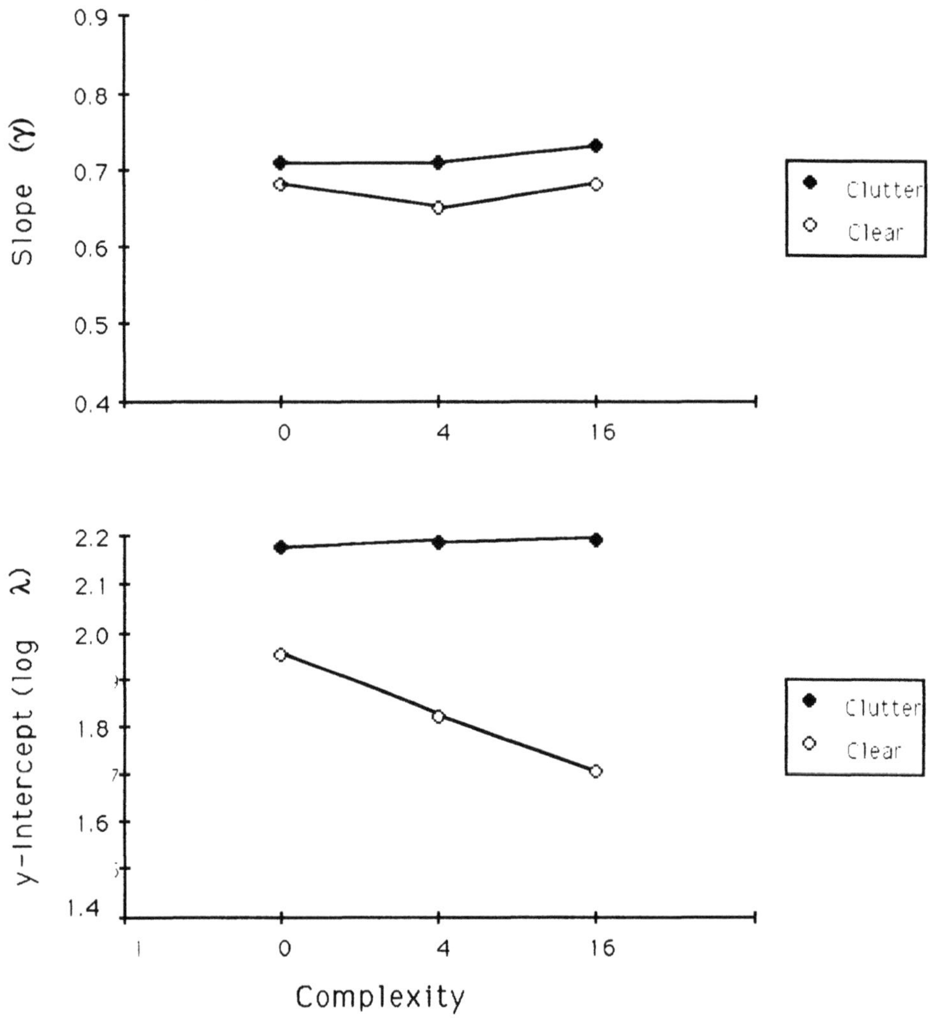

Figure 7.8: Clutter and clear vanishing-point exponents and multiplicative constants as a function of object complexity (level of surface detail). Exponents are in the top panel and multiplicative constants are in the bottom panel. After Figure 5 in Hubbard and Baird (1991).

of four buildings, two on each side of the railroad track. For both partial-clutter conditions, the objects were to be imaged at a location approximately halfway between the observer's station point and the horizon. Exponents for both symmetric and asymmetric partial clutter conditions were very similar to the exponents found previously in the clutter condition. There are at least two possible reasons: (a) perhaps clutter acts in a threshold manner, and that once a threshold is passed, additional clutter has no influence on the exponent, (b) with extreme clutter, the cognitive demands are too high and so the image or estimation process breaks down, resulting in a plateau (or perhaps even in the lower and middle portions of a curvilinear relationship) between clutter and the psychophysical exponent. The relationship between clutter and y-intercept was clearer, as both partial-clutter conditions exhibited y-intercepts intermediate between the y-intercepts measured in the clutter and clear conditions.

One interesting possibility, albeit speculation, is that a partial clutter (either symmetric or asymmetric) is closest to what occurs naturally in subjects' images. In Hubbard et al (1989), subjects were given a list of objects which they were to image. After imaging an object, they reported the imaged distance (a first-sight distance) and the imaged context, if any, which spontaneously surrounded the object in their image. Examination of these reports suggest that a "clear" condition was relatively rare. Only 3 out of 180 items contained no context, e.g., were "floating in space." Similarly, few of the contexts could be regarded as highly detailed; a partial clutter or intermediate level of context seemed to be preferred. Perhaps this preference is linked to the value of the exponents; for example, subjects may prefer an intermediate level because it is closest to a linear function, or perhaps the intermediate level is closest to a linear function because it is most used or preferred. These possibilities await further investigation.

What do these results tell us about the structure of visual imagery? The use of psychophysical techniques in the assessment of first-sight, overflow, and vanishing-point distances led to the discovery of several properties of visual images. Metric information is contained within an image (first-sight distance), but such information cannot account solely for the apparent structural regularities of images, such as the constant overflow angle. A power function with an exponent less than 1 for a vanishing-point function is consistent with the idea that the grain at any given point in a visual image is not constant or at least that grain size may not be a critical parameter of information storage in visual images. In Hubbard and Baird (1991) we discuss several ways in which the idea of a constant grain size can be salvaged, but the main point here is that this aspect of visual images might not have been discovered were it not for the application of psychophysical techniques. Additionally, the presence of other objects in a visually imaged scene (i.e., clutter) can subtly influence both the psychophysical exponent and the y-intercept of the function relating imaged vanishing point to referent object size.

VII. Conclusions

Psychophysics provides many tools for the assessment of perceived intensity, and to the extent that perception, imagery, and memory are similar, we should be able to adapt these tools to investigate imaged or remembered intensity. Shepard and Podgorny (1978) pointed out that many cognitive processes resemble perceptual processes, and they suggest that techniques developed for the study of perception might be fruitfully adapted to the study of cognition. As we have seen in this and other chapters in this volume, such an adaptation has indeed been fruitful. Although our focus here has been on scaling of imaged and remembered quantities, the successful application of psychophysical theory to the study of mental representation goes beyond mere scaling; for example, by conceptualizing imaged vanishing-point distance as a type of threshold, an entire new literature within classical psychophysics becomes relevant to the study of imagery, thus helping to achieve a deeper understanding about how distance is portrayed in visual images.

By incorporating the concepts of imagery and memory within psychophysics, the scope of psychophysics is broadened considerably. Such an idea is hardly new, however. As early as 1960, Björkman, Lundberg, and Tarnblom observed that psychophysical techniques could also be used to investigate memory. They proposed that "A generalized psychophysics ... has to take into account magnitudes of two subjective continua (spaces): the perceptual (immediate experiences) and the memory continuum (past experiences)." These authors went so far as to generalize the psychophysical law (Equation 1) to include relationships between stimulus intensity, perceived magnitude, and memory magnitude:

$$P = \lambda S^{\gamma} \tag{3}$$

$$M = \pi P^{\beta} \tag{4}$$

$$M = \phi S^{\eta} \tag{5}$$

Equation 3 gives the relationship between perceived magnitude (P) and stimulus intensity (S) and is identical to the law proposed by Stevens (Equation 1). Equation 4 shows the relationship between remembered magnitude (M) and perceived magnitude, and Equation 5 shows the relationship between remembered magnitude and stimulus intensity. In these equations π and ϕ are the multiplicative constants, and β and η are the exponents.

In Björkman et al's formulation, what differs between the description of remembered and perceived magnitude is not the functions themselves, but their parameter values (the exponents and multiplicative constants). This, then, is an early version of a functional equivalence hypothesis between memory and perception. When we take a contemporary view of functional equivalence, we can expand Björkman et al.'s ideas to include imagery as well (granting, of course, that the parameter values may be more similar between memory and imagery than they are between imagery or memory and perception).

The hypothesis of functional equivalence between imagery and perception is important for the psychophysics of imagery. Scaling of the relationships between remembered or imaged magnitude and physical intensity and between perceived magnitude and physical intensity both result in power functions. This functional similarity offers some support for the functional-equivalence hypothesis. Although it is possible that different processes operate in both cases and just coincidentally produce similar functions, it is more parsimonious to accept that hypothesis, being the simplest explanation which accounts for the majority of the data (cf. Finke & Shepard, 1986). That such equivalence is partial is reflected in the fact that the exponents for memory and perception generally differ (see Algom, this volume). Had equivalence been complete, we would have found highly similar functions with similar exponents.

The functional equivalence hypothesis and the wealth of theory and data in classical psychophysics makes it tempting to rush into the large unexplored territory of the psychophysics of imagery and memory. Application of psychophysical techniques and theory to all questions concerning cognitive representation would be foolhardy, however, because some perceived dimensions are not well treated by psychophysical methods. For example, the mel scale of pitch (see Stevens & Volkman, 1940) assumes pitch is a unitary dimension, but several later papers (e.g., Krumhansl & Shepard, 1979; Shepard, 1982, 1983) argue that the cognitive representation of pitch is multidimensional. Thus, we would not expect unidimensional psychophysics to be appropriate for studies of the representation of pitch in memory (Hubbard & Stoeckig, in press). If the methods of classical psychophysics are clearly not appropriate for the scaling of some perceptual dimension, it is probably inappropriate to adapt those techniques to scale analogous mental continua.

Psychophysical theory and techniques can lead to further development of cognitive psychology by providing a familiar guide to the quantification of mental experience. Cognitive psychology can also lead to further development of psychophysics by providing new domains for exploration. As our discussion of magnitude estimation in the investigation of the structural properties of visual imagery reveals, psychophysical methods can easily be adapted to the more general questions of cognition, especially when the cognitive experience seems to resemble the perceptual experience. Strict resemblance is not required, however; psychophysical methods can also be applied to such cognitive domains as aesthetics (Merrill & Baird, 1980; see also Merrill & Baird, 1987), assessment of attitudes (Thurstone, 1959), vigilance and signal detection (Green & Swets, 1966). We anticipate future applications of psychophysics to even more varied psychological phenomena.

References

Algom, D., Wolf, Y., & Bergman, B. (1985). Integration of stimulus dimensions in perception and memory: Composition rules and psychophysical relations. *Journal of Experimental Psychology: General*, **4**, 451-471.

Ames, A. Jr. (1946-1947). *Nature and origin of perception: Preliminary laboratory manual for use with demonstrations disclosing phenomena which increase our understanding of the nature of perception*. Hanover, N.H.: Institute for Associated Research.

Anderson, J.R. (1978). Arguments concerning representations for mental imagery. *Psychological Review*, **85**, 249-277.

Baird, J.C. (1963). Retinal and assumed size cues as determinants of size and distance perception. *Journal of Experimental Psychology*, **66**, 155-162.

Baird, J.C. (1964). Size of retinal image as a perceptual cue. *Perceptual & Motor Skills*, **21**, 115-124.

Baird, J.C. (1970). *Psychophysical Analysis of Visual Space*. New York: Pergamon Press.

Baird, J.C., & Brier, J.M. (1981). Perceptual awareness of energy requirements of familiar objects. *Journal of Applied Psychology*, **66**, 90-96.

Baird, J.C., Merrill, A.A., & Tannenbaum, J. (1979). Cognitive representation of spatial relations: II. A familiar environment. *Journal of Experimental Psychology: General*, **108**, 92-98.

Baird, J.C., Noma, E., Nagy, J.N., & Quinn, J. (1976). Predicted and observed activity patterns in campus settings. *Perception & Motor Skills*, **43**, 615-624.

Baird, J.C., & Noma, E. (1978). *Fundamentals of Scaling and Psychophysics*. New York: Wiley.

Bisiach, E., & Luzzatti, C. (1978). Unilateral neglect of representational space. *Cortex*, **17**, 129-133.

Brooks, L. (1968). Spatial and verbal components of the act of recall. *Canadian Journal of Psychology*, **22**, 349-368.

Björkman, M., Lundberg, I., & Tarnblom, S. (1960). On the relationship between percept and memory: A psychophysical approach. *Scandinavian Journal of Psychology*, **1**, 136-144.

Coltheart, M. (1970). The effect of verbal size information upon visual judgments of absolute distance. *Perception & Psychophysics*, **5**, 143-144.

Cooper, L.A. (1976). Demonstration of a mental analog of an external rotation. *Perception & Psychophysics*, **19**, 296-302.

Coren, S., & Ward, L. (1979). Levels of processing in visual illusions: The combination and interaction of distortion-producing mechanisms. *Journal of Experimental Psychology: Human Perception & Performance*, **5**, 324-335.

Da Silva, J.A. (1985). Scales for perceived egocentric distance in a large open field; Comparison of three psychophysical methods. *American Journal of Psychology*, **98**, 119-144.

Epstein, W. (1967). *Varieties of Perceptual Learning.* New York: McGraw-Hill.

Epstein, W., Park, J., & Casey, A. (1961). The current status of the size-distance invariance hypothesis. *Psychological Bulletin*, **58**, 491-514.

Farah, M.J. (1984). The neurological basis of mental imagery: A componential analysis. *Cognition*, **18**, 245-272.

Farah, M.J. (1985). Psychophysical evidence for a shared representational medium for mental images and percepts. *Journal of Experimental Psychology: General*, **114**, 91-103.

Farah, M.J. (1988). Is visual imagery really visual? Overlooked evidence from neuropsychology. *Psychological Review*, **95**, 307-317.

Fechner, G.T. (1876). *Vorschule der ästhetik.* Leipzig: Breitkopf & Härtel.

Finke, R.A. (1980). Levels of equivalence in imagery and perception. *Psychological Review*, **87**, 113-132.

Finke, R.A. (1985). Theories relating mental imagery to perception. *Psychological Bulletin*, **98**, 236-259.

Finke, R.A. (1989). *Principles of Mental Imagery*. Cambridge, Mass.: MIT Press.

Finke, R.A., & Kosslyn, S.M. (1980). Mental imagery acuity in the peripheral visual field. *Journal of Experimental Psychology: Human Perception and Performance*, **6**, 244-264.

Finke, R.A., & Kurtzman, H.S. (1981). Area and contrast effects upon perceptual and imagery acuity. *Journal of Experimental Psychology: Human Perception and Performance*, **7**, 825-832.

Finke, R.A., & Pinker, S. (1982). Spontaneous imagery scanning in mental extrapolation. *Journal of Experimental Psychology: Learning, Memory, and Cognition*, **8**, 142-147.

Finke, R.A., & Pinker, S. (1983). Direction scanning of remembered visual patterns. *Journal of Experimental Psychology: Learning, Memory, and Cognition*, **9**, 398-410.

Finke, R.A., & Shepard, R.N. (1986). Visual functions of mental imagery. In K.R. Boff, L. Kaufman, and J.P. Thomas (Eds.), *Handbook of Perception and Human Performance*, New York: Wiley.

Furlong, E.J. (1951). *A Study in Memory*. London: T. Nelson.

Gescheider, G.A. (1985). *Psychophysics: Method, Theory, and Application* (2nd ed.). Hillsdale, NJ: Erlbaum.

Goldston, D.B., Hinrichs, J.V., & Richman, C.L. (1985). Subjects' expectations, individual variability, and the scanning of mental images. *Memory & Cognition*, **13**, 365-370.

Green, D.M., & Swets, J.A. (1966). *Signal detection theory and psychophysics*. New York: Wiley.

Hubbard, T.L. (1991). Where is the "image" in models of "mental imagery?" Manuscript submitted for publication.

Hubbard, T.L., & Baird, J.C. (1988). Overflow, first-sight, and vanishing point distances in visual imagery. *Journal of Experimental Psychology: Learning, Memory, and Cognition*, **14**, 641-649.

Hubbard, T.L., & Baird, J.C. (1991). The effects of size, clutter, and complexity on vanishing-point distances in visual imagery. Unpublished manuscript.

Hubbard, T.L., Kall, D., & Baird, J.C. (1989). Imagery, memory, and size-distance invariance. *Memory & Cognition*, **17**(1), 87-94.

Hubbard, T.L., & Stoeckig, K. (1988). Musical imagery: Generation of tones and chords. *Journal of Experimental Psychology: Learning, Memory, and Cognition*, **14**, 656-667.

Hubbard, T.L., & Stoeckig, K. (in press). The representation of pitch in musical imagery. In D. Reisberg (Ed.), *Auditory Imagery*. Hillsdale, NJ: Erlbaum.

Intons-Peterson, M.J. (1983). Imagery paradigms: How vulnerable are they to experimenters' expectations? *Journal of Experimental Psychology: Human Perception and Performance*, **9**, 394-412.

Intons-Peterson, M.J., & White, A.R. (1981). Experimenter naivete' and imagined judgments. *Journal of Experimental Psychology: Human Perception and Performance*, **7**, 833-843.

Jackendoff, R. (1987). *Consciousness and the Computational Mind*. Cambridge, MA: MIT Press.

Johnson, M.K. (1988). Reality monitoring: An experimental phenomenological approach. *Journal of Experimental Psychology: General*, **117**, 390-394.

Johnson, M.K., & Raye, C.L. (1981). Reality monitoring. *Psychological Review*, **88**, 67-85.

Jolicoeur, P., & Kosslyn, S.M. (1983). Coordinant systems in long-term memory representations of three-dimensional shapes. *Cognitive Psychology*, **15**, 301-345.

Jolicoeur, P., & Kosslyn, S.M. (1985). Is time to scan visual images due to demand characteristics? *Memory and Cognition*, **13**, 320-332.

Kosslyn, S.M. (1975). Information representation in visual images. *Cognitive Psychology*, **7**, 341-370.

Kosslyn, S.M. (1978). Measuring the visual angle of the mind's eye. *Cognitive Psychology*, **10**, 356-389.

Kosslyn, S.M. (1980). *Image and Mind.* Cambridge, MA: Harvard University Press.

Kosslyn, S.M. (1981). The medium and the message in mental imagery: A theory. *Psychological Review*, **88**, 46-66.

Kosslyn, S.M. (1987). Seeing and imaging in the cerebral hemispheres. *Psychological Review*, **94**, 148-175.

Kosslyn, S.M. (1990). Mental imagery. Chapter in D.N. Osherson, S.M. Kosslyn, & J.M. Hollerbach, (Eds.) *Visual Cognition and Action: An Invitation to Cognitive Science*, Vol. 2. Cambridge, Mass.: MIT Press, p. 73-97.

Kosslyn, S.M., Ball, T.M., & Reiser, B.J. (1978). Visual images preserve metric spatial information: Evidence from studies of image scanning, *Journal of Experimental Psychology: Human Perception and Performance*, **4**, 46-60.

Kosslyn, S.M., & Pomerantz, J.R. (1977). Imagery, propositions, and the form of internal representations. *Cognitive Psychology*, **9**, 52-76.

Krumhansl, C.L., & Shepard, R.N. (1979). Quantification of the hierarchy of tonal functions within a diatonic context. *Journal of Experimental Psychology: Human Perception and Performance*, **5**, 579-594.

Levine, D.N., Warach, J., & Farah, M.J. (1985). Two visual systems in mental imagery: Dissociation of "what" and "where" in imagery disorders due to bilateral posterior cerebral lesions. *Neurology*, **35**, 1010-1018.

Luce, R.D. (1986). *Response Times: Their Role in Inferring Elementary Mental Organization*. New York: Oxford University Press.

Luria, S.M., Kinney, J.A.S., & Weisman, S. (1967). Distance estimates with filled and unfilled space. *Perceptual & Motor Skills*, **24**, 1007-1010.

Marr, D. (1982). *Vision*. San Francisco, CA: Freeman.

Marschark, M., Richman, C.L., Yuille, J.C., & Hunt, R.R. (1987). The role of imagery in memory: On shared and distinctive information. *Psychological Bulletin*, **102**, 28-41.

Merrill, A.A., & Baird, J.C. (1980). Perception and recall of aesthetic quality in a familiar environment. *Psychological Research*, **42**, 375-390.

Merrill, A.A., & Baird, J.C. (1987). Semantic and spatial factors in environmental memory. *Memory & Cognition*, **15**(2), 101-108.

Mitchell, D.B., & Richman, C.L. (1980). Confirmed reservations: Mental travel. *Journal of Experimental Psychology: Human Perception and Performance*, **6**, 58-66.

Moyer, R.S., Bradley, D.R., Sorenson, M.H., Whiting, J.C., & Mansfield, D.F. (1978). Psychophysical functions of perceived and remembered size. *Science*, **200**, 330-332.

Neisser, U. (1967). *Cognitive Psychology*. New York: Appleton-Century-Crofts.

Paivio, A. (1971). *Imagery and Verbal Processes*. New York: Holt, Rinehart, & Winston.

Paivio, A. (1986). *Mental Representations: A Dual Coding Approach*. New York: Oxford University Press.

Podgorny, P., & Shepard, R.N. (1978). Functional representations common to visual perception and imagination. *Journal of Experimental Psychology: Human Perception and Performance*, **4**, 21-35.

Pastore, N. (1971). *Selective History of Theories of Visual Perception: 1650-1950*. New York: Oxford University Press.

Pinker, S., Choate, P.A., & Finke, R.A. (1984). Mental extrapolation in patterns constructed from memory. *Memory and Cognition*, **12**, 207-218.

Pressey, A.W. (1974). Age changes in the Ponzo and filled-space illusions. *Perception & Psychophysics*, **15**, 315-319.

Pylyshyn, Z.W. (1973). What the mind's eye tells the mind's brain: A critique of mental imagery. *Psychological Bulletin*, **80**, 1-24.

Pylyshyn, Z.W. (1981). The imagery debate: Analog media versus tacit knowledge. *Psychological Review*, **87**, 16-45.

Pylyshyn, Z.W. (1984). *Computation and Cognition*. Cambridge, MA: MIT Press.

Reisberg, D., & Chambers, D. (1985). Can mental images be ambiguous? *Journal of Experimental Psychology: Human Perception and Performance*, **11**, 317-328.

Rock, I. (1983). *The Logic of Perception*. Cambridge, MA: MIT Press.

Saarinen, T.F. (1976). *Environmental Planning: Perception and Behavior*. Boston: Houghton Mifflin.

Sacks, O. (1990). *The Man Who Mistook His Wife for a Hat*. New York: Harper Perennial.

Sedgwick, H.A. (1986). Space Perception. In K.R. Boff, L. Kaufman, & J.P. Thomas (Eds.), *Handbook of Perception and Human Performance:* Vol. 1 (pp.21.1-21.57). New York: Wiley.

Segal, S.J., & Fusella, V. (1970). Influences of imaged pictures and sounds on detection of visual and auditory signals. *Journal of Experimental Psychology*, **83**, 458-464.

Shepard, R.N. (1981). Psychophysical complementarity. In M. Kubovy, & J.R. Pomerantz (Eds.), *Perceptual Organization*. Hillsdale, NJ: Erlbaum, pp. 279-341.

Shepard, R.N. (1982). Geometrical approximations to the structure of musical pitch. *Psychological Review*, **89**, 305-333.

Shepard, R.N. (1983). Structural representations of musical pitch. In D. Deutsch (Ed.), *The Psychology of Music*. New York: Academic Press, pp. 344-390.

Shepard, R.N., & Chipman, S. (1970). Second-order isomorphism of internal representations: Shapes of states. *Cognitive Psychology*, **1**, 1-17.

Shepard, R.N., & Cooper, L.A. (1982). *Mental Images and Their Transformations*. Cambridge, MA: MIT Press.

Shepard, R.N., Kilpatric, D.W., & Cunningham, J.P. (1975). The internal representation of numbers. *Cognitive Psychology*, **7**, 82-138.

Shepard, R.N., & Podgorny, P. (1978). Cognitive processes that resemble perceptual processes. In W.K. Estes (Ed.), *Handbook of Learning and Cognitive Processes* (Vol. 5). Hillsdale, NJ: Erlbaum.

Sherman, R.C., Croxton, J., & Giovanatto, J. (1979). Investigating cognitive representations of spatial relationships. *Environment and Behavior*, **11**, 209-216.

Stevens, S.S. (1975). *Psychophysics: Introduction to Its Perceptual, Neural, and Social Prospects*. New York: Wiley.

Stevens, S.S., & Volkman, J. (1940). The relation of pitch to frequency: A revised scale. *American Journal of Psychology*, **53**, 329-353.

Thorndyke, P. (1981). Distance estimation from cognitive maps. *Cognitive Psychology*, **13**, 526-550.

Thurstone, L.L. (1959). *The Measurement of Values*. Chicago: University of Chicago Press.

Tulving, E. (1983). *Elements of Episodic Memory*. New York: Oxford University Press.

Weist, W.M., & Bell, B. (1985). Stevens' exponent for psychophysical scaling of perceived, remembered, and inferred distance. *Psychological Bulletin*, **98**, 457-470.

Psychophysical Approaches to Cognition
D. Algom (Editor)

8

MEMORY PSYCHOPHYSICS: AN EXAMINATION OF ITS PERCEPTUAL AND COGNITIVE PROSPECTS[1]

Daniel Algom
Bar-Ilan University

[1] Preparation of this chapter was supported in part by grant 89-00460 from the US-Israel Binational Science Foundation. I thank Ella Gindi and Avi Szanto for excellent technical assistance.

Table of Contents

I. Introduction

Psychophysics is the science that explicates the functional relations between physical stimuli and the resulting sensory responses. Memory psychophysics, or mnemophysics (Algom & Marks, 1989), is the branch of psychophysics that treats the functional relations between physical stimuli and their *remembered* sensory responses. Memory psychophysics derives from the two branches of experimental psychology that its name comprises. Both psychophysicists and memory researchers are interested in the quantitative measurement of the correspondence between the objective properties of the stimulus and their subjective counterparts in the human cognitive system. Despite de facto similarity in their ultimate epistemological objectives (Algom, Wolf, & Bergman, 1985), however, the study of memory and psychophysics have developed independently, using separate methods of experimentation and analysis. The realization that the full arsenal of modern psychophysical methods (notably, ratio scaling analyses and multivariate models of measurement) can profitably be applied to study memorial reactions -- at no cost of extra manipulations to the experimenter -- has come fairly lately (Algom, 1988b; Hubbard, 1991a). An encompassing, data-driven examination of the prospects of memory psychophysics forms the theme of the present chapter.

First, I examine some historical roots with an eye on timing: Why has memory psychophysics emerged at the time it did? Hopefully, this places mnemophysical pursuits in a richer context that also enables one to gauge their merit against some common yardsticks. Then I present the main hypotheses that have been suggested to account for the (rather small body) of empirical findings. A survey of results follows, classifying studies in terms of modality, design and concomitant theoretical ramifications. I conclude with a discussion of several outstanding methodological issues.

How do remembered sensory magnitudes relate to the referent physical stimuli? Do they follow a lawful relation, and, if so, is the relation mathematically the same as that characterizing perceptual functions? Importantly, do the principles of stimulus construction and organization in memory mirror those used for stimulus integration in perception? The cognitive processes underlying such transformations are fundamental, yet still poorly understood. Data are sparse and not readily generalizable. Delineating the major issues may help to start to answer some of the intriguing questions germane to the psychophysical exploration of human memory.

II. Some Historical Antecedents and Conjectures

The idea that memory is based on images, on seeing of internal pictures, can be traced back to at least Aristotle, if not Plato. The notion of *eikon* is used throughout Plato's discussions of memory in Cratylus, Phaedo, Phaedrus, Shopist, Republic, Theaetetus, Timaeus, as well as in other places. Although the exact meaning of the term and whether it was used consistently by Plato are the subject of some controversy (Sorabji, 1972), there is widespread agreement that *eikon* refers to a copy or an image that holds considerable similarity to the original. Plato suggests that memory involves a sort of imprint that later philosophers and present-day psychologists have interpreted as a mental or even a physical image. Theaetetus' simile of the block of wax has proved especially influential in promoting a perceptual or analog conceptualization of memory.

However, the analog account of memory is but one conjecture in Plato's theory of knowledge and probably not the dominant explanation. Given the inferior status of empirically derived or sensory information in that theory this should come as no surprise. Indeed, Theatetus contains the simile of the aviary as well, portraying memory as a storehouse. Note that his simile does not specify the nature of the things stored, which permits one to posit that not all memories are images. St. Augustine did just that, as do modern propositional theories of memory and imagination. Most important, although *eikones* may be involved in the process of recollecting the Forms (eternally true ideas or pure knowledge that we apprehend before birth), higher modes of thinking and reasoning dispose of *eikones* altogether.

Aristotle, in contrast, holds that all human thinking comprises images. This conclusion emerges clearly in Sorabji's (1972) translation and interpretation of Aristotle's little-read treatise De Memoria. The present discussion draws heavily on Sorabji's exposition (and the reader is well advised to consult that source for detailed references). Aristotle's theory of remembering requires an image that is "causally derived from the past act of perceiving and from the corresponding object of perception" (p. 3). Hence, the memory image must resemble the perceptual image which, in turn, must resemble the referent physical stimulus. In other words, memory requires an *eikon*, and "whether one is remembering may depend on whether one's image is an *eikon*" (p. 3).

The reason for Aristotle's departure from his teacher's doctrine appears in De Memoria, and is summarized succinctly by Sorabji (p. 6):

> Objects of though must be housed somewhere. Plato has supposed that the objects of dialectical thought were ideal Forms, which exist separately from the sensible world. But Aristotle believes that very few things can exist separately from the sensible world. So objects of thought need a sensible vehicle. And a convenient vehicle is the sensible form, which exists in external physical objects, and which during perception is transferred to one's sense-organs. An example of such a sensible form would be the colours of the external objects, colours which are taken on by one's eye-jelly during perception. These colours, first in the external object, then in the eye-jelly, provide a vehicle for the object of thought. And after perception is over, it is the resulting image that provides the vehicle.

All thinking and memory thus involve images. The latter, however, requires a special kind of image -- an eikon -- one that is like what the person is thinking of. That attribute, namely, the correspondence between memory images and their respective physical and perceptual referents is fundamental, and the reason Aristotle provides in De Memoria carries a striking affinity to modern ways of construing memory-percept interactions. Aristotle suggests that, when thinking of certain magnitudes, people rely on small-scale models in their mind. Similarly, "when one remembers an event, and remembers how long ago it was, then too one makes use of images which are small-scale models. These images serve as a source of information about the length of the time that has elapsed" (p. 7). Because memory images both represent the thing remembered and locate it in time, they must preserve proportional information about the source. As Sorabji (1972) states, an "impressionistic image of David and Goliath would not serve the purpose" (p. 7). Nor would simple versions of symbolic encoding or propositional networks provide the kind of isomorphism inherent in eikones.

How does one distinguish between perception and memory, especially as both are subserved by images that are supposed to entail a copy or likeness of the physical referent? Here, too, Aristotle's account has an unmistakably modern ring. Logically, one must be aware that one is remembering, i.e., surmise veridically that one had encountered the imaged thing before, and, therefore, assume that what one is experiencing is a copy. Many later philosophers have developed versions of this position including William James who, in The Principles of Psychology, talked of referring one's image to the past (cf. Sorabji, 1972).

Psychologically, the dynamics of memory images itself may provide clues for dating their referent in the past. Strikingly, Aristotle suggests a mechanism used in thinking about spatial magnitudes. There, the sizes of objects are represented by images that serve as small-scale models; the larger image corresponds to the larger object. Likewise, the larger of two (or more, otherwise equivalent) memory images implies a shorter time period or a more recent physical referent. But the scaling of remembered sizes and the corresponding distances in time is accomplished on a finer than ordinal level. According to a probable interpretation, Aristotle suggests that "one does not statically view the imaged diagram, but moves in one's mind along the lines that compose it at a standard pace determined by human physiology" (p. 20). Based on the time required to traverse the image mentally, one can calculate the time period implied. One cannot help but be reminded of the modern experiments on scanning of images by Kosslyn and his coworkers (e.g., Kosslyn, Ball & Reiser, 1978; see Finke, 1989, for a summary of relevant research).

These succinct observations do not nearly summarize Aristotle's theory of memory and recollection portrayed in his De Anima and De Memoria. Nevertheless, we cannot miss the mark by far stating that Aristotle had a representational or even perceptual account for at least certain kinds of memory. Anachronistically speaking, Aristotle proposed an analog-spatial representation underlying memories of scenes and events. The spatial images undergo continuous transformation that enable the person to date the original events in the past. A shrinkage over time in the size of the memory images is implied. In several places, the text comes remarkably close to suggesting a reperceptual theory of memory, anticipating the modern mnemophysical hypothesis bearing that name.

Sorabji's (1972) commentary offers an interesting distinction which reinforces the previous conclusion. It relates to Aristotle's reflections on retrieval, to notions that are usually regarded as the first statement of the laws of association (p. 42). Notably, Aristotle applied these notions solely to memory. Schacter (1982) has stressed the fact that, when Aristotle's ideas were incorporated into the philosophical systems of the British empiricists, they were applied to a wider range of phenomena than Aristotle had originally intended. That *association* is currently associated mainly with learning is the legacy of the British associationists, but it does not reflect accurately Aristotle's original account. The latter underscores the role perceptual variables play in elucidating processes of retrieval.

A largely unexpected precursor of modern mnemophysical ideas is Fechner, the founder of psychophysics. That Fechner entertained psychophysical theories of higher mental processes such as memory is revealed at once by the title of his little-read article from 1882, "Some thoughts on the psychophysical representation of memories" (Fechner, 1882/1987). Fechner argues that both perception and memory, as well as other mental activities and structures, are subject to the "oscillation principle." Memories are *not* "pictures," images, or "stable" particles stored at individual loci (cells or ganglions) in the brain, but rather depend on oscillations in the entire population of nerve fibers and on relatively permanent changes in the configuration of oscillating corpuscles. Memory rests in neural networks created by perception and is retrieved by the resonance principle. In Scheerer's (1987) words, "The oscillatory patterns underlying sensations leave behind more or less permanent changes in the configuration of corpuscles, which enable them to resonate with incoming stimuli, provided they share the same oscillatory pattern" (p. 201).

Fechner's ideas anticipate several recent developments in psychophysics and cognitive psychology, including the principle of distributed representation, holographic theory of memory, and signal detection theory. From the present vantage, we should take note of Fechner's construal of memory as mere perception albeit one that is altered -- actually, made possible -- by a previous act of perception. Of course, neither the mathematics nor high-speed computers were available to "old" Fechner to couch these ideas in appropriate quantitative fashion.

Other pioneers of psychology, too, were interested in exploring the possibility of a psychophysics applied to memory. The following paragraph in E.B.

Titchener's (1906) An Outline of Psychology, may serve as an illustration bound to convince even the skeptic:

> Since the raw material of sensory-ideas consists in every case, of centrally aroused sensations, it is natural that memory should obey Weber's law in every instance where the law holds for the corresponding peripheral sensations. Thus our memory for brightness is *relative*; the distribution of light and shade in a painting is accepted as a correct representation of reality, although the landscape painted was, absolutely, very much brighter than anything on the painted canvas can be. Our memory of a melody is also relative (§ 50); we recognize it, as is now played, although it may be played in a different key from that in which we have heard it rendered on former occasions. On the other hand our memory of color is *absolute* (pp. 286-287).

Not only does Titchener acknowledge the possibility of a discipline of mnemophysics but, characteristically perhaps, he seems to endorse a strong version of memory psychophysics. Psychophysical laws apply regardless of the mode of cognitive generation, i.e., regardless of whether stimuli are perceived or re-membered. The hinted classification of sensory continua, too, anticipates modern developments and the implications surface in current mnemophysical research.

Wundt was not as committed or explicit as his student, yet his psychology of consciousness clearly allows for, if not actually invites, the perceptual study of memory. A key distinction to recall is the one that Wundt draws between *apprehension* (or perception) and *apperception*. The former refers to the automatic or passive experience of the physical stimulation present, whereas the latter is the result of focal attention directed at selective portions of the perceptual field. Apperception is active, voluntary, and creative, able to synthesize elements of sensation. Apperception is important in Wundt's system because it is also responsible for the higher mental activities of judgment, reasoning and certain forms of memory called recollection. Recollection involves reconstruction as does apperception. In Leahey's (1987) rendition of Wundt, "One cannot reexperience an earlier event, for ideas are not permanent. Rather one reconstructs it from current cues and certain general rules" (p. 186). Other forms of memory, subsumed under the term recognition, are also related to sensation -- to "passive" apperception or mere perception. Although it has not been worked out in sufficient detail by Wundt, the psychological infrastructure capable of subserving a memory psychophysics clearly is extant.

Finally, let me take a quick look at the work of Hermann Ebbinghaus, the founder of the experimental study of memory. His pioneering role as well as his famous retention curve are widely acclaimed in current psychological texts. Less frequently mentioned, however, is the fact that the shape of that curve is basically logarithmic and that, almost certainly, it's derivation was inspired by Fechner's prior work in psychophysics. Allegedly, while in Paris, Ebbinghaus came across a copy of Fechner's Elemente der Psychophysik and the book sparked his interest in the quantitative study of psychological processes. It is widely believed that "Essentially, he started to study memory in the same manner that Fechner studied sensations" (Brennan, 1986; p. 161). Remarkably, then, Ebbinghaus, the architect of modern memory research was influenced by Fechner's psychophysics, whereas Fechner had sought to apply psychophysical premises in the study of memory. The advent of memory psychophysics may thus signal the closing of a full circle in the history of psychology.

I do not wish to convey the false impression that these allusions represent a coherent development, the sporadic instances of direct treatment notwithstanding. Much less do they tap a concerted effort at the realization of an explicit discipline of memory psychophysics. Nevertheless, the examples, however incomplete, do correctly portray the intellectual atmosphere around the turn of the century. In that period, the emergence of a memory psychophysics was quite probable as a natural outgrowth of popular scientific doctrines. Why did it fail to materialize? Why did we have to await psychology's centennial for the science of mnemophysics to emerge? To achieve a satisfactory answer one must examine the status of memory theory in a broad historical context.

As we have seen, Aristotle's theory of memory was couched in perceptual terms. Properly speaking, memory denoted but a special class of perceptual processes. The so-called laws of association referred solely to the problem of retrieval conditions (Schacter, 1982). Aristotle's notions remained essentially undeveloped until the 17th century. Then, in the hands of the British empiricists, Aristotle's ideas -- in particular, his laws of association -- underwent considerable elaboration to account for a wide range of psychological phenomena. The associationists drew no sharp distinctions among the host of cognitive phenomena subsumed under the laws of association. Their real interests lay in following the course of the associations. Nevertheless, over successive ramifications, the British empiricists came to ascribe prime importance to encoding processes that have become known as learning in modern psychology. A largely unnoticed by-product of these developments was the minority role assigned to memory. Memory has turned into a pale and rather neglected companion to the major psychological field of learning.

Ebbinghaus' epoch making study of memory underscored these developments. His remarkable achievement notwithstanding, Ebbinghaus' approach also helped to entrench memory more firmly in the set of learning-dependent phenomena. Following Schacter (1982) we can partition the system called human memory into three basic processes. *Encoding* is the process by which incoming information is registered, *storage* refers to the conservation of encoded information, and *retrieval* concerns the events that occur when one attempts to utilize previously acquired information. Ebbinghaus addressed the first (and, to a lesser degree, the second) of these processes. In Schacter's words, "Ebbinghaus painted an empirical picture of memory that ignored retrieval factors. The effects of repetition and the temporal characteristics of storage can be revealed, of course, only through the act of retrieval; but Ebbinghaus neither experimentally investigated nor theoretically addressed either the conditions, functions, or processes of retrieval in his influential studies" (p. 153). Unwittingly perhaps, Ebbinghaus thus fortified the alliance of memory and learning.

The subsequent direction of memory research, due to the tremendous impact of Ebbinghaus' methods, was closely tied to the development of learning theory. Consequently, major causal status was ascribed to events occurring at the input stage of memory. The enfolding of memory research during the ensuing decades cannot be outlined here, but the general picture is of a dynamic, quantitative field, one that, nonetheless, is strongly linked to (not to say, overshadowed by) the primary field of learning.

The net result of the developments that I have sketched in rough outline is clear: Despite it's close ties to sensation in antiquity, memory theory became separated from perceptual discourse to the point of irrelevance. Most introductory psychology students and many seasoned psychologists to date "know" that memory is a subsidiary of learning. Some of our current textbooks purvey the same learning-memory affinity. And that "knowledge," recent yet resilient, explains why the merger of memory and perception could not come forth as psychological science earlier. The reasons for the delayed appearance of memory psychophysics fit into a much larger vista of science.

The vicissitudes of memory theory by no means exhaust the historical underpinnings of memory psychophysics. Psychophysics, too, must bear the onus for the late recognition of mnemophysics. True, it's pioneers might well have entertained the possibility of a psychophysics applied to various cognitive processes besides perception. Yet the subsequent preoccupation of psychophysics with the measurement of thresholds during the first half of this century made it an unlikely candidate for any joint pursuit of cognitive phenomena. That preoccupation, coupled with the virtual exclusion of retrieval from memory theory, rendered a perception-memory alliance impracticable.

The advent of memory psychophysics was made possible by two, fairly independent developments. One is the "liberation" of psychophysics via the application of new, ratio-level, methods to an increasingly challenging repertoire of problems. Scaling became prominent and, as rule, was used to characterize entire perceptual systems. The approach is frequently dubbed "the new psychophysics" (cf. Marks, 1974). The other development, occurring at about the same time, is the so-called cognitive revolution of the late sixties. The sweeping changes in our construal of human cognition subsumed under that title (cf. J. Anderson, 1985) need no documentation here. From the present vantage, the most important development was the broader perspective on the nature of memory: it was approached as an information processing system. Significantly, retrieval processes regained their prominence in the elucidation of human recollection. Memory psychophysics really is the offspring of parallel movements of reformation in it's parent disciplines. As a result, neither memory nor psychophysics remain the purview of isolated groups of specialists.

III. Modern Beginnings

Bjorkman, Lundberg, and Tarnblom (1960) were probably the first modern psychophysicists to contemplate the possibility of a memory psychophysics seriously. They proposed a psychophysics that was larger in scope, comprehending "magnitudes of two subjective continua (spaces): the perceptual (immediate experiences) and the memory continuum (past experiences)." Bjorkman et al. asked subjects to judge the ratio between the magnitudes of a perceived stimulus (one presented physically) and a remembered stimulus (one represented by a name learned earlier). Despite the involvement of memory-based subjective magnitudes, data were coherent and permitted the derivation of psychophysical functions (for circle area and weight). Unfortunately, mixing perceptual and memorial information was not conductive towards disentangling the two modes of cognitive generation. Bjorkman et al's ideas proved influential, although not their experimental method.

The former bore fruit fairly early as Dornic (1968), working, too, at the Stockholm laboratory, became the first researcher to apply Stevens' power law to remembered stimuli. Dornic even proposed a preliminary explanation for the finding that power function exponents for remembered distance are usually smaller than exponents for perceived distance (cf. Wiest & Bell, 1985). Closely linked to these early mnemophysical forays was the more general concern of Swedish psychophysicists with quantitative cognitive analysis. Ekman and Bratfish (1965) and Dornic (1967) asked subjects to assess intercity distances such as that between Paris and Athens. Other researchers (e.g., Lowrey, 1970; Briggs, 1973) treated judgments of intracity distances that may or may not be viewable (barriers can prohibit direct viewing). Wiest and Bell (1985) comment duly that "Both intra- and intercity distance estimation may be considered to be forms of cognitive psychophysics inasmuch as the stimulus or referent for the estimated distance is frequently linked only ambiguously to specifiable previous visual stimulation. Estimated distances in such cases may be considered to be inferences based on verbal representation, visual representation, or both" (p. 458). Note that the term "cognitive psychophysics" is *not* an ex post facto description coined of late. As early as 1970, Baird, a veteran associate of the Stockholm laboratory, proposed a cognitive theory of psychophysics (Baird, 1970a, 1970b). Thus, the notion of a mental psychophysics was unmistakably in the air during the sixties, mainly due to the interest of Scandinavian researchers. It is also true, however, that much of this effort was exploratory and tentative, and, consequently, wielded little influence.

A decade after the Bjorkman et al. study, Shepard and Chipman (1970) coined the term "second-order isomorphism" to represent the relations between external objects and their internal representations. They asked subjects to compare states of the continental United States for geometric similarity. In one condition, subjects gave comparative judgments of all 105 possible pairs made of the outline of 15 states. In a second condition, subjects performed the same task, but were presented with names of the states (rather than with the relevant visual information). Notably, the ratings according to shapes and those according to names were quite similar. From these results Shepard and Chipman concluded that internal representations or mental images are second-order isomorphic to the referent physical stimuli.

A simple isomorphic relationship entails a direct, one-to-one correspondence between external objects and their internal representations. Shepard and Chipman, however, propose a one-to-one relationship between external and internal *relations*. The following summary helps clarify their position: "When someone says 'I am imagining a green square', he is not telling us that there is anything that is literally either green or square going on in his head. What he is really telling us is that whatever is going on is functionally similar to what usually goes on when he is confronted with the kind of external object to which we have all associated the words 'green' and 'square'" (p. 16). In a more formal fashion, "the proposed equivalence between perception and imagination implies a more abstract or 'second-order' isomorphism in which the functional relations among objects as imagined must to some degree mirror the functional relations among the same objects as actually perceived" (Shepard, 1978, p. 131).

These provided powerful ideas, as influential as the set of experimental findings developed by Shepard and his colleagues to support them. Certainly, the notion of corresponding subjective and physical *relations* carries a special flavor with psychophysicists. It evokes at once a particular class of possible psychophysical functions. Although serious examination of psychophysical functions for memory had to await yet another decade, a cogent argument for doing so has been provided by Shepard's ingenious research.

Another landmark on the way toward the appearance of a palpable science of mnemophysics is the study by Robert Moyer (1973) on the psychophysical contingency called (later) the *symbolic distance effect*. The phenomenon is fairly common: It is easier to tell from an image that an elephant is larger than a dog, for example, than to tell that a dog is larger than a cat. Moyer presented subjects with pairs of animal names and asked them to choose the name indicating the larger animal. He found that the response time for indicating the larger of the two animals decreased as the difference in size between the animals increased. This finding mirrors the perceptual relation, where reaction time is inversely related to stimulus difference (Curtis, Paulus, & Rule, 1973; Johnson, 1939; see Woodworth & Schlosberg, 1954).

Moyer's interpretation of the findings was as challenging as it was novel. He surmised that subjects convert the names to analog, size-preserving representations (i.e., they form mental images), then perform the required comparison by making an "internal psychophysical judgment." Which is why mental comparisons involve the same difficulties of discrimination that are encountered in making perceptual comparisons. Along with Shepard's "second-order isomorphism," Moyer's maxim underscored the potential of a psychophysical attract in unravelling features of internal representations. Subsequent studies showed similar effects for mental judgments of time (Holyoak & Walker, 1976), digits from the set of 1 to 9 (Buckley & Gillman, 1974; see also Moyer & Landauer, 1967), and all kinds of objects besides animals (Paivio, 1975). These studies make a further, quantitative point. In all of the cited studies, reaction time was a linear function of the *logarithm* of the ratio of the two names (or digits). In Moyer's (1973) original study, for example, equal ratios (but *not* equal differences) of estimated animal-size yielded equal increments of decrements in response time. This provided another quantitative constraint for the looming mnemophysics to reckon with.

Ultimately, it was 1978 that ushered in the new discipline of memory psychophysics. Two independent studies in prestigious journals (*Memory & Cognition* and *Science*) appeared, deriving psychophysical functions for remembered stimuli. The one by Moyer and his coworkers may serve to illustrate the method and principal results of both, as well as those of subsequent investigations. Moyer, Bradley, Sorensen, Whiting, and Mansfield (1978) had separate groups of subjects estimate the size of perceived and of remembered one-, two-, and three-dimensional objects. Subjects in the memory conditions were told to imagine (rather than view) each stimulus as its prelearned name was called out, and then to assign a number in accord with standard magnitude estimation instructions (Stevens, 1975). Perceptual and memorial estimates were well fit by power functions, but the exponent for memory-based judgments was reliably smaller. For example, perceptual area related to physical area by a power function with an exponent of 0.64, whereas remembered area related to physical area by a power function with an exponent of 0.46. The reappearance of the power function for remembered magnitudes is especially remarkable. It implies that remembered stimuli map onto physical values the same way as do perceived stimuli, supporting the view that internal processes -- of memory or imagery -- mirror processes of perception given the same task and stimulus characteristics. On a more general level, the results may be interpreted as displaying lawful and long-enduring constraints on internal representation of perceptual knowledge (Shepard, 1984; Wolf & Algom, 1987).

The advent of a full-grown memory psychophysics opened up a new avenue for cognitive research, permitting investigators to answer some unaddressed questions relating to people's implicit knowledge of perceptual experience, its long-term representation, and the rules governing its composition. How do remembered sensory magnitudes depend on referent physical intensities? Do memory scale values map onto their physical referents by means of the same functional relation (power transform) as do perceptual scale values? If so, do the same parameters (exponents) govern perceptual and memory functions? Univariate research designs (i.e., studies testing values along but a single stimulus dimension) used in the first mnemophysical investigations can already address many of the outstanding issues. Factorial designs, used later, invite examination of an equally intriguing class of questions. How do remembered representations of components (e.g, the height and width of a rectangle) interact -- or fail to interact -- to produce an integrated, memorial representation of the global stimulus (e.g., the rectangle's area)? What cognitive processes underlie such mental combination, where the only available information comprises symbols representing the original physical components? How do the (presumably tacit) rules of memorial concatenation compare with the rules of integration that operate in perception? And, in general, do the same rules of organization and synthesis govern combinational operations in perception and memory?

Note the comprehensive nature of these questions, blurring the boundaries between quantitative and qualitative aspects of sensory representation.

Mnemophysical investigations entail some sort of a numerical magnitude response for both perception and memory. Hence, standard psychophysical methods and analyses can be used with both types of judgments. Yet, beneath those judgments, general properties of perceptual and memorial functioning surface.

I conclude this section with a short discussion of an often asked question (in classrooms, not yet in textbooks) about the relation(s) between memory psychophysics and research done on mental imagery. In point of fact, both fields are young, fruits of the "cognitive revolution" of the sixties and have been flourishing since. Substantively, much is common to the two lines of research. Virtually all studies of mental imagery rely on the subject's memory of materials presented at an early stage of the experiment. Conversely, subjects in mnemophysical experiments are often explicitly instructed to image. Investigators in both fields aimed at elucidating the notion of *functional equivalence* of percepts, memories, and images (Finke, 1980; Finke & Shepard, 1986). Consider, for example, the principle of mental imagery called "perceptual equivalence" (Finke, 1989): "Imagery is functionally equivalent to perception to the extent that similar mechanisms in the visual system are activated when objects or events are imagined as when the same object or events are actually perceived" (p. 41). Many psychophysicists, I believe, would subscribe to this principle, or, in fact, prefer a weaker version than the one espoused by Finke.

Empirically, too, large portions of the research conducted under the rubric of mental imagery have psychophysical underpinnings. Traditionally, however, these studies have not been identified with psychophysics, or have their findings cast in psychophysical terms. A good example is the study by Kosslyn (1978) on the point of "overflow" in visual images. The term "overflow" was defined as that subjective distance where all parts of an image cannot be glanced by the "mind's eye" at the same time. Subjects were first asked to form an image of a given object, then to imagine walking toward the object until its image overflowed. The estimated distance at which overflow occurred increased in proportion to the stated size of the object (along its largest axis). Kosslyn concluded that the "mind's eye" is characterized by a fairly constant visual angle. The ingenuity and theoretical significance of Kosslyn's study need no documentation here. His use of memory-based judgments of subjective distance does! Plotting estimated distance against stimulus diagonal is a (memory) psychophysical function in all but name. As Hubbard (1991a) notes, Kosslyn's "use of a psychophysical scaling technique to examine a cognitive construct produced new data that led to theoretical breakthroughs which might not be otherwise attainable" (p. 23). Indeed Hubbard and Baird (1988; Hubbard, Kall, & Baird, 1989; see also their chapter in this volume) have extended Kosslyn's findings and their implications by applying techniques borrowed from classical psychophysics. Incidentally, Hubbard and Baird have also reaffirmed the affinity of memory psychophysics and mental imagery.

The close linkage is most conspicuous and has been fruitfully exploited in the study of subjective distance. I defer discussion of the mnemophysics of distance to a later section; here I wish to sketch briefly contributions to the mental imagery of distance. In the now-classic "map-scanning" experiment by Kosslyn, Ball, and Reiser (1978), subjects learned the locations of seven objects on a fictional map. They imagined each object as it was named, then scanned mentally to a second object to verify that it was also on the map. Subjects performed the mental scanning by imaging a small black "speck" moving in a direct path from the first object to the second. Strikingly, response time increased with interobject distance in a strictly linear fashion ($r = 0.97$). These results suggest that images can preserve two-dimensional distances on actual maps (cf. Finke, 1989). Pinker (1980) extended the Kosslyn et al method and findings to three-dimensional arrays. First, subjects learned the locations of small toys suspended in an open box; then, with closed eyes, they imagined scanning the distance between a given pair of objects along a straight line. Pinker found that scanning time was highly correlated with interobject distance in three-dimensional space, but *not* with interobject distance in a two-dimensional projection of the objects. Instructing subjects to scan the latter (e.g., telling them to imagine that there is glass plate covering the front/side of the box), however, results in response time that does depend on two-dimensional distance -- as seen from the appropriate vantage point. Evidently, people can produce images that preserve three-dimensional distances, then change them voluntarily, for example, by the removal of depth.

Mental imagery is not limited to mental scanning, mental construction, or even the whole class of "mental imagery" tasks. It informs judgmental processes of perceptual psychophysics as well. There is evidence that people judge distances by imagining that they are laying out a mental "ruler" of constant length (Hartley, 1977, 1981; see also Finke, 1989). In Hartley's experiments, subjects reported that they laid off a mental image of the standard line (provided by the experimenter) along the comparison line to be estimated. Consistent with Hartley's image-based model of mental measurement was his finding of a linear relation between the *time* required to make the judgment and the *magnitude* of the estimate. Longer lines -- and greater estimates -- were associated with increased response times, suggesting a dependence on the number of times the standard was mentally laid off against the comparison . Commensurably, too, increasing standard size produced shorter response times. Kerst and Howard (1983) replicated Hartley's main result, and found a strong linear relation between response time and estimated length. Because they used a sequential procedure, Kerst and Howard concluded that Hartley's mental measurement effect operates with (short-term) memory images too. Patently, "Unknown distances might therefore be estimated by measuring out the distances in imagination" (Finke, 1989, p. 88).

Why then is it still the case that memory psychophysics and mental imagery are often considered separate disciplines by their own practitioners?

Finke's (1989) recent book, Principles of Mental Imagery, is a case in point. It does not mention the term memory psychophysics, and devotes less than a full page to a description of a single mnemophysical study. Shared goals and history notwithstanding, the precise connection between mental imagery and memory psychophysics is likely to be fairly complex. Investigators of the two fields use distinct methods of experimentation and analysis. Studies of mental imagery typically test discrete stimuli (animals, all kinds of objects, symbols), usually paired for a comparative judgment (e.g., which is longer, a minute or a month?). The main (often exclusive) response measure is reaction time. Analyses of results follow, as a rule, the mental chronometry tradition used in related cognitive domains. Comparisons with perception are qualitative in nature, despite the use of reaction time. Mnemophysical studies, by contrast, allow for independent estimates of parameters with continuous variables. Stimuli comprise relatively large sets of values on the stimulus dimension(s) tested. Numerical magnitude judgments are used with both memory and perceptual stimuli. In fact, the full arsenal of psychophysical scaling techniques can be deployed to characterize both sets of data. Hence, memory-percept comparisons are strictly quantitative. Whether the differences in method and general theoretical outlook betray deeper contrasts remains to be seen.

IV. Theories of Memory-based Magnitude Judgments

Two general findings have emerged from the early studies of memory psychophysics. First, remembered stimuli relate to their corresponding physical stimuli via power transforms, much the same way that do perceptual values. Second, systematically smaller exponents characterize the judgments from memory. Two main hypotheses have been suggested to account for the parameter difference. According to the reperception hypothesis (Kerst & Howard, 1978; Moyer et al., 1978) perception and memory perform identical transformations on the input data. Therefore, two transformations intervene between the memorial estimate and the physical stimulus. For perception, a simple two-parameter power function describes how psychological magnitude increases with physical magnitude (Stevens, 1975). Thus,

$$R = aS^b \quad , \qquad (1)$$

where R is perceived magnitude, S is physical magnitude, and a and b are constants. The exponent is given by b, whereas a is a scale modulus determined by the choice of units. For memory, judgment is again a power function of the input with the same value of exponent. However, the proper input for memory-based estimates is not the original stimulus magnitudes S, but rather their perceptually transformed scale values R. Therefore,

$$M = a'R^b \quad , \qquad (2)$$

where M is remembered magnitude, and a' is an arbitrarily determined measurement modulus as a in Equation 1. Substituting for R yields

$$M = AS^{b^2} , \qquad (3)$$

where A is the new scaling factor. The reperceptual hypothesis predicts perforce a square relation between a given pair of perceptual and memorial exponents.

The alternative uncertainty hypothesis attributes the lower exponent in memory to the greater vagueness inherent in such tasks. According to one version (Kerst & Howard, 1978), subjects constrict their range of responses as a result of increased uncertainty. A second version (Algom et al., 1985) holds that it is the stimulus dimension (rather than the response continuum) that undergoes changes under the rather fuzzy memory-based judgment condition. In this version, the attenuated memory exponent constitutes a special case of a general psychophysical principle, namely, the inverse relation between dynamic response range and power function exponent (Teghtsoonian, 1971, 1973). In either case, the effect of uncertainty is to lower the value of the memorial exponent.

For *compressive* sensory continua (i.e., perceptual dimensions characterized by exponents smaller than unity), both theories predict an even more compressive memory exponent. For *expansive* continua (dimensions characterized by exponents greater than unity), however, different predictions exist. The reperceptual hypothesis predicts a steeper memory function in this case because the memory exponent should equal the square of the greater than 1 perceptual exponent. The uncertainty hypothesis, on the other hand, still predicts an attenuated memory exponent, regardless of the value of the corresponding perceptual exponent. Unfortunately in this respect, most data to date have been garnered on continua belonging to the nondiagnostic compressive class.

Although the two theories fulfilled a valuable service, guiding early research, they suffer both from a substantial limitation. They address results deriving from univariate designs only, ones that call on subjects to judge stimuli varying along a single dimension (e.g., lines of differing length, different-size rectangles). Indeed, the great bulk of work in memory psychophysics is based on unifactor stimulus designs in conjunction with direct scaling techniques for obtaining the response. Such work and those theories cannot deal with the organizational principles in memory being examined in current cognitive research. Aside from the limited scope, these theories are beset by a fundamental difficulty that also plagues perceptual psychophysics: The validity of numerical responses such as magnitude estimates relies on the questionable assumption that putative numerical ratios reflect actual ratios of subjective magnitudes (e.g., Algom & Marks, 1984; Anderson, 1970, 1981, 1982; Torgerson, 1961). In the absence of criteria for validation, one cannot be sure that the numbers proferred by the subjects faithfully reflect the magnitudes of their memorial or perceptual representations.

As a partial remedy -- no comprehensive solution is possible within a unidimensional scheme -- Algom and Marks (1989) have recently suggested a two-stage model, modifying the reperception hypothesis, that can account for some discordant data too. According to their two-stage model of judgment (e.g., Algom & Marks, 1984, 1990), the sizes of the measured exponents b_p (perception) and b_m (memory) vary because of response transformations imposed by nonlinear judgmental processes (transformations by a power function with exponent c). Mathematically, for perception, Equation 1 then can be specified as:

$$R = aS^{v \times c} \tag{4}$$

where v is the underlying unbiased exponent, and the measured perceptual exponent becomes:

$$b_p = v \times c \quad . \tag{5}$$

For memory, Equation 3 similarly changes to:

$$M = AS^{v \times v \times c} \tag{6}$$

where the measured memorial exponent is:

$$b_m = v \times v \times c \quad . \tag{7}$$

The ratio of the measured exponents

$$b_m \,/\, b_p = v \times v \times c \,/\, v \times c = v \tag{8}$$

yields the "true" perceptual exponent. This exponent v should be distinguished from the observed exponent b which <u>is</u> confounded by nonlinear biases.

V. Unidimensional Mnemophysics

Virtually all studies followed a common methodology regardless of the continuum under test. Experiments comprised two sessions. In a first session, subjects learned to associate symbolic codes (such as colors or CVCs) with each of the different stimuli on the tested dimension. After an interval (of usually 24 h), subjects returned for a judgment session. In the perceptual conditions, actual stimuli were presented, one at a time, for magnitude judgment. In the memorial conditions, stimuli were represented by their codes. Subjects had to imagine each stimulus and estimate its magnitude from memory. Again, standard psychophysical methods and analyses can be used with both types of judgments, the only procedural difference being that stimuli are in the one case physically presented, in the other, symbolically represented. In the following, I classify studies along modality and assess the bearing of the results on the theories of memorial judgment.

Visual Length and Distance

The aforementioned study by Moyer et al. (1978) included an experiment on judgments of line length that probably comprises the first mnemophysical investigation of visual extent. Magnitude estimates were well fit by power functions for both the perception and memory conditions. Exponents for the two groups were 0.87 and 0.70, respectively. A corresponding study conducted in this laboratory by Barak-Mayer (1985) yielded very similar results: The respective exponents for perception and memory were 0.87 and 0.63. In yet another study of line length in my laboratory, Sarfaty (1986) obtained a mean exponent of 0.92 for perception and an insignificantly greater value of 0.96 for memory. Kerst and

Howard (1984) reported a similar exponent for perception, 0.93, but an exponent of 0.84 for memory.

In a developmental study of memory psychophysics, Wolf and Algom (1987, Experiment 4) used chocolate bars (at a fixed width) to elicit judgments of visual extent ("amount to eat") with children. For the 6-year-olds, exponents were 1.11 for perception and 1.23 for memory. For the 10-year-olds, perceptual judgments yielded a power function exponent of 1.30, whereas judgments made from memory resulted in an exponent of 0.82.

Other studies used maps, veridical and fictitious, as stimuli. Kerst and Howard (1978) had subjects judge interstate distances based on the prior (memory group) or the continuous (perception group) study of a map of the continental United States. They obtained perceptual and memorial exponents of 1.04 and 1.10 for these judgments of visual length. Da Silva, Ruiz, and Marques (1987) obtained magnitude estimates of the distances among the state capitals of Brazil under three experimental conditions. Subjects judged distance while viewing a map (perceptual condition), or from memory based on the prior study of the map (memory condition); in a third condition, the judgments were based on general geographic knowledge only (inferred distance condition). The exponents were 1.05, 0.86, and 0.76, respectively, for perceived, remembered and inferred distance. Replication of the entire experiment a month later produced similar results: corresponding exponents equalled 1.06, 0.72, and 0.68. Kerst, Howard, and Gugerty (1987) used a map of a fictitious college to obtain magnitude estimates (and map-sketching assessments) of distance. Perceptual estimates (given with the map in clear view) obeyed a power function characterized by an exponent of 1.09. A group responding immediately after the removal of the map from view obtained a mean exponent of 0.77, whereas a second memory group -- responding 24 h after the map's removal -- obtained an exponent of 0.66.

The use of an "inferred distance" condition by DaSilva et al (1987) merits some comments. Examination of judgments of this nature was inspired by the cognitive psychophysics studies by several Swedish precursors of memory psychophysics. The task became popular (see, Canter, 1977), although "inferred" judgments are largely eschewed by psychophysicists. The reason has recently been stated by Hubbard (1991a): "Inferred conditions are operationally distinguished from memory or perception conditions by not showing subjects the stimuli. Unfortunately, the origin of inferred knowledge is not known .... In any event, the unconstrained nature of inferred distance renders it useless in delimiting a psychophysical theory of mental representation" (p. 10). A recent meta-analytic review of 70 studies of distance estimation (Wiest & Bell, 1985) found average power function exponents of 1.08, 0.91, and 0.75 for perception, memory, and inference, respectively.

A mnemophysical study conducted in a natural setting was reported by Bradley and Vido (1984). Their subjects learned the locations (and names) of objects viewed from the top of a mountain. After an interval of 24 h, the subjects in the perception group made judgments of distance from the same mountain site, whereas the subjects serving in the memory condition proffered their judgments of remembered distance from a laboratory. Power function exponents were 0.81 for perception and 0.60 for memory.

How do these results speak to the question of deciding between the alternative theories of memory-based magnitude judgment? Collectively, they favor none of the proposed accounts in an unequivocal fashion. Although earlier studies (notably those by Moyer et al., 1978; and Kerst & Howard, 1978) lent support for the reperception hypothesis, discordant results are too many to be disregarded. That memorial exponents are often greater than corresponding perceptual exponents conflicts with the predictions of the uncertainty hypothesis. Algom and Marks' two-stage model can handle such results with ease, but some of the studies yield unbiased exponents that deviate extensively from unity -- the "expected" value for visual extent (Baird, 1970c; see also Wiest & Bell, 1985).

Visual Area

I have already cited the results obtained by Moyer et al. (1978) on perceptual and memorial judgments of area: exponents of 0.64 and 0.46, bearing the square relation prescribed by the reperception hypothesis. Kerst and Howard (1978) found a similar relation, 0.79 and 0.60, whereas a slightly modified version of their study (Chew & Richardson, 1980) yielded exponents of 0.79 and 0.64. In yet another study of visual area, DaSilva, Marques, and Ruiz (1987) reported almost identical exponents for perception and memory, but a smaller value (of approximately 0.50) for their additional condition of "inferred area." Kemp's (1988) study of visual area (European countries and islands) included multiple delays, ranging from responding 2 minutes after removal of the (map) stimuli to a week. Subjects in a perception condition responded with the stimuli in view, whereas subjects in a control group gave responses of area inferred from their geographic knowledge. Results of the perceptual group could be described by a power function with an exponent of 0.82. Memorial judgments were also governed by power functions but with smaller exponents: 0.67, 0.65, and 0.54 for delays of 2 min., 90 min., and 1 week, respectively. Again, the control condition yielded a much smaller exponent, 0.43. These five studies used geographic area of states or countries -- presented via outline maps -- as stimuli.

Algom et al. (1985) asked subjects to judge areas of rectangles. The perceptual and memorial exponents were 0.78 and 0.66. The developmental study by Wolf and Algom (1987) also used rectangular shapes for judgments of area with children at 6, 8, and 10 years of age. The respective exponents for the three age groups in the perception condition were 0.88, 0.98, and 1.00. The corresponding exponents from the memory condition were 0.84, 0.87, and 0.83. Noteworthy is the near uniformity of exponents for the youngest children; perceptual and memorial psychophysical functions became discriminantly different at older age only. The use of rectangular stimuli entails a valuable bonus for the student of memory psychophysics. Because these are multidimensional stimuli (height and width can be manipulated independently), we were able to bypass the upper bound of 5-7 items (Miller, 1956) imposed on the recognition (and, consequently, the recollection of) unidimensionally varying stimuli. The latter, incidentally, may not sufficiently constrain the form and fit of the psychophysical function (see also Hubbard, 1991a). In contradistinction, subjects in the Algom et al. (1985) study, for example, experienced no difficulty acquiring names to 16 different rectangles (all subjects passed the fairly stringent criterion of 300% overlearning).

Circle area, it may be recalled, was the dimension of choice in Bjorkman et al.'s (1960) pioneer research of memory psychophysics (another dimension tested in that study was weight). Based on indirect procedures, these authors conjectured that the psychophysical function for remembered area may be expansive. By contrast, a tightly controlled experiment on circle area conducted in this laboratory (Sarfaty, 1986) yielded traditional results: exponents of 0.79 and 0.68, respectively, for perception and memory. Fantini (1984) reported similar results, with the memorial exponent approximating the square perceptual exponent. Moyer, Sklarew, and Whiting (1982) obtained exponents of 0.96 and 0.79, respectively, for perception and memory of circle size. Recently, Algom (1991) had 7 groups of subjects estimate circular areas. The investigation included four memory delays, ranging from responding immediately after the learning of symbolic codes to the different circles to 24 h. To control for the effects of familiarity and time of testing, the study also included three perceptual conditions: judgments of *physically* presented stimuli either without associative learning or with immediate or an earlier (24 h before testing) associative learning.

Results of the three perceptual groups could be described by power functions with exponents of 0.68, 0.66, and 0.68, respectively. Memorial judgments were also governed by power functions, but with smaller exponents: 0.42, 0.49, 0.50, and 0.45 for delays of 0, 10 min., 180 min., and 24 h, respectively. These results imply that, within the span tested, the magnitude of delay does not materially influence memory-based judgments of visual area (but see Hubbard, 1991b).

Let me relate to the problem of stimulus choice again. With artificial stimuli varying along a single dimension subjects are not able to remember more than about seven stimuli. With multidimensional stimuli such as rectangles we can bypass that limitation, but another problem arises. Subjects may respond -- perceptually as well as from memory -- by mental calculation, i.e., commit the "stimulus error" (e.g., they may judge area by multiplying height and width). One way to circumvent that problem is to use natural stimuli (e.g., countries) that are both multidimensional and irregular in shape. Mental calculations are highly unlikely with such stimuli. However, these stimuli presuppose familiarity, and familiarity entails at least ordinal information. That ordinal knowledge suffices to produce acceptable memorial functions -- independent of any experimental manipulation of memory (see also Hubbard, 1991a,b). Psychophysical functions for "inferred" area or distance were generated, I suspect, just by such ranking, not by resorting to memorial representations.

Artificial stimuli of irregular shape are beset less by these problems. Kemp (1988, Experiment 2) used such items -- configuration of yellow on red background -- as stimuli. The exponent of the power function relating perceived to actual area was 0.82. Data of three memory groups were characterized by the following exponents: 0.72, 0.69, and 0.58, respectively, for delays of 2 min., 90 min., and 1 week. Reassuringly perhaps, the pattern of data replicate that found for "conventional" geographic stimuli under comparable conditions. Kerst and Howard (1984) used computer-generated irregular polygons as stimuli. They found exponents of 0.77 and 0.61 for perception and memory, respectively. Again, these results replicate those found for cartographic area by the same investigators (0.79 and 0.60, Kerst & Howard, 1978).

Overall, the collective data on visual area is quite (though perhaps not fully) consistent with the predictions of the reperception hypothesis. As visual area is a compressive sensory dimension, however, many of the same results also are in accord with the premises of the uncertainty hypothesis. And, again, the lack of a satisfactory criteria for validation plagues these data as it does all judgments deriving from unconstrained univariate designs.

Visual Volume

Moyer et al.'s (1978) study contained an experiment on judgments of volume (of familiar spherical objects). Perceptual and memorial exponents were 0.729 and 0.527. Wolf and Algom (1987) presented 6-year-olds and 10-year-olds with solid parallelepipeds and asked them to assess their volume. Neither perceptual nor memory-based judgments were well fit by power functions (although the same data-sets yielded clear metric structures). One possible reason for the failure of the power fit was restricted range: a ratio of 8:1 between the biggest and smallest stimuli.

Brightness

Barak-Mayer (1985) obtained exponents of 0.40 and 0.32, respectively, for perceived and remembered brightness (of small luminous circles). Moyer, Bradley, and Cutcomb (1977) and Hubbard (1991a) reported that their preliminary data on brightness were also incongruent with the reperception hypothesis (but did not elaborate). Data on brightness, though extremely sparse, are valued because early proponents of the reperception hypothesis (Kerst & Howard, 1978; Moyer et al., 1978) conjectured that it applies to extensive continua, but not to intensive continua such as brightness.

Loudness

Barak-Mayer (1985) used pure tones at several frequencies and found power function exponents of 0.34 and 0.24 for perception and memory. Sarfaty (1986) used pure tones at 2 kHz and obtained an exponent of 0.47 for perception, and a greater exponent of 0.55 for memory. Recently, Algom and Marks completed another study on the perception and memory of loudness at the Pierce laboratory at Yale University. Perceptual and memory-based judgments both were governed by power functions with exponents of 0.46 and 0.43. The study included two additional groups that underwent the same learning (to associate symbols to sounds), but were tested only on a sample of the original set of sounds. For these subjects, the softest and loudest SPLs were dropped from the judgment session, thereby truncating range substantially. Perceptual and memorial exponents were 0.47 and 0.45. There is a slight trend for increased exponents with constricted range (e.g., Algom & Marks, 1990; Teghtsoonian, 1971, 1973); notably, the contingency applies to memorial judgments to at least the same extent as it does to perceptual judgments.

The collective results of these three studies are inconsistent with the predictions of the reperception hypothesis as in no case do memorial exponents approximate the square of the respective perceptual exponents. This outcome may or may not be related to the fact that, like brightness, loudness is an intensive judgment continuum.

Auditory Volume

We can describe several qualitatively different experiences arising from sound stimuli. They include not only pitch and loudness but also volume -- the sense in which the sound fills space and seems large or small. Volume increases with intensity and decreases with frequency, such that listeners must add to the intensity of high-pitched tones in order to keep their volume constant (Stevens, 1934, 1975). Barak-Mayer (1985) used Thomas' (1949) equal-volume-contours to derive a relatively large set of sounds (pure tones of varying intensity and frequency). Because of channel limitations, subjects learned names to random subsets only of these stimuli. Partial overlap among the subsets permitted normalization of data across subjects and stimuli, and, consequently, the derivation of psychophysical functions for volume. Figure 8.1 presents the perceptual (left panel) and memorial (right panel) psychophysical functions for volume at several sound frequencies.

First, consider the family of perceptual functions. Volume grows with intensity at a faster rate at high frequency than at low frequency causing the family of power functions to converge at 143 dB. This value, at which all sounds have the same perceived volume, agrees with the one derived by Terrance and Stevens (1962) on a different set of stimuli (140 dB). Next, consider the data on remembered volume. Remembered volume too relates to sound intensity by a power function governed by a frequency-specific exponent: the higher the frequency the greater the exponent. However, memorial exponents differ from the perceptual exponents characterizing the same frequencies. As a result, memorial functions converge at a much lower value, 125 dB, where all remembered sounds have the same volume. Therefore, compared with the perception of volume, the mind's ear is characterized by a more constrained space, just as the mind's eye is characterized by a more limited visual angle (Kosslyn, 1978).

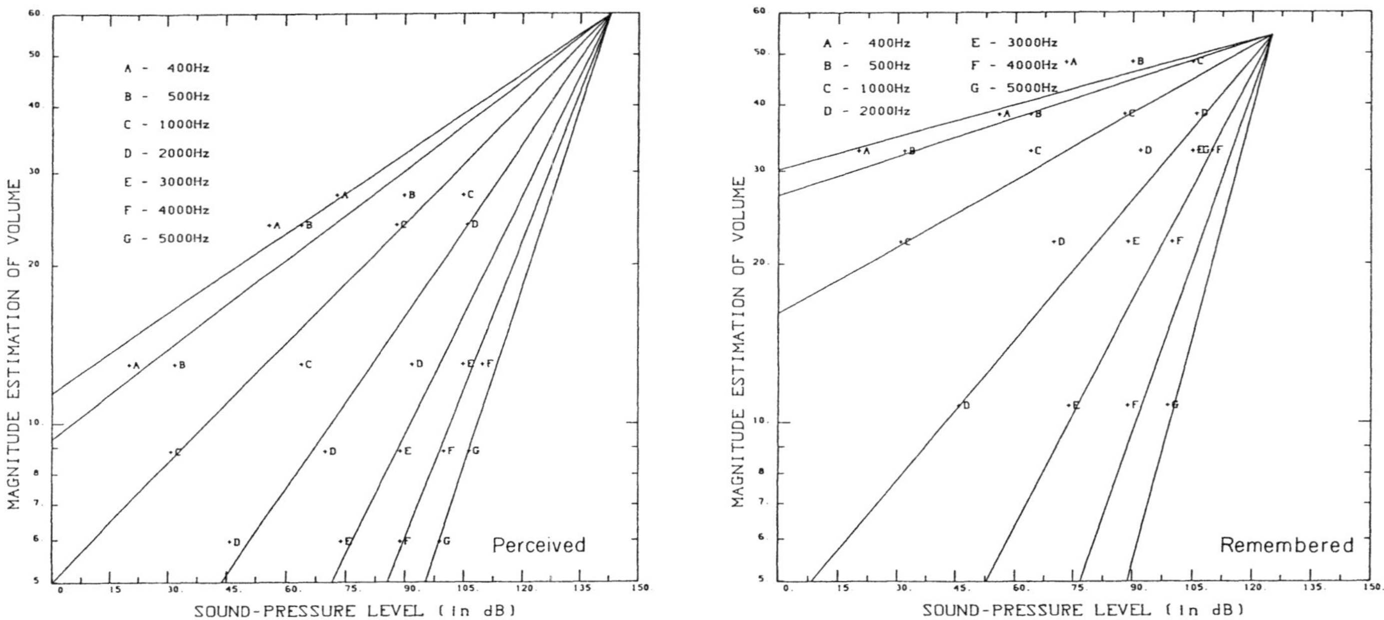

Figure 8.1: Magnitude estimates of auditory volume as a function of sound pressure level. A different function is drawn for each frequency. The points of convergence are calculated analytically. Data are presented for perceptual (left panel) and memorial (right panel) judgments.

Because perceived volume and remembered volume both are power functions of the referent intensities, one set of estimates should be a power function of the other. Plotting the judgments from memory against the respective perceptual judgments resulted indeed in a power function governed by an exponent of 2.01. That outcome is exactly the one predicted by the reperception hypothesis. In fact, this finding confers on the theory its strongest support yet. Unlike other reports relating to a pair of exponents, Barak-Mayer's results depict a functional relation between sets of perceptual and memorial exponents. (To be sure, the actual values did not bear the prescribed square relation, as the intercept of the power function relating the two sets differed from zero).

A final comment is in order. Barak-Mayer used the same sounds in her aforementioned experiment on loudness (exponents of 0.34 and 0.24, for perception and memory). Importantly, then, a common set of stimuli served to derive estimates on intensive (loudness) and extensive (volume) judgment continua. Results were inconsistent with the reperception hypothesis with the former stimuli, but bore out the theory's predictions with the latter. These results reinforce the notion that different memorial processes may apply to intensive and extensive continua.

Weight

I am aware of only four mnemophysical studies probing this dimension. Moyer et al (1982) report exponents of 1.15 and 1.04, respectively, for perception and memory. In a second experiment with a larger range of stimuli, the exponents were 0.88 and 0.62 (all values based on reading of their figure 7). In this laboratory, Sarfaty (1986), using an intermediate range, obtained perceptual and memorial exponents of 0.91 and 0.82. Bjorkman et al (1960) tested apparent heaviness using an indirect procedure and concluded (tentatively) that the mnemophysical contingency might be expansive.

Roughness

Moyer et al. (1982) report results of two studies on perceived and remembered roughness (of paper stimuli). The respective exponents for perception and memory were 1.10 and 1.48 in the first experiment, and 1.08 and 1.26 in the second (the last two values are approximations based on their figure 6).

Haptic Extent

Sukenik (1985), working in this laboratory, obtained exponents of 1.03 and 1.07 for perception and memory of linear haptic extent. Sarfaty (1986) found perceptual and memorial exponents of 0.99 and 0.85. Mnemophysical work on weight, roughness, and haptic extent was inspired by reports of greater than unity exponents for perception in these continua. These reports, in turn, nourished hopes for performing diagnostic experiments, ones that could decide among the alternative accounts of memorial judgment. Apparently, these expectations were largely premature.

Taste

In a recent study (Algom & Marks, 1989), subjects made quantitative judgments of various concentrations of sucrose perceptually or from memory. Perceived and remembered intensities related to referent concentrations by power functions with similar exponents. Actually, the memorial exponent was slightly greater than the perceptual exponent (0.87 versus 0.70), though not reliably so.

Moyer et al (1982) have similarly found an insignificant difference between functions for perceived and remembered sweetness of sucrose (exponents of 1.21 and 1.1). For sweetness of saccharine, Moyer et al. report exponents of 0.93 and 0.7, respectively, for perception and memory. (These and the previous values are approximations based on their figure 8).

Odor

Algom and Cain (1991a,b; see also Algom, Marks, & Cain, 1989) used the banana-smelling substance amyl acetate (five discriminantly different suprathreshold concentrations) as the stimulus. Mean exponents were 0.33 for perception and 0.36 for memory; the difference was not significant. Osaka (1987) reported exponents of 0.38 for perception and 0.52 for memory for the smell of pyridine. That study suffers from several weaknesses, however, providing a caveat with regard to the methodology to be adhered to in mnemophysical investigations. Osaka used a within-subject design, that is, the same subjects participated in perception and memory. Thus, subjects might have recalled their perceptual *judgments* rather than their perceptual experiences. Hence, validity of the memory-based judgments is suspect. In addition, no criterion for the acquisition of the smell-color associations was set (the two stimulus presentations could hardly have provided the needed learning-base for the 10 day retention interval). Patently, mnemophysical investigations call for between-subjects designs coupled with extensive and testable acquisition procedures.

Data on chemosensation is still sparse. Yet the uniformity of corresponding perceptual and memorial exponents demonstrated in current studies contrasts with typical results reported for extensive visual continua. Neither the reperception nor the uncertainty hypothesis can accommodate these data. Therefore, we must reject these traditional formulations as a *general* account of memorial judgment (even if either of them proves adequate for extensive continua in vision and in other sensory departments). By contrast, the two-stage model can, in principle, account for the chemosensory data as well. Applying this model to the taste data collected by Algom and Marks (1989), for example, yields a value of 1.26 that fares well with exponents for sweetness of sucrose reported in the literature (often in the vicinity of 1.3; e.g., Stevens, 1969; see also Moyer et al., 1982). The model, however, seems less conclusive in other cases. It predicts a theoretical exponent of 1.09 when applied to the odor data of Algom and Cain (1991b); although exponents greater than unity have been reported for smell (Laing, Panhuber, & Baxter, 1978), that value certainly is not typical.

Electrocutaneous pain

Psychophysical studies relating subjective magnitude to the current or voltage of electric pulses abounded in the last two decades (see Algom, Raphaeli, & Cohen-Raz, 1986, and Rollman & Harris, 1987, for succinct summaries of this literature; see too the chapter by Rollman in this volume). This research confirmed the heralded status of painful electric stimulation as the prototype of expansive psychophysical relations, where the rate of growth of the sensory variable exceeds that of the physical one. For memory psychophysics, nociception held the promise of providing a diagnostic criterion-dimension to decide between the alterative accounts of remembered information.

Sukenik (1985) used three groups in a first mnemophysical investigation of pain. There were two perceptual conditions: subjects judged the painfulness of shocks either with or without prior learning (to associate symbols to the shocks). Hence the former but not the latter were familiar with the pulses delivered to the undersite of the wrist. In the memory condition, subjects judged pain based on symbolic representations of the original stimuli. Results showed that the psychophysical functions for both perceived and remembered pain approximate power functions. The exponent for memory-based judgments of pain was 1.33, whereas the respective exponents for the simple and familiarized perceptual groups were 1.06 and 0.81. A salient characteristic of these data is the steeper memorial function. Notable too is the effect of familiarity with the stimulus. People react differently to aversive stimuli experienced in the past and to novel noxious stimuli. Algom (1991) and Algom et al (1985) found no effect of familiarity for judgments of area. Obviously, the case for nociception differs, compromising an explanation of the results in terms of the reperception hypothesis.

Sarfaty (1986) found exponents of 1.74 for perception and 1.17 for memory of painful electrical shocks. Recently, Algom, von Schwarze, and Shakuf completed a mnemophysical study of electrical shock on separate groups of males and females. For the former, perceptual and memorial exponents were 2.21 and 1.8; for the latter, the respective exponents were 1.61 and 1.65. Neither cognitive mode nor gender was statistically significant.

The paucity of research notwithstanding, extant studies do not support the reperception hypothesis. Neither have these studies helped adjudicate the theoretical disagreements. These failures may be interpreted in two ways. For one, they cast doubt on the validity of the traditional formulations as genuine explanations of memorial judgment. Alternatively, the failures merely reflect on the status of electrocutaneous pain as an intensive judgment continuum; as was suspected by their proponents, the formulations might apply to extensive continua only.

Labor Pain

Labor offers a particularly penetrating way of looking at pain. It combines the natural, endogenous quality of clinical pain (assuring external validity) with precise control and measurement characteristic of laboratory pain (assuring internal validity). Taking advantage of standard medical equipment and practices, Algom and Lubel (1989; see also Algom, 1988a) related pain judgments of individual uterine contractions to the biometrically measured magnitude (peak pressure) of those contractions. Different groups of women estimated the painfulness of sets of irregularly selected contractions either immediately (perceptual condition) or at time intervals varying from 8 to 48 h after their completion (memorial conditions). In the latter groups, women were told to imagine each contraction as the codes (associated with the contractions upon their occurrence in labor) were shown and then estimate its painfulness. Note that, as pains were self generated, intrauterine pressure values differed as a matter of course across women. Nevertheless, the functional relations between the pain stimulus and sensation could be compared across subjects and conditions.

Perceptual and memorial judgments were governed by power functions. Mean exponents were 1.4 for perception, and 1.63, 2.0, and 1.75 for memory, for delays of 8 h, 24 h, and 48 h, respectively. These results suggest a consistently higher exponent for memory-based judgments. A one-tailed perception versus memory test indeed yielded a marginally significant effect ($t = -1.48$, $df = 44$, $p < 0.10$). Reducing variance by a logarithmic transform gave a significant difference ($t = -1.698$, $df = 44$, $p < 0.05$).

Psychophysical functions for remembered pain were, therefore, more expansive than that for perceived pain, and could be characterized by an exponent of 1.79 (the geometric average of memory data over all time delays).

There was no indication of a change in exponent as a function of delay; only the mode of response (perceptual or memorial) counted. It follows that for a contraction to feel twice as painful as a second contraction, its intensity would need to be about 1.64 as great. Yet for one contraction to be *remembered* twice as painful as another, the ratio of physical intensities would need to be no greater than 1.47. Remembered labor pain grows at a faster rate than does instantaneous labor pain. Although memorial judgments of labor pain were dependable (as evidenced by good fits), the underlying psychophysical contingency is markedly nonlinear, characterized by a positively accelerated function.

The reperception hypothesis is the alternative favored by these data. Commensurate with its predictions, the memory functions are steeper than the already expansive perceptual function. Although the numerical values deviate somewhat from the expected square relation ($1.4^2 = 1.96 \neq 1.79$), the deviation is not great. Moreover, the memorial exponents remained largely invariant across the different time delays.

I have no ready answer for the question why the data on labor support the reperception hypothesis whereas the electrocutaneous data are equivocal. There seems to be no obvious difference between shocks and contractions in terms of their space fulfilling properties, although such a difference is a possibility to reckon with. On the surface, both types of pain are examples of intensive judgment continua. Be this as it may, the field study of Algom and Lubel must carry a special weight when deciding among the theoretical alternatives.

In summary, this survey provides qualified support for the reperception and the uncertainty hypotheses (in that order) for extensive (primarily visual) continua. These continua -- characterized by compressive psychophysical functions -- are not diagnostic, however, and cannot decide between the two rival hypotheses. Expansive psychophysical dimensions are diagnostic, yet the (few) continua studied were intensive, and the hypotheses may possibly apply to extensive continua only. The two-stage model of judgment suggested by Algom and Marks (1989) can accommodate the various data-sets, but some applications are more plausible than others. Finally, all models are vulnerable on counts of validity, a problem insolvable within the confines of the univariate designs reviewed.

Nevertheless, to offer a balanced perspective, I wish to conclude this review on a positive note. Despite the modulating effect of the structural limitations, the cumulative results emerging from this research are encouraging. They suggest that "memory for continuous magnitudes is far from crude, but instead preserves much of the information present in the physical scale; that is equal stimulus ratios correspond to equal ratios of subjective magnitude estimates at all locations on the scale" (Kerst & Howard, 1984, p. 517). The good fits to the memory functions obtained throughout the different studies affirm that more than just ordinal information is conserved. Such data, in turn, offer a promising basis to start confronting the intriguing questions of memory psychophysics.

VI. Multidimensional Mnemophysics

As I have alluded, the methods of memory psychophysics become perhaps most powerful when applied to multidimensional stimuli. First, subjects are able to remember a greater number of such stimuli (especially those composed of separable dimensions). Second, response validity is tractable because the rules by which the components integrate -- evidenced in the resulting metric structures -- provide the necessary constraints to validate the psychophysical functions (Anderson, 1970, 1981, 1982; Krantz & Tversky, 1971; see also Anderson's chapter in this volume). Third and most important, this allows examination of a whole new class of questions relating to organizational principles in perception and memory.

Consider the approach advocated over the past three decades by Norman Anderson, designated *functional measurement*. It handles explicitly the rules used when people combine information from different stimulus components. Such rules, it should be recognized, are ubiquitous as virtually any behavior is the integrated outcome of multiple determinants. Accordingly, the theory focuses on uncovering the exact form of concatenation of subjective components into a unitary overt response. Specification of the metric structure that underlies the overt judgments provides the logical base to validate these judgments. Therefore, the functional model contains the scale -- the psychophysical function -- as its natural derivative.

Functional measurement has been applied throughout different domains in psychology, notably to probe perceptual processes. Nothing inherent to the method, however, prevents its application to memory. The latter may actually

provide a novel tool of exploration in the attempt to render memorial phenomena experimentally tractable. Only by recognizing the full system characteristics of memory can we address the primary concerns of integration and synthesis. Applications of the information integration approach to memory have nonetheless been few and selective. The modest body of research notwithstanding, results to date demonstrate the great potential of this approach. Insights into the quality of sensory knowledge and representations have been gained and, in turn, led to the unraveling of a general-purpose strategy of cognitive action.

The methodology used in multidimensional explorations of memory psychophysics is straightforward. Values of one component variable are combined factorially with values of another component variable to produce the experimental stimuli. For example, in vision, one can combine 4 values of height with 3 values of width to produce a matrix of 12 rectangles, or, in olfaction, pure concentrations of two different substances can be combined to yield all possible binary mixtures. As with unidimensional stimuli, the experiment typically comprises two phases: a learning phase and a judgment phase. During the former, subjects learn to associate symbols to physical stimuli; in the latter, subjects estimate the stimuli either perceptually or from memory. Unlike the univariate case, however, the experimenter in the multidimensional investigation has several options as to what stimuli to present the subjects in the initial learning session. That choice carries important theoretical ramifications to the examination of which I turn now.

To help make sense of the various alternatives, I will suggest a new terminology to delineate the implied processes. It is possible to distinguish between four classes of pertinent mnemophysical phenomena. First, the experimenter may elect to present the global, multidimensional stimuli themselves (e.g., rectangles, mixtures) for associative learning and, subsequently, for judgment. We can designate that condition as *remembered stimuli* (e.g., remembered rectangles, remembered mixtures). On the surface, this condition replicates that used in the univariate studies. There is, however, a crucial difference. Here stimuli are multidimensional, allowing for the specification of the rule(s) of integration in perception and memory. Alternatively, subjects may be presented with components only of the to-be-judged stimuli. Thus, for example, subjects can learn CVCs to several horizontal and vertical line stimuli. At a subsequent judgment session, the experimenter may covary the CVCs in a factorial design. Presented with a pair of CVCs, subjects are instructed to form an imaginary rectangle whose sides are made of the referent line stimuli. I use the phrase *mental stimuli* (e.g., mental rectangles, mental mixtures) to refer to the processes of mental construction that presumably operate under such conditions. A slight variation on the previous procedure yields another condition. The experimenter may choose to present one variable via prelearned symbols, but the other component physically. For example, subjects may be presented simultaneously with a color standing for one substance and the actual smell of another and try to form an image of the appropriate binary mixture. The term *semimental stimuli* refer to these instances (e.g., semimental rectangles, semimental mixtures). Finally, one can focus on the fate of the individual components in the integrated memory stimulus rather than on the process of synthesis that creates it. For example, subjects can smell an odorant while viewing a color standing for a second odorant and imagine the two mixed together. Then, subjects may try to assess the intensity of the second (coded) odorant -- as it would smell in the imagined mixture. I coin such conditions *mental analysis*. Each of these aspects of memory psychophysics is illustrated in the following survey of empirical results.

Visual Area

Algom et al. (1985) used the methods of functional measurement in a first study of multidimensional mnemophysics. Separate groups of observers estimated the area of perceived, remembered, mental, and semimental rectangles.

A multiplicative Area = Height x Width composition rule underlay the perceptual judgments. The crucial finding of our study, however, was the reappearance of the normative Height x Width pattern in memorial estimates of area. Subjects used the same cognitive algebra in judgments of area when those judgments were based on imaginary constructs. The way in which the relevant information was conveyed -- perceptually or memorially, with or without presentation of the global physical referent (i.e., actual rectangles) -- mattered little to the composition of area (see Figure 8.2).

The multiplicative rule found throughout the perceptual and memorial conditions allowed derivation of validated psychophysical functions. As I have mentioned, the exponents were largely consistent with the predictions of the reperception hypothesis: memorial exponents were smaller than the already compressive perceptual exponents. We concluded perforce that the pervasive multiplicative model acts on *different* sets of implicit values in perception and memory. The latter set is nonlinearly related to the former set of scale values.

The discovery of across-mode invariance for the form of the composition rule (though not for the parameter governing the psychophysical function) entails a general cognitive principle of vast importance. It means that perceptual organization and capacities pose tight constraints on people's inner world of memory and imagery. The latter seem to obey the very rules used in constructing people's physically bound perceptual world. However, the invariance finding derived from a single model of integration based on the results of one study. Hence, the implied constancy may not have been general. To rectify that situation, Wolf and Algom (1987) undertook a developmental study on the mnemophysics of visual area.

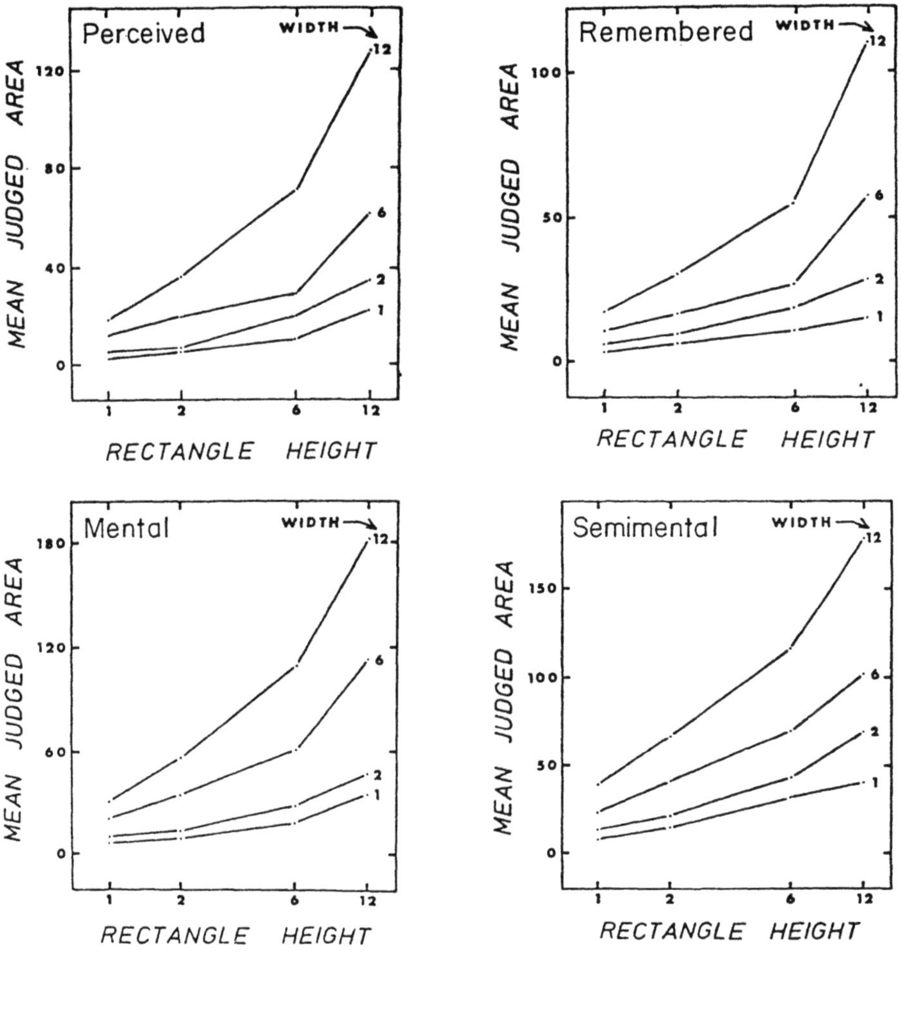

Figure 8.2: Magnitude estimates of area as a function of rectangle height. The parameter is rectangle width. The different panels depict results for perceived, remembered, mental, and semimental rectangles. After Algom et al., 1985.

Children's judgments of size offer a convenient tool for explicating the memory psychophysics of area. Several studies (e.g., Anderson & Cuneo, 1978; Wilkening, 1979) demonstrated a clear developmental trend in the perception of area. Between the ages of 6 and 10, there is a transition from an initial additive, Area = Height + Width rule to the final, normative, multiplicative model. The fact that children use different algebraic rules at different ages enables one to test the complementary integration models for remembered area. We followed just this tactic in our mnemophysical investigation.

Children at three different ages (means of 6, 8, and 10 years) made judgments of physically presented (perceptual estimation) or symbolically represented (memorial estimation) rectangles. Memorial data obeyed the same integration rules that operated in the original perceptual judgments even when younger children and older children used different combination models. Where, in the course of development, perceptual algebra changes (from addition to multiplication), so too does the corresponding memorial algebra. The developmental study thus yielded additional support for a "law of across-representation invariance" coined by Wolf and Algom (1987).

An important, though largely unexpected, result of that study concerns the psychophysical functions. For the 8-year-olds and the 10-year-olds, psychophysical functions for memory were markedly more compressive than those for perception. In that respect, these older children behaved the same way as adults do. By contrast, for the 6-year-olds, memorial and perceptual functions had virtually identical exponents. At this age, then, perceptual and memorial processes act both on practically equivalent sets of implicit values. For 6-year-olds, one can speak of a *first-order isomorphism* between physical and mental relations in that, at this age, the cognitive algebra and valuation operation both assume the same form in perception and memory.

Visual Volume

The Wolf and Algom (1987) study included an experiment on judgments of volume. Six-year-olds and 10-year-olds were presented with three-dimensional solid objects (rectangular cardboard blocks) to obtain perceptual and memorial judgments of volume (in separate groups). The perceptual data for the 6-year-olds conformed fairly well to an overall additive, Volume = Height + Width + Depth model. The perceptual data for the older children could be characterized by a compound adding-multiplying model. Failure of the normative Height x Width x Depth pattern to appear in the latter set of data is surprising from a developmental perspective. However, the most striking feature of the results was the close correspondence, at each age, of perception and memory (see Figure 2.11). The findings of this experiment verify and generalize the equivalence of cognitive algebra used in perception and memory, across different rules of integration and stimulus dimensionality.

Odor

Algom and Cain (1991a,b) used binary mixtures of the banana smelling amyl acetate and the crushed-grass-smelling leaf alcohol as stimuli. Separate groups of observers judged the intensity of perceived, remembered, mental, and semimental banana-grass mixtures. The results from the perceptual condition displayed many of the documented features of (odor) mixture perception. Salient were the so-called "masking" or suppression phenomena (e.g., Cain, 1988) resulting in a noted tendency of the family of functions to convergence at the upper right corner. Adding a low level of one stimulus component to a low level of the other augmented odor sensation considerably, but adding a low level to a high level effected virtually no change in smell intensity.

The most striking feature of the various sets of the memorial data was that they too evidenced masking and convergence. The results showed that even for the intensity of mental mixtures -- stimuli composed wholly subjectively -- the rule of integration was the same one that operated in physical mixture perception. The data were intriguing because they demonstrated mutual suppression even for symbolically represented *nonsmelled* constituents of mentally composed mixtures. In displaying an invariance in the principle of multidimensional integration olfaction joins the visual continua of area and volume (see Figure 8.3).

The reappearance of the original -- perceptual -- pattern in memorial estimates of mixture intensity carries further implications. These results suggest that olfactory memory and imagery are lawfully related to the chemo-physical properties of the odoriferous environment. People may well possess large reservoirs of implicit knowledge about odors and the rules governing their composition. All of which explain the main conclusion we have drawn based on the collective data: People display far deeper olfactory knowledge than they either are aware of or can intelligently articulate.

Finally, consider the condition in the Algom and Cain (1991b) study designated mental analysis. There, we sought to tap the psychological parallels not of chemical synthesis but rather of the complementary process of chemical analysis. How well can people analyze mixtures psychologically? Can they tell the fate of a familiar odorant once it is mixed with another familiar odorant? With physical mixtures, a constituent in a mixture feels less intense than the same constituent smelled alone. The phenomenon is labelled mutual masking or mixture suppression. Does masking or suppression characterize constituents of mental mixtures -- mixtures constructed subjectively and which lack chemical or sensory interaction of components?

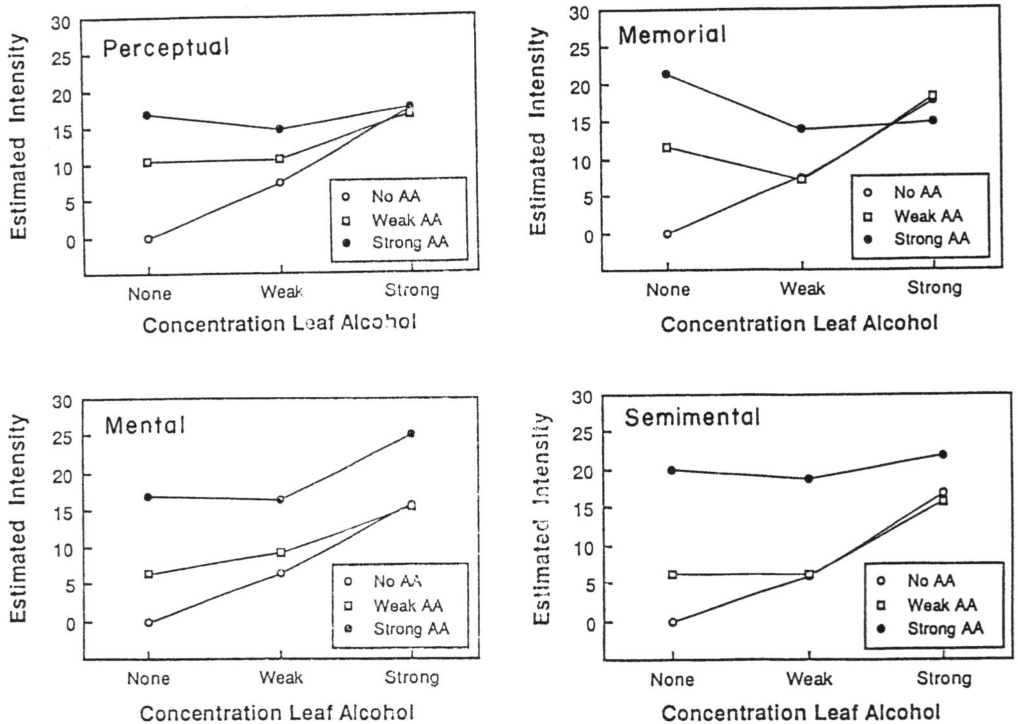

Figure 8.3: Mean intensity estimates of odor mixtures. Magnitude judgments are plotted as a function of the concentration of leaf alcohol; the parameter is concentration of amyl acetate (AA). The different panels depict results for perceived, remembered, mental, and semimental mixtures. After Algom and Cain, 1991b.

Results showed that, quite expectedly, subjects in a perceptual condition experienced considerable masking. In the physical mixtures, the target constituent felt stronger when accompanied by a lower concentration of the masker. Strikingly, subjects in a memory condition also seemed to "experience" masking. Although these subjects never smelled the relevant mixtures (the semimental mixtures comprised a symbolized target and a smelled masker), they did assess the target correctly, its intensity depending functionally on the concentration of the masker. Apparently, people are able to analyze mixtures mentally vis-a-vis concentrations of their components and, remarkably, their analysis of mental mixtures is basically sound -- using actual smelling as our yardstick. That the pattern of analysis remains invariant reinforces the notion that people carry an underlying core of ecologically valid chemosensory knowledge.

Odor and Taste

Recently, Algom, Marks, and Cain (1991) sought to expand chemosensory mnemophysics by testing heteromodal odor-taste mixtures. We selected smell-taste mixtures, taking advantage of a compelling illusion of localization (Cain, 1988): Even sophisticated observers tend to misperceive orally presented odors as tastes. The mixtures stimulate two modalities, and the effects combine through a multimodal process. But to the naive observer, mixtures of an odorant and a tastant, through mislocalization of the odorant, are cognized as homomodal (taste) mixtures. With homomodal mixtures, as we have just seen, a salient characteristic is mutual suppression expressed as interaction of components. With heteromodal mixtures, on the other hand, the perceptual rule is not interactive but additive: mixture intensity approximates the sum of the intensities of the unmixed components. We presented the mixtures intraorally. Hence, our subjects "believed" they were experiencing homomodal stimuli where, in fact, they sensed heteromodal ones. In a second group, no physical mixtures were presented;

mixtures were instead constructed subjectively by mixing mentally the remembered representations of the odor and taste components.

In the perceptual group, results demonstrated additivity of the odor and taste components -- the illusion of localization notwithstanding. Strikingly, in the memorial group, the pattern of combination was also additive. Given separately presented taste and odor components, the mental mixtures nevertheless mirrored the rule used when the global stimulus was presented physically (and hence the physical mixtures were processed bimodally). Counterintuitively perhaps, even under the present conditions, the rule of memorial combination followed the original perceptual pattern dictated by actually experiencing the solutions.

These results illustrate the pervasiveness of a chemosensory "deep structure" of perceptual knowledge that may prove to be not explicit but tacit, and therefore cognitively impenetrable.

Pain

In a recent study conducted in the author's laboratory, Lindenberg (1987) combined painful electric shocks and disagreeably loud tones in a factorial design (see Algom, Raphaeli, & Cohen-Raz, 1986, 1987, for a fuller description of such designs). Separate groups of observers judged the painfulness of perceived, remembered, and mental tone-shock mixtures. In the latter condition, for example, subjects first learned names to separate electric and auditory stimuli. In a second session, the experimenter covaried factorially the names to produce imagery mixtures. Presented with a pair of names, the subjects imagined the appropriate noxious compound produced by the referent shock and tone components, then judged its painfulness. Results are presented in Figure 8.4.

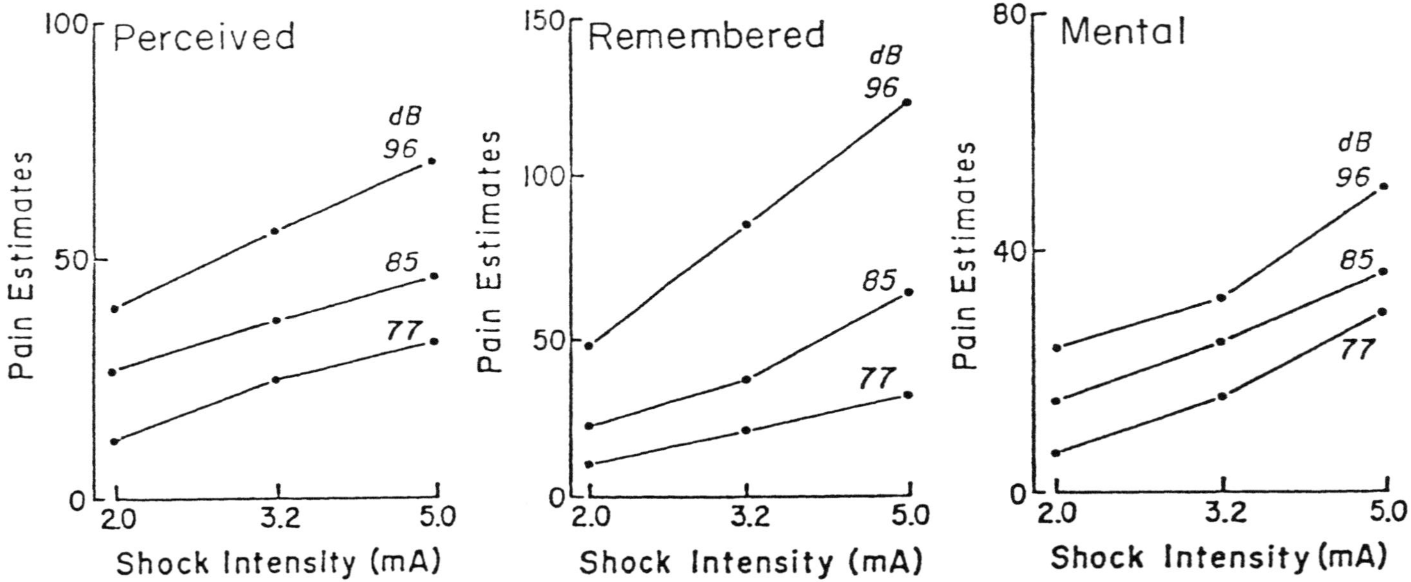

Figure 8.4: Integration of perceived, remembered, and mental pain.

The additive structure evident in the perceptual estimates of concurrent pain (left panel) provides a further replication of similarly parallel patterns obtained in previous studies of pain integration (e.g., Algom et al., 1986, 1987; Jones, 1980; Jones & Gwynn, 1984; Gracely & Wolskee, 1983; see also Algom, 1987, 1992). Next consider the judgments of mental compounds in the right panel. Clearly, the additive structure reappeared in that condition. Thus even for judgments of mental pain -- events constructed wholly subjectively -- the integration rule is one of linear summation of component scale values. Additivity fails, however, for remembered noxious compounds (middle panel). Why do perceptual estimates of pain add linearly but remembered values of the same components obey a nonlinear rule of concatenation? I do not have a ready explanation for this single violation of the invariance principle. The finding may be fortuitous or a result of the influence on painful memories of affective factors. More research is clearly needed. But the same is true for virtually any aspect of memory psychophysics.

In summary, the few multidimensional studies of memory psychophysics attest already to the great potential of this approach. Although mnemophysical methods can measure directly a person's memory for intensity (neglected in current cognitive research), they also make possible to probe underlying sensory processes and representations when applied to multidimensionally constructed arrays of stimuli. These applications enable one to uncover properties of cognitive predispositions in the relevant domains. Two such properties of general significance emerged. First, people carry a core of ecologically valid sensory knowledge which is cognitively impenetrable. Second, consequently, people's memorial and imaginary representations obey the same rules used in constructing their perceptual responses. In a strict sense, there are not two worlds available for humans, one perceptual and physically oriented, the other imaginal and detached from reality. Far from being detached, people's world of make-believe is governed by the same combinational principles that form their physically-bound sensory world.

VII. Methodological Problems

I have hinted at several vexing problems confronting research in memory psychophysics. Unless they are addressed in a serious manner no real breakthrough in the field can be expected. Actually, the very possibility of pursuing memory psychophysics then becomes suspect (see also Hubbard, 1991a).

Stimulus Choice

If we seek guidance from existing research, it is clear, I think, that multidimensional stimuli should always be preferred. One should use rectangles, complex sounds, and mixtures rather than lines, tones or pure odorants. Information regarding the latter can still be recovered -- but only if they comprise a variable within the framework of an appropriate factorial design. The choice of multidimensionally constructed stimuli is dictated primarily by methodological considerations pertaining to a limitation on the number univariate items and to validity. However, as we have seen, their use is to be preferred based on substantive, cognitive considerations as well.

Of course, many more questions remain. A noxious compound is different from an odor mixture which, in turn, differs from a rectangle. All multidimensional stimuli do not yield psychologically comparable products. Thus an odor mixture may produce a new smell that is different from the elements that made it up; in fact, the smells of the unmixed constituents may turn undetectable once the constituents combine in a mixture. By way of contrast, although there exists an over-all feeling of pain, the different noxious components are nonetheless available to perception. In general, a stimulus mixture can be synthetic or analytic, depending on whether its components comprise integral or separable dimensions

(Garner, 1974). The former, incidentally, may be plagued by some of the methodological problems that affect univariate mnemophysics. Be it as it may, memory psychophysics can profitably deal with issues of dimensional interaction. Cognitive psychology reaped substantial gains confronting the same questions (see Melara's chapter in this volume).

Familiarity poses another challenge. We are familiar with many odorants, tastants, cartographic shapes, or sounds, some of which may serve as stimuli in the mnemophysical experiment. Familiarity was shown to affect results in the related field of symbolic comparison (e.g., Banks, 1977). It entails ordinal knowledge already capable of producing memorial functions with good fits (Parker, Casey, Ziriax, & Siberberg, 1988). Arbitrary stimuli, on the other hand, may invite responses based on mental calculation rather than on authentic sensation or memory. Even if we grant that both types of stimuli produce valid judgments, familiarity can still make a difference.

Response Validity

The use of factorial designs settles the fundamental validation problem, but several uncertainties remain. How do we know that, instructed to imagine a given stimulus, the subject does in fact remember the stimulus? He or she may respond in a random fashion or report the intensity of another stimulus erroneously taken for the experimental one. Large r^2s characterizing the memory functions may provide one pause, but they come short of a real remedy. Needed are measures of memory that reflect directly on the accuracy of recollection. After providing their memorial judgments, subjects can be tested by such classic methods as relearning, recognition, or free recall. Moreover, we can enrich the arsenal of dependent measures by using responses such as sketching, matching of magnitudes, or reaction time aside from the vital magnitude judgments.

Elimination of responses based on faulty memory could create more homogeneous sets of data.

Data-driven Classifications

I have identified five separate procedures germane to memory psychophysics. They include perceived, remembered, mental, and semimental stimuli, as well as mental analysis. The conditions are defined solely in terms of the experimental designs used to establish the context of response evocation. Clearly, much research is needed to delineate experimentally the cognitive processes that presumably underlie behavior in the different conditions. The "law of across-representation invariance" denotes one strategy common to all conditions. Other strategies, however, may apply selectively. That classification (as well as future ones) may afford a unique opportunity for exploring the cognitive potential of memory psychophysics.

Time Delay

The temporal intervals between learning the stimuli and judging them from memory used in mnemophysical research have been fairly limited. Most studies used delays ranging between 0 and 24 h, but some tested memory after 2 days or even 1 week. Results are discordant as some studies (Hubbard, 1991b; Kemp, 1988) report a decrease in the value of the memorial exponent with increased retention interval, whereas another study (Algom, 1991) failed to detect a systematic trend. The effect on the exponent of varying the extent of delay has yet to be systematically investigated. It also remains to be seen whether extant findings and theories apply to much longer intervals of say weeks and months.

Exponent Magnitude Versus Response Magnitude

The almost exclusive concern of mnemophysical studies related to the exponent of the memorial function. Needed are data on the magnitude of the memorial judgments themselves, vis-a-vis the magnitude of the corresponding perceptual judgments. Several studies (e.g., Algom & Marks, 1989; Barker & Weaver, 1983) indicated smaller absolute judgments for memory. The comparison is a difficult one to make, however, given the between-subjects designs used. Clever experimental maneuvers are needed to redress the situation and marshal new data both on response magnitude and its relation to other mnemophysical indices.

Instructions

Whether subjects are instructed to judge the "objective" or "subjective" area of geometrical shapes affects their judgments as well as the resulting psychophysical functions (e.g., M. Teghtsoonian, 1965; Baird, 1970c). Do instructions affect mnemophysical performance as well? And, in general, how does the exact form of instructions for the memory-based judgments effect statistical properties of those judgments? Again, new data are badly needed.

Stimulus Coding

A final issue to be considered is the manner in which the stimuli are coded. Obviously, one must use unordered codes such as nonsense syllables or colors, so as not to provide subjects with ordinal information for their memorial judgments. Beyond that requirement, however, virtually nothing is known about the effects on memory of the various features of the learning procedure. Should stimuli and codes be presented simultaneously or sequentially? What durations and inter-stimulus-intervals should be used? How does learning (i.e., repeated preexposure to the to-be-judged stimuli) affect *perceptual* judgments of those stimuli? What criterion should acquisition meet? Experimental resolution of these issues should eventually narrow down the range of possible explanations for the findings of mnemophysical experiments. Ultimately, the debates surrounding memory psychophysics will be decided by how successful we are in removing the whimsicalities that still mark this young field of inquiry.

References

Algom, D. (1987). Pain: A functional approach. In M. Teghtsoonian & R. Teghtsoonian (Eds.), *Fechner Day '87* (pp. 53-54). Durham NH: International Society for Psychophysics.

Algom, D. (1988a). *Psychophysics in the field: Perceptual and memorial psychophysical functions for labor pain.* Paper presented at the Twenty-ninth Annual Meeting of the Psychonomic Society, Chicago, IL.

Algom, D. (1988b). Tephisa vedimuy: Meaffyenim meshutaphim (Perception and imagery: Some common features). *Psychologia*, **1**, 5-10.

Algom, D. (1991). Memory psychophysics for area: Effect of length of delay. *Perceptual Motor Skills,* **72**, 296.

Algom, D. (1992). Psychophysical analysis of pain: A functional perspective. In H.G. Geissler, S.W. Link, & J.T. Townsend (Eds.), *Cognition, information processing, and psychophysics: Basic issues.* Hillsdale, NJ: Erlbaum.

Algom, D. & Cain, W.S. (1991a). Chemosensory representation in perception and memory. In S.J. Bolanowski, Jr., & G.A. Gescheider (Eds.), *Ratio scaling of psychological magnitude.* Hillsdale, NJ: Erlbaum.

Algom, D. & Cain, W.S. (1991b). Remembered odors and mental mixtures: Tapping reservoirs of olfactory knowledge. *Journal of Experimental Psychology: Human Perception and Performance,* **17**, 1104-1119.

Algom, D. & Lubel, S. (1989). *Memory and perception of clinical and laboratory pain: Psychophysical relations and rules of integration.* Unpublished manuscript, Bar-Ilan University.

Algom, D. & Marks, L.E. (1984). Individual differences in loudness processing and loudness scales. *Journal of Experimental Psychology: General,* **113**, 471-493.

Algom, D. & Marks, L.E. (1989). Memory psychophysics for taste. *Bulletin of the Psychonomic Society,* **27**, 257-259.

Algom, D. & Marks, L.E. (1990). Range and regression, loudness scales and loudness processing: Toward a context-bound psychophysics. *Journal of Experimental Psychology: Human Perception and Performance,* **16**, 706-727.

Algom, D., Marks, L.E., & Cain, W.S. (1989). *Memory psychophysics for smell and taste.* Poster presented at the Eleventh Annual Meeting of the Association for Chemosensory Sciences, Sarasota, FL.

Algom, D., Marks, L.E., & Cain, W.S. (1991). *Memory psychophysics for chemosensation: Perceptual and mental mixtures for smell and taste.* Unpublished manuscript, Pierce Laboratory and Yale University.

Algom, D., Raphaeli, N., & Cohen-Raz, L. (1986). Integration of noxious stimulation across separate somatosensory communication systems: A functional theory of pain. *Journal of Experimental Psychology: Human Perception and Performance*, **12**, 92-102.

Algom, D., Raphaeli, N., & Cohen-Raz, L. (1987). Pain combines additively across different sensory systems: A further support for the functional theory of pain. *Perceptual and Motor Skills,* **54**, 619-625.

Algom, D., Wolf, Y., & Bergman, B. (1985). Integration of stimulus dimensions in perception and memory: Composition rules and psychophysical relations. *Journal of Experimental Psychology: General,* **114**, 451-471.

Anderson, J.R. (1985). *Cognitive psychology and its implications.* New York: Freeman.

Anderson, N.H. (1970). Functional measurement and psychophysical judgment. *Psychological Review,* **77**, 153-170.

Anderson, N.H. (1981). *Foundations of integration information theory.* New York: Academic Press.

Anderson, N.H. (1982). *Methods of integration information theory.* New York: Academic Press.

Anderson, N.H., & Cuneo, D.O. (1978). The height + width rule in children's judgments of quality. *Journal of Experimental Psychology: General,* **107**, 335-378.

Baird, J.C. (1970a). A cognitive theory of psychophysics. I. *Scandinavian Journal of Psychology,* **11**, 35-46.

Baird, J.C. (1970b). A cognitive theory of psychophysics. II. *Scandinavian Journal of Psychology,* **11**, 89-103.

Baird, J.C. (1970c). *Psychophysical analysis of visual space.* Oxford: Pergamon Press.

Banks, W.P. (1977). Encoding and processing of symbolic information in comparative judgments. In G.H. Bower (Ed.), *The psychology of learning and motivation Vol. 11* (pp. 101-159). New York: Academic Press.

Barak-Mayer, N. (1985). *Perceptual and memorial psychophysical functions for intensive and extensive continua.* Unpublished M.A. Dissertation, Bar-Ilan University.

Barker, L.M., & Weaver, C.A. III. (1983). Rapid, permanent loss of memory for absolute intensity of taste and smell. *Bulletin of the Psychonomic Society,* **21**, 281-284.

Bjorkman, M., Lundberg, U., & Tarnblom, S. (1960). On the relationship between percept and memory; a psychophysical approach. *Scandinavian Journal of Psychology*, **1**, 136-144.

Bradley, D.R., & Vido, D. (1984). Psychophysical functions for perceived and remembered distance. *Perception,* **13**, 315-320.

Brennan, J.F. (1986). *History and systems of psychology* (2nd edition). Englewood Cliffs, NJ: Prentice-Hall.

Briggs, R. (1973). Urban cognitive distance. In R.M. Downs & D. Stea (Eds.), *Image and environment: cognitive mapping and spatial behavior* (pp. 361-390). Chicago: Aldine.

Buckley, P.B., & Gillman, C.B. (1974). Comparison of digits and dot patterns. *Journal of Experimental Psychology,* **103**, 1131-1136.

Cain, W.S. (1988). Olfaction. In R.C. Atkinson, R.J. Herrnstein, G. Lindzey, & R.D. Luce (Eds.), *Stevens' handbook of experimental psychology: Vol I. Perception and motivation* (pp. 409-459). New York: Wiley.

Canter, D. (1977). *Psychology of place.* London: The Architectural Press.

Chew, E.I., & Richardon, J.T.E. (1980). The relationship between perceptual and memorial psychophysics. *Bulletin of the Psychonomic Society,* **16**, 25-26.

Curtis, D.W., Paulos, M.A., & Rule, S. (1973). Relations between disjunctive reaction time and stimulus difference. *Journal of Experimental Psychology,* **99**, 167-173.

DaSilva, J.A., Marques, S.L., & Ruiz, E.M. (1987). Subject differences in exponents of the psychophysical power functions for inferred, remembered, and perceived area. *Bulletin of the Psychonomic Society,* **25**, 191-194.

DaSilva, J.A., Ruiz, E.M., & Marques, S.L. (1987). Individual differences in magnitude estimates in inferred, remembered, and perceived geographical distance. *Bulletin of the Psychonomic Society,* **25**, 240-243.

Dornic, S. (1967). Subjective distance and emotional involvement: A verification of the exponent invariance. *Reports from the psychological laboratories, Report No. 237* (pp. 1-7). The University of Stockholm.

Dornic, S. (1968). Perception and memory in distance estimation. *Reports from the psychological laboratories, Report No. 242* (pp. 1-6). The University of Stockholm.

Ekman, G., & Bratfish, O. (1965). Subjective distance and emotional involvement: A psychological mechanism. *Acta Psychologica,* **24**, 430-437.

Fantini, d.A. (1984). *Psychophysical functions for the size judgments of seen and remembered circles.* Paper presented at the Fifty-fifth Annual Meeting of the Eastern Psychological Association, Baltimore, MD.

Fechner, G.T. (1882/1987). Some thoughts on the psychophysical representations of memories. *Psychological Research,* **49**, 209-212.

Finke, R.A. (1980). Levels of equivalence in imagery and perception. *Psychological Review*, **87**, 113-132.

Finke, R.A. (1989). *Principles of mental imagery.* Cambridge, MA: The MIT Press.

Finke, R.A., & Shepard, R.N. (1986). Visual functions of mental imagery. In K.R. Boff, L. Kaufman, & J. Thomas (Eds.), *Handbook of perception and human performance, Vol. II.* New York: Wiley.

Garner, W.R. (1974). *The processing of information and structure.* Potomac, MD: Erlbaum.

Gracely, H.R., & Wolskee, P.J. (1983). Semantic functional measurement of pain: Integrating perception and language. *Pain*, **15**, 389-398.

Hartley, A.A. (1977). Mental measurement in the magnitude estimation of length. *Journal of Experimental Psychology: Human Perception and Performance*, **3**, 622-628.

Hartley, A.A. (1981). Mental measurement of line length: The role of the standard. *Journal of Experimental Psychology: Human Perception and Performance*, **15**, 309-317.

Holyoak, K.J., & Walker, J.H. (1976). Subjective magnitude information in semantic ordering. *Journal of Verbal Learning and Verbal Behavior*, **15**, 287-299.

Hubbard, T.L. (1991a). *Memory psychophysics.* Unpublished manuscript.

Hubbard, T.L. (1991b). *Temporal aspects of memory psychophysics.* Unpublished manuscript.

Hubbard, T.L., & Baird, J.C. (1988). Overflow, first-sight, and vanishing point distances in visual imagery. *Journal of Experimental Psychology: Learning, Memory, and Cognition*, **14**, 641-649.

Hubbard, T.L., Kall, D., & Baird, J.C. (1989). Imagery, memory, and size-distance invariance. *Memory & Cognition*, **17**, 87-94.

Johnson, D.M. (1939). Confidence and speed in the two-category judgment. *Archives of Psychology*, **241**, 1-52.

Jones, B. (1980). Algebraic models for integration of painful and nonpainful electric shocks. *Perception & Psychophysics*, **28**, 572-576.

Jones, B., & Gwynn, M. (1984). Functional measurement scales of painful electric shocks. *Perception & Psychophysics*, **35**, 193-200.

Kemp, S. (1988). Memorial psychophysics for visual area: The effect of retention interval. *Memory & Cognition*, **16**, 431-436.

Kerst, S.M., & Howard, J.H. (1978). Memory psychophysics for visual area and length. *Memory & Cognition*, **6**, 327-335.

Kerst, S.M., & Howard, J.H. (1983). Mental processes in magnitude estimation of length and loudness. *Bulletin of the Psychonomic Society*, **21**, 141-144.

Kerst, S.M., & Howard, J.H. (1984). Magnitude estimation of perceived and remembered length and area. *Bulletin of the Psychonomic Society*, **22**, 517-520.

Kerst, S.M., Howard, J.H., & Gugerty, L.J. (1987). Judgment accuracy in pair-distance estimation and map sketching. *Bulletin of the Psychonomic Society*, **25**, 185-188.

Kosslyn, S.M. (1978). Measuring the visual angle of the mind's eye. *Cognitive Psychology*, **10**, 356-389.

Kosslyn, S.M., Ball, T., & Reiser, B.J. (1978). Visual images preserve metric spatial information: Evidence from studies of image scanning. *Journal of Experimental Psychology: Human Perception and Performance*, **4**, 47-60.

Krantz, D.H., & Tversky, A. (1971). Conjoint-measurement analysis of composition rules in psychology. *Psychological Review*, **78**, 151-169.

Laing, D.G., Panhuber, H., & Baxter, R.I. (1978). Olfactory properties of amines and n-butanol. *Chemical Senses and Flavor*, **3**, 149-166.

Leahey, T.H. (1987). *A history of psychology*. Englewood Cliffs, NJ: Prentice-Hall.

Lindenberg, Z. (1987). *Perceptual and memorial psychophysical functions for electrocutaneous and auditory pain: The integration of noxious stimulation across different bodily sources*. Unpublished M.A. Dissertation, Bar-Ilan University.

Lowrey, R.A. (1970). Distance concepts of urban residents. *Environment and Behavior*, **2**, 52-73.

Marks, L.E. (1974). *Sensory processes*. New York: Academic Press.

Miller, G.A. (1956). The magical number seven, plus minus two: Some limits on our capacity for processing information. *Psychological Review*, **63**, 81-97.

Moyer, R.S. (1973). Comparing objects in memory: Evidence suggesting an internal psychophysics. *Perception & Psychophysics*, **13**, 180-184.

Moyer, R.S., Bradley, D.R., & Cutcomb, S. (1977). *Memory psychophysics*. Paper presented at the Forty-eighth Annual Meeting of the Eastern Psychological Association, Boston.

Moyer, R.S., Bradley, d.R., Sorensen, M.H., Whiting, J.C., & Mansfield D.P. (1978). Psychophysical functions for perceived and remembered size. *Science*, **200**, 330-332.

Moyer, R.S., & Landauer, T.K. (1967). Time required for judgments of numerical inequality. *Nature*, **215**, 1519-1520.

Moyer, R.S., Sklarew, P., & Whiting, J.C. (1982). Memory psychophysics. In H.G. Geissler, & P. Petzold (Eds.), *Psychophysical judgment and the process of perception* (pp. 35-46). Berlin: VEB Deutcher Verlag der Wiessenschaften.

Osaka, N. (1987). Memory psychophysics for pyridine smell scale. *Bulletin of the Psychonomic Society*, **25**, 56-57.

Paivio, A. (1975). Perceptual comparisons through the mind's eye. *Memory & Cognition*, **3**, 635-647.

Parker, S., Casey, J., Ziriax, J.M., & Silberger, A. (1988). Random monotone data fit simple algebraic models: Correlation is not confirmation. *Psychological Bulletin,* **104**, 417-423.

Pinker, S. (1980). Mental Imagery and the third dimension. *Journal of Experimental Psychology: General*, **109**, 354-371.

Rollman, G.B., & Harris, G. (1987). The detectability, discriminability, and perceived magnitude of painful electric shock. *Perception & Psychophysics*, **42**, 257-268.

Sarfaty, O. (1986). *Perceptual and memorial psychophysical functions in different sensory domains.* Unpublished M.A. Dissertation, Tel-Aviv University.

Schacter, D.L. (1982). *The stranger behind the engram.* Hillsdale, NJ: Erlbaum.

Scheerer, E. (1987). The unknown Fechner. *Psychological Research*, **49**, 197-202.

Shepard, R.N. (1978). The mental image. *American Psychologist*, **33**, 125-137.

Shepard, R.N. (1984). Ecological constraints on internal representation: Resonant kinematics of perceiving, imaging, thinking, and dreaming. *Psychological Review*, **91**, 417-447.

Shepard, R.N., & Chipman, S. (1970). Second-order isomorphism of internal representations: Shapes of states. *Cognitive Psychology*, **1**, 1-17.

Sorabji, R. (1972). *Aristotle on memory.* London: Duckworth.

Stevens, S.S. (1934). The volume and intensity of tones. *American Journal of Psychology,* **46**, 397-408.

Stevens, S.S. (1969). Sensory scales for taste intensity. *Perception & Psychophysics*, **6**, 302-308.

Stevens, S.S. (1975). *Psychophysics*. New York: Wiley.

Sukenik, M. (1985). *Memorial and perceptual psychophysical functions for intensive and extensive, and for expansive and compressive dimensions.* Unpublished M.A. Dissertation, Bar-Ilan University.

Teghtsoonian, M. (1965). The judgment of size. *American Journal of Psychology,* **78**, 392-402.

Teghtsoonian, R. (1971). On the exponent of Stevens' law and the constant in Ekman's law. *Psychological Review*, **78**, 71-80.

Teghtsoonian, R. (1973). Range effects in psychophysical scaling and revision Stevens' law. *American Journal of Psychology*, **86**, 3-27.

Terrace, H.S., & Stevens, S.S. (1962). The quantification of tonal volume. *American Journal of Psychology*, **75**, 596-604.

Thomas, G.L. (1949). Equal volume judgments of tones. *American Journal of Psychology*, **62**, 182-201.

Titchener, E.B. (1906). *An outline of psychology*. London: Macmillan.

Torgerson, W.S. (1961). Distances and ratios in psychological scaling. *Acta Psychologica*, **19**, 201-205.

Wiest, W.M., & Bell, B. (1985). Stevens' exponent for psychophysical scaling of perceived, remembered, and inferred distance. *Psychological Bulletin*, **98**, 457-470.

Wilkening, F. (1979). Combining stimulus dimensions in children's and adult's judgments of area: An information integration analysis. *Developmental Psychology*, **15**, 25-33.

Wolf, Y., & Algom, D. (1987). Perceptual and memorial constructs in children's judgments of quality: A law of across-representation invariance. *Journal of Experimental Psychology: General*, **116**, 381-397.

Woodworth, R.S., & Schlosberg, H. (1954). *Experimental psychology*. New York: Holt, Reinhart, & Winston.

Psychophysical Approaches to Cognition
D. Algom (Editor)

9

COGNITIVE EFFECTS IN PAIN AND PAIN JUDGMENTS

Gary B. Rollman
University of Western Ontario

Table of Contents

I. Introduction

Near the beginning of "Les Belles Soeurs," a black comedy by Quebec playwright Michel Tremblay, a very elderly woman is heard, offstage, to fall out of her wheelchair. One woman asks her daughter-in-law, "She's not hurt, I hope," and receives the reply, "Oh no, she's used to it."

The exchange is predicated on the assumptions that pain can be measured or assessed and that cognitive variables, such as those incorporating previous pain experiences, can modulate or influence current pain.

The reader may take the first of these assumptions as a given, but prominent experts have challenged the foundations of a pain psychophysics. Wall (1979) writes:

> The delight of psychophysicists is their ability to establish thresholds of sensation and to measure lawful relations between stimulus intensity and the strength of sensation. They have obviously been very successful in vision and hearing. No such psychophysics exist for sensations such as hunger or thirst but there have been persistent attempts to establish thresholds and scales relating experimental stimuli to evoked pain. The results are farcical in their wild variability when compared to vision, hearing, smell, task and touch. The persistent failure of subjects to relate stimulus intensity to pain intensity is one of the strongest reasons to question the classical attempt to group pain with the familiar sensations evoked by external sources.

Researchers in the common senses have come to appreciate that their data, too, are often marked by "wild variability" in inter-subject and intra-subject judgments. Rollman and Harris (1987) reviewed studies in audition, vision, olfaction, and somesthesis. Thresholds for pure tones had a standard deviation of 5.7 to 10.7 dB for frequencies between 80 Hz and 15 KHz (Dadson & King, 1952). Vibration sensitivity on the finger tip had standard deviations on the order of 10 dB (Goff, Rosner, Detre, & Kennard, 1965). Thresholds of a group of dark-adapting subjects varied over a 4-fold range (Hecht & Mandelbaum, 1948). After correction for stimulus noise and measurement errors, olfactory sensitivity still spanned a 20-fold range (Rabin & Cain, 1986).

Ippolitov (1972) tested thresholds in a variety of modalities for a large group of observers. Careful examination of those most consistent in their performance still revealed a 28-fold range of scotopic visual threshold, a 15.5 dB range in pure-tone threshold, a 3.5 fold range in mechanical pressure threshold using von Frey hairs, and a 6-fold range in electrocutaneous threshold for constant voltage stimulation.

Consequently, the 8-fold range for pain threshold induced by constant current stimulation or the similar range for pain tolerance (Rollman & Harris, 1987) seemed quite comparable. The sensory and cognitive factors which underlie signal detection theory procedures (Green & Swets, 1966) are certain to apply to the traditional five senses and to pain.

Is Pain a Special Sense?

Pain has, however, often stood apart from the traditional five senses. Boring (1942) noted that pain had generally been classified as a *Gemeingefuhl* rather than a component of touch; part of the "classificatory catch-all for everything that did not fit the *Tastsinn*." The view that "all intense stimuli are painful" irrespective of modality was widely debated during the 19th Century, with challenge coming from those who directly stimulated the optic nerve to yield a very bright, but painless, flash or those who felt that surgical intervention in the spinal cord differentially interrupted the experience of pain and touch.

The debate became even more lively in the late 1890's when Blix and Goldscheider first claimed to have found distinct pain spots on the skin and, later, reversed their positions and declared that pain is common sensibility. Meanwhile, von Frey argued that pain is a separate skin modality, with multiple pain spots served by free nerve endings (Boring, 1942). Von Frey's theory has been discredited on anatomical and psychological grounds (Melzack & Wall, 1962), but its simplicity, coupled with the logical appeal of a direct, linear pain system extending from the periphery to the cortex, gave it credence in medical textbooks until the present day.

II. The Gate Control Theory

The advent of Melzack and Wall's (1965) gate control theory challenged the traditional model, replacing a linear system with one possessing multiple nodes of interaction. Melzack and Wall recognized a number of difficulties with a straight-through pain model. First, it predicts that interruption of ascending pain tracts abolishes the experience of pain, but surgical experience failed to confirm that. Second, it associates increased peripheral activity with increased pain, yet common responses to pain involve rubbing or massaging the affected area or applying heat or cold - methods which increase afferent input but *reduce* the pain experience. Third, anecdotal and clinical evidence suggested that severe injury can often occur without severe pain. There are many accounts of athletic injuries, wounds sustained during military battles, or civilian trauma in which major tissue damage is sustained without immediate pain. Likewise, distraction, expectation, emotion, and suggestion can modulate the pain experience.

In order to incorporate the failure of surgical interruption of ascending tracts, Melzack and Wall (1988) had to consider the possibility of multiple ascending pathways, the establishment of new connections, and the notion that the absence of normal tonic input to central structures may be as disruptive to central processing as an abundance of peripheral activity.

To account for the paradoxical inhibition of pain by mechanical or thermal input, the gate control model suggested a complex interplay of inputs from small peripheral fibers (which respond to noxious inputs and are consequently labelled nociceptors) and from larger myelinated fibers which have lower thresholds and faster conduction velocity. As shown in Figure 9.1, which represents a modification of the original gate control model (Melzack & Wall, 1988), the activity transmitted in small diameter fibers is proposed to have facilitatory effects on

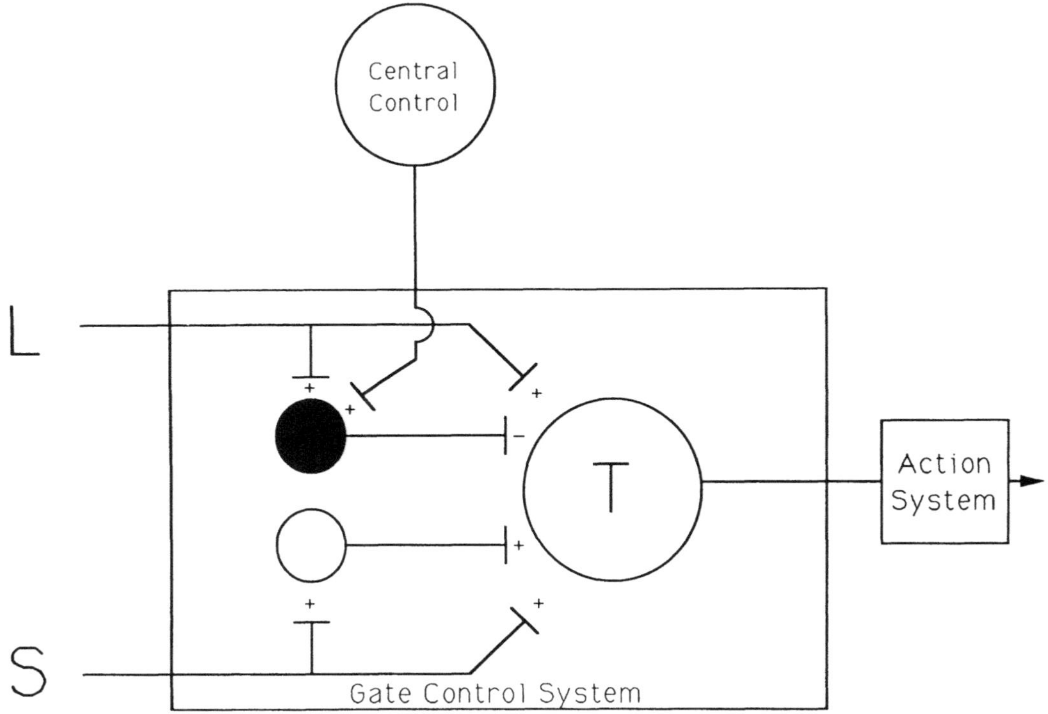

Figure 9.1: A schematic representation of Melzack & Wall's (1988) revised gate control model. The solid and open circles show cells in the substantia gelatinosa of the dorsal horn which exert inhibitory (solid circle) and the excitatory (open circle) influences on nearby transmission cells (T) after activation of large (L) and small (S) diameter afferent fibers. The input from the central control areas depicts the modulating influence of higher nervous system activity.

transmission cells in the dorsal horn of the spinal cord, both directly and via excitatory interneurons in the nearby substantia gelatinosa. The model also proposes that the large fibers, because of their connections to inhibitory interneurons in the substantia gelatinosa, are capable of modifying, by pre- and post-synaptic inhibition, the firing level of the T cells and, consequently the nature of the message sent to more central sites.

This gating mechanism, whereby large fiber inputs can modulate the transmission of nociceptor signals, allows for peripheral inputs to influence activity at the spinal cord level. It suggested that electrical stimulation of large fibers could reduce pain experiences and the subsequent confirmation of this in laboratory and clinical settings led to the development of commercially available transcutaneous electrical nerve stimulation (TENS) devices (e.g., Eriksson, Rosen, & Sjolund, 1985).

The evidence concerning the profound effects of distraction, suggestion, expectation, and emotion on pain experiences indicted that pain is not only the purview of anatomists, neurophysiologists, and medical personnel. It made clear that both the study and treatment of pain is very much in the domain of psychology.

The gate model provided for a vague "central control" trigger which descends from the brain to provide further modulation of T cell activity. While the physiological and neurochemical nature of such descending controls was unknown in 1965, it is now known that electrical and chemical activation of cells in such areas as the hypothalamus, the periaqueductal grey of the midbrain, and the nucleus raphe magnus of the medulla, can exert powerful analgesic effects. The subsequent discovery of endogenous opioid peptides in the hypothalamus, midbrain, medulla, and spinal cord, and evidence that they could be released by factors as diverse as physical activity (Colt, Wardlaw, & Frantz, 1981; Janal, Colt,

Clark, & Glusman, 1984), stress (Maier, Laudenslager, & Ryan, 1985), and cognitive mechanisms (Bandura, O'Leary, Taylor, Gauthier, & Gossard, 1987) provided further testimony to the decisive role of descending inhibitory mechanisms and their dependence on psychological factors.

The Nature of Pain

The Oxford English Dictionary defines pain as "A primary condition of sensation or consciousness, the opposite of pleasure; the sensation which one feels when hurt (in body or mind)" and "a distressing sensation of soreness (usually in a particular part of the body)." Aside from problems related to the imprecise operational nature of the first definition ("feels when hurt") and the fact that such a rigid linkage is untrue and to the circular nature of the second definition (pain is soreness and soreness is pain), it is also improper that pain should be considered simply a "sensation."

Melzack and Casey (1968) observed that "pain has a unique, distinctly unpleasant, affective quality that differentiates it from sensory experiences such as sight, hearing, or touch." While aficionados of Old Master paintings, Puccini operas, or silk bed sheets may take issue with the notion that sight, hearing, or touch lack affective quality, they may well agree with Melzack and Casey's further observation, "To consider only the sensory features of pain, and ignore its motivational and affective properties, is to look at only part of the problem."

Melzack and Casey (1968) declared that it is erroneous to consider a sequential model of pain perception in which primary "pain sensation" is followed by secondary "reactions to pain" which involve motivational (driving "the organism into activity aimed at stopping the pain as quickly as possible") and cognitive processes. Were that the case, pain sensation could be blocked by cognitive mechanisms, producing the "paradox of nonpainful pain." They considered it more reasonable to say that noxious inputs could be "blocked or modulated by cognitive activities before it could evoke the motivational-affective processes that are an integral part of the total pain experience."

Citing the capacity of brain activities to "influence the gate control system through central control efferent fibers," Melzack and Casey proposed, among other things, that "neocortical or higher central nervous system processes, such as evaluation of the input in terms of past experience, exert control over activity in both the discriminative and motivational systems."

The components of their conceptual model are presented in Figure 9.2. The "action system" of the original gate control model is replaced with a detailed system of mutually interactive elements, with the "sensory-discriminative" component of pain mediated by the neospinothalamic projection system, the "motivational-affective" component tapping into reticular and limbic structures, and what has come to be called the "cognitive-evaluative" component (although here was labelled simply "central control processes") being served by "higher central nervous system" activities.

Melzack and Casey (1968) incorporated a host of data under the "central control" rubric: effects on pain of anticipation, anxiety, attention, suggestion, placebos, cultural background, evaluation of meaning, hypnosis, early experience, and prior conditioning. They provided for the central control processes to modify the spinal gate and to influence (and be influenced by) the motivational-affective and sensory-discriminative systems. As well, they noted that cognitive variables underlying such effects as suggestion and placebos may "modulate the motivational-affective dimension and leave the sensory-discriminative dimension relatively undisturbed," a notion to which we'll return below.

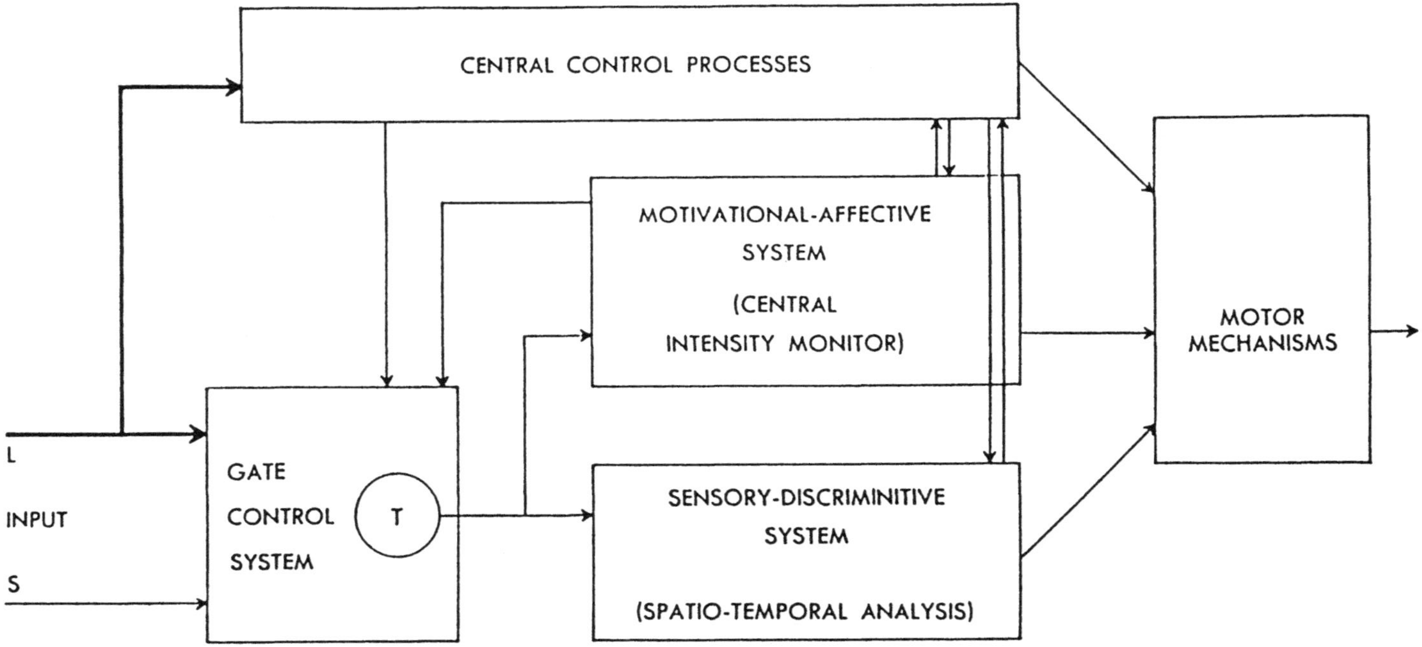

Figure 9.2: A conceptual model of sensory-discriminative, motivational-affective, and central control components of pain and their interactions suggested by Melzack and Casey (1968) (from R. Melzack & K.L. Casey 1968, Sensory, motivational, and central control determinants of pain: A new conceptual model. In D. Kenshalo (Ed.), The skin senses pp. 423-443, reprinted by permission).

Implications of the Melzack and Casey Model

Although elements of the gate control theory were challenged on a number of physiological grounds, the conceptual model proposed by Melzack and Wall (1965) and extended by Melzack and Casey (1968) provided considerable heuristic value in thinking about the components of the pain experience, the neural elements underlying them, and the possible therapeutic implications of a variety of treatments targeted at sensory, emotional, or cognitive systems.

Moreover, the expanded model led to a widely used (although still debated) definition of pain, adopted by the Subcommittee on Taxonomy of the International Association for the Study of Pain (Merskey, 1986): "Pain is an unpleasant sensory and emotional experience associated with actual or potential tissue damage, or described in terms of such damage." The definition gives relatively short shrift to cognitive variables, making passing reference to processes of association or description, but it clearly broadens the domain of pain beyond a pure sensory experience.

Melzack and Torgerson (1971) broadened the domain in another manner. Scanning the clinical literature relating to pain, they selected 102 words which were used to describe the phenomenon. The adjectives were classified into smaller groups, falling into 3 major classes and 13 subclasses. Subsequently, they were scaled as to how much pain each word represents. Based upon the results of this analysis, Melzack (1975) devised the McGill Pain Questionnaire, an adjective scale used to assess the multiple components of the pain experience. Other attempts to quantify such distinctions will be examined below.

Cognitive Manipulation of Pain

Another major outcome of the broadened conception of pain was a growing realization that traditional analgesic procedures, which generally utilized pharmacological or surgical interventions aimed at altering sensory transmission or analysis, were often inadequate in dealing with pain problems. Consequently, techniques which had been applied with success to problems of depression (Meichenbaum, 1977) began to be employed in the treatment of chronic pain, under the heading of "cognitive behavioral therapy" (Tan, 1982; Turner & Chapman, 1982a; Turk, Meichenbaum, & Genest, 1983). As Turner and Chapman (1982b) noted, "A basic assumption is that the cognitions (attitudes, beliefs, and expectations) people maintain in certain situations can determine their emotional and behavioral reactions to those situations. As cognitive (e.g., distraction, significance of the pain for the individual) and emotional variables (e.g., anxiety) influence the experience of pain, it seems logical that the modification of cognitions could be used to alter the pain experience."

Tan (1982) added, "Cognitive methods are those which attempt directly to modify thought processes in order to attenuate pain. The underlying assumption of these approaches is that a person's 'cognitions' or appraisals of his environment are critical determinants of his experiences and emotions. Hence faulty 'cognitions' lead to negative experiences, including exacerbation of anxiety, depression and pain. By altering such 'cognitions' to more adaptive ones, negative experiences may be attenuated."

A number of strategies have been utilized by cognitive-behavioral therapists: relaxation, imagery, relabelling sensations, education, self-monitoring, thought-stopping, information, distraction, and calming self-statements. As this list shows, cognitive and behavioral methods are frequently blended in a treatment package.

The cognitive strategies were first tested in laboratory settings, utilizing pain induced by immersion of the arm in ice water or exposure to shock, pressure, heat, or muscle ischemia. Turk, Meichenbaum, and Genest (1983) distinguish between strategies that attempt to alter the appraisal of the painful situation and those that attempt to divert attention away from the pain. Attention diversion strategies include:

1. **Imaginative inattention** - ignoring the pain by establishing a mental image of a scene or activity that is incompatible with the experience of pain. ("I am frolicking in the surf at Waikiki").
2. **Imaginative transformation of pain** - interpreting the sensations as something other than pain or treating them as trivial or unreal ("My arm is numbed by local anesthetic or is mechanical").
3. **Imaginative transformation of context** - the noxious sensation is acknowledged, but the setting is altered ("A foreign agent is attempting to interrogate me").

Whereas the first three called upon the production of an image to divert attention, the following three involve a refocusing of attention.

4. **Focusing attention on physical characteristics of the environment** - diversion of attention to external objects such as counting ceiling tiles or studying the composition of a nearby object.
5. **Mental distractions** - diversion of attention to self-generated thoughts such as doing mental arithmetic or singing the words of a song.
6. **Somatization** - focusing attention on the body part exposed to noxious stimulation in an "objective, rather than subjective, manner." The subject is told to analyze the sensations as if preparing to write a scientific report.

The data from a large number of laboratory studies utilizing such techniques to increase pain threshold or tolerance or to decrease pain report are, as Tan (1982) noted, "inconsistent and often contradictory." In somewhat more than half of the studies, greater effects were observed for subjects asked to utilize specific strategies than for control subjects (some of whom, presumably were using self-generated strategies).

Tan (1982) and Turk, Meichenbaum, and Genest (1983) pointed to a number of methodological and procedural differences which may have contributed to the equivocal results. These include different pain induction techniques, different dependent pain measures, different instructions, motivational differences among subjects, the use of pre-tests, and the spontaneous use of self-generated strategies.

Harris and Rollman (1985) exposed 40 subjects to three forms of experimentally-induced pain: trains of constant current electrical pulses delivered to the volar forearm, the cold pressor test in which the arm is inserted into a tank of circulating ice water, and a constant pressure algometer, which applies a weighted wedge against the forefinger. After baseline measures, subjects were given strategies for attention diversion, dissociation, transformation of the sensation, and imaginative diversion. Significant increases occurred in tolerance levels for all three stressors, but the largest increases occurred for those subjects whose baseline tolerance was already high. If one can extend this to a clinical setting, those who needed the greatest assistance from the cognitive intervention benefitted the least.

One possible reason is that the observers with a high baseline tolerance were already using self-initiated coping strategies before they received instruction in the specific techniques of the study. Indeed, a coping strategies questionnaire revealed that those subjects who had used such strategies showed larger changes in tolerance for the stressors. Use of a coping strategy in the pretest did not preclude an increase in later tolerance. If anything, it facilitated the benefit.

Cognitive-behavioral strategies for pain control have also been examined directly within a clinical context. For acute pain, there is considerable evidence of the efficacy of such techniques in dealing with post surgical pain, dental pain, headaches, burn treatments, and labor pain (Turk, Meichenbaum, & Genest, 1983). For chronic pain, cognitive-behavioral approaches have surpassed control or relaxation training conditions in studies of recurrent headache (Bakal, Demjen, & Kaganov, 1981), low back pain (Turner & Clancy, 1986), pain of the facial temporomandibular joint (Stam, McGrath, & Brooke, 1984), and rheumatoid arthritis (Bradley, Young, Anderson, Turner, Ggudelo, McDaniel, Pisko, Semble, & Morgan, 1987), among others.

Three points should be noted. First, these cognitive-behavioral approaches go beyond the imagery and attention diversion techniques mentioned earlier. The therapeutic packages typically also include training in stress-coping, elimination of "catastrophic thoughts" and "irrational cognitions," counteracting attitudes of helplessness, and self-monitoring (Prkachin & Cameron, 1990). Few studies (e.g., Vallis, 1984) have attempted to separate the various components of such programs in order to see which cognitive interventions are necessary or sufficient in order to achieve significant pain reduction. Second, the clinical studies have generally been conducted over a relatively brief time span. There is little evidence about the long-term utility of cognitive interventions aimed at reducing clinical pain. Finally, descriptions of "cognitions" involved in altering pain experiences need to be broadened to include concepts such as "self-efficacy" (Bandura, 1977), even when applied to behavioral analyses. As Prkachin and Cameron (1990) observed, "self-efficacy refers to individuals' belief in their ability to perform requisite behaviors. Individuals must acquire a sense of self-efficacy if they are to attempt and persist in coping behaviors. The effectiveness of different procedures in bringing about behavior change is proportional to their ability to induce expectations of personal efficacy."

III. Laboratory Assessment of Pain

Laboratory studies of pain have typically given considerable attention to stimulus and response variables and less attention to intervening cognitive factors. Even in selecting a stimulus, however, cognitive factors deserve consideration. Smith and Andrew (1970) described six characteristics of a satisfactory pain source:

1. A severity comparable to a surgical incision, or, even better, comparable to a muscle splitting incision.
2. Controllable as to severity, so pain intensity could be decreased or increased as desired.
3. Ends instantly when desired.
4. No tissue injury produced.
5. Repeatable with good degree of uniformity of results.
6. No startle component.

The major items on Gracely's (1989) list of properties of an ideal pain stimulus are, for the most part, similar:

1. Rapid onset.
2. Rapid termination.
3 Natural.
4. Repeatable with minimal temporal effects.
5. Similar sensitivities in different individuals.
6. Excite a restricted group of primary afferents.

Smith and Andrew's quest led them to a ramped train of electrical pulses while Gracely concluded that thermal stimuli come closest to his ideal. There is room for debate on such lists of appropriate noxious stimuli. An intensity comparable to a "surgical incision" is certainly not necessary for all pain studies, nor is a "natural" stimulus (ruling out electrical pulses that bypass receptors and excite afferent nerve fibers [Higashiyama & Rollman, 1991; Rollman, 1975]) or one that activates only a single class of nociceptors. Among the four common classes of noxious stimuli: electrical, thermal, mechanical, and chemical, the last group has typically been avoided because of the problems, among others, of stimulus control, rapid termination, tissue damage, and repeatability, but each of the others have been widely used.

Harris and Rollman (1983) measured pain threshold and pain tolerance for trains of electrical shocks, the cold pressor task (in which the arm is immersed in a container of ice water), and a mechanical device which applies a constant pressure against a small area of skin on the second phalanx of the finger. The correlations between the threshold and tolerance measures for each of the stressors were examined using multitrait-multimethod analysis (Campbell & Fiske, 1959). Strong evidence was found for both convergent and discriminant validity. The high correlations between measures for cold and pressure confirm the earlier results of Brown, Fader, and Barber (1973) and Davidson and McDougall (1969). Cold and pressure, as applied here, increase with the passage of time, induce deep pain, and are highly familiar experiences. Pain produced by electrical shock has different sensory qualities, and, perhaps more important here, is unfamiliar and often accompanied by reports of anxiety and stress. Thus, while thermal and mechanical stimuli may produce qualitative effects closer to many clinical pains than do electrical stimuli, significant alterations in affective and evaluative dimensions produced by shock may cause it to be preferred in assessing the effects of cognitive manipulations.

The evidence for discriminant validity in the Harris and Rollman (1983) study came from the finding that pain thresholds and pain tolerance levels across stressors correlated more highly with each other than did correlations for the two measures within a stress condition. Thus, for example, cold threshold and presser threshold levels had a correlation of 0.88, whereas cold threshold and cold tolerance had a correlation of only 0.28. Threshold and tolerance measures, then, represent different components of the pain experience, with the former, perhaps, reflecting the discrimination of nociceptive quality from non-nociceptive (sensations such as touch, warmth, or cold), while the latter indicates an unwillingness to receive more intense stimulation. Tolerance should be more susceptible to cognitive manipulations, a concept supported by findings as diverse as Sternbach and Tursky's (1965) report that tolerance was appreciably more influenced by ethnic group membership than was threshold, by Harris' (1981) observation that tolerance changed more than threshold after cognitive-behavioral therapy, and by Turk and Kerns' (1983) finding that catastrophic thoughts about the possible damage to the limb caused by immersion in ice water had enormous influences on pain tolerance but little on pain threshold.

Classical Pain Measures

Beecher (1959) said, "Pain is measured in terms of its relief." For clinical pain states, this is often the case, but for induced pain, pain relief is generally measured only indirectly. If an analgesic agent raises pain threshold or pain tolerance, one assumes that a stimulus presented at the baseline threshold or tolerance level will now be less painful than before and that pain relief has been achieved. Direct scaling procedures allow more direct examination of this issue.

Beecher (1959) realized that both pain threshold and tolerance reflect important cognitive contributions. "Pain does not 'occur' in the periphery," he wrote; "it is a phenomenon of the central nervous system. Evidence has been accumulating that consciousness of pain has more to do with the cortex than was once believed." He went on to cite Bishop's (1946) observation, "it is not clear whether the increased perceptual threshold under drugs, etc., is in effect a result of changed mental attitude, lack of attention, interest, or less careful discrimination." Likewise, Cattell (1943) said, "It may well be that the threshold raising effect [of analgesics] is secondary to influences on the mental state of the subject, who otherwise is likely to be preoccupied with the painful experiences. Just as environmental distractions cause a rise in pain threshold, so do mood changes or the interference with mental processes through drug action. The rise in threshold which may accompany analgesia must then be looked upon as incidental to the changes in mental function, with awareness of pain not necessarily altered."

Pain threshold and tolerance measures reflect a combination of sensory and response bias components. Although neither is a "pure" measure of any of the components of the pain experience, they can still be of considerable value in identifying whether a manipulation has an effect on pain or whether two groups differ in some respect in their pain behaviors. As noted earlier, threshold and tolerance measures have discriminant validity. There is evidence for reliability both within and across repeated sessions. While direct scaling methods may have a greater precision (gained after appreciably longer testing sessions), they are not independent of the traditional measures.

Rollman and Harris (1987) found that the exponents of individual power functions for a group of 40 subjects had a significant negative rank order correlation (rho = -.60) with the pain sensitivity range (the range between pain threshold and tolerance). Individuals with a small dynamic range had steep power functions, suggesting that they may be mapping a constant response range onto individually differing stimulus ranges (Teghtsoonian, 1971). This relation between the response continuum and the dynamic range lends support to the notion that threshold and tolerance measures, particularly the latter, reflect interindividual differences in pain judgments similar to those underlying scaling performance.

Limitations of Threshold and Tolerance Measures

Taub and Campbell (1974) measured pain threshold by determining the displacement of a needle pressed onto the skin just maximal to the nailbed until "pain was first reported." Two sessions were run with each observer: one baseline and one while stimulating the finger with continuous 100 Hz electrical current at one of the two currents. The lower current had no effect on pain threshold; the higher current raised it significantly. These findings, coupled with reductions in the averaged compound action potential, led the authors to conclude that the current caused peripheral blockade of smaller myelinated fibers, the A-delta nociceptors, creating nearly full analgesia to pinprick.

Bobey and Davidson (1970) had subjects rehearse the experience of exposure to radiant-heat pain on separate days, followed by actual application of the heat. Rehearsal increased the duration of exposure before subjects reported tolerance. Since rehearsal did not affect tolerance when an intervening day was not provided, Neufeld and Davidson (1971) suggested that the extended period may have provided "extended opportunity for the person to invoke strategies of coping with the impending harm."

In the first of these experiments, the authors interpreted the change in pain threshold as a sensory alteration. In the second study, cognitive mechanisms were invoked. Threshold and tolerance measures, alone, don't readily distinguish between the two.

Blitz and Dinnerstein (1971) asked one group of subjects to immerse their hands in ice water and report pain threshold. A second group was given instructions to "focus your attention and concentrate on the cold and try to ignore or focus away from the component of discomfort or pain," while a third group was told, "imagine that it is a very hot day and that the water is refreshing and pleasantly cool." The attentional redirection groups both showed large elevations in pain threshold. Blitz and Dinnerstein raised an essential question, "was the change in pain threshold a reflection of changes in perception, or might it simply reflect a change in the subjects' reporting of pain in an attempt, for example, to please the experimenter?" They noted that "the present data cannot differentiate between those alternatives" but indicated that questioning of their subjects suggested a sensory alteration in that "most subjects felt that on the instruction trials the pain was less intense."

Overview

The threshold and tolerance data reported above demonstrate that these variables can provide data indicating a change in pain behavior, but they don't distinguish between sensory and response alterations. Two very different approaches, sensory decision theory methods and differential scaling of intensity and affect have attempted to provide greater insight into the nature of such behavior shifts.

IV. Sensory Decision Theory Methods

At first blush, sensory decision theory or signal detection theory (SDT) (Green & Swets, 1966) techniques might seem optimum for separating sensory from response bias changes in pain reports. The SDT approach provides a means of independently measuring two components of an observer's performance when detecting a stimulus or discriminating between two different ones: sensitivity and response bias, therefore separating the sensory and cognitive factors responsible for the person's responses.

Common SDT experiments in psychoacoustics or vision investigate detection processes, examining the confusion between signal and noise. Pain studies, however, require intense levels of stimulation, but the presentation of strong electrical, mechanical, or thermal stimuli mixed with blank trials would not create the uncertainty needed to extract the sensitivity and criterion measures (Rollman, 1977). Consequently, pain researchers using SDT methodology have had to present pairs of intense stimuli of somewhat different intensity and to ask the observer to distinguish between them.

Typically, pain researchers have had their observers using rating scales, so that "5" means strong pain, "3" means "warmth" and "1" means "nothing." Although this marks a departure from the usual discrimination procedure (in which "5" means certainty that the presentation was stimulus A, "3" means uncertainty, and "1" means certainty that the presentation was stimulus B), the ability to partition responses to two stimuli into several classes makes it possible to use cumulating procedures and plot receiver operating characteristic curves and to determine sensitivity and criterion parameters.

Rollman (1977) reviewed a series of studies which examined the effects of placebos, drugs, age, sex, verbal suggestions, exposures to models, acupuncture, dorsal column stimulation, and transcutaneous electrical nerve stimulation (TENS). The literature was marked with inconsistencies, methodological inadequacies, and questionable interpretation of the data.

In prototypical experiments, subjects rated the subjective pain levels produced by several levels of radiant heat before, during, or after acupuncture (Clark & Yang, 1974) or various currents of tooth pulse stimulation before and after acupuncture (Chapman, Gehrig, & Wilson, 1975). Clark and Yang found that subjects assigned lower numbers to the thermal stimuli. However, since sensitivity parameter for the discrimination of adjacent levels did not change after acupuncture, while the criterion parameter was higher, they concluded that acupuncture had no sensory effects and that "the sole effect of acupuncture was to cause the subjects to raise their pain criterion in response to the expectation that acupuncture works." Consequently, they attributed acupuncture analgesia to cognitive alterations.

Chapman et al. (1975) reported that subjects reduced the discriminability of adjacent stimulus pairs and that acupuncture also reduced the criterion for describing the stimulus as painful. Thus, they concluded that the treatment caused a true sensory loss plus a change in response bias.

Rollman (1977) examined the assumptions underlying such interpretations [e.g., i) a reduction in neural activity will produce a reduction in d' and ii) a reduction in d' indicates a reduction of neural activity]. He challenged the first assumption, noting that an analgesic which reduces neural activity at a peripheral or central site could reduce the activity produced by *both* the weaker and the stronger of a stimulus pair, shifting their distributions to the left along a sensation continuum, as shown in Figure 9.3, but leaving the distance between them, and the sensitivity parameter, unchanged. As a consequence, a strict interpretation of signal detection theory parameters would lead to an erroneous conclusion. Under the above conditions, where the neural activity produced by each of the noxious stimuli is modulated by a putative analgesic, the sensitivity parameter (which reflects the ability to discriminate between the stimuli, not their level of painfulness) is unchanged but the criterion parameter is increased.

Such an apparent change in the criterion parameter can arise even though the criterion has not changed. The distributions of the two noxious stimuli may have shifted relative to a constant criterion, leaving the spurious outcome of a seeming criterion shift. It is then inappropriate to conclude that acupuncture produces a placebo-like effect.

Signal detection theory methods fail to permit an unequivocal separation between changes in pain responsiveness cause by sensory modulation and those due to changes in criterion or response bias. Both can appear to produce alterations in the "criterion" parameter. Moreover, even when the "sensitivity" parameter is reduced, it is impossible to conclude that a true analgesic effect has occurred, since all one can say with certitude is that the stimuli are less easily distinguished. They may be less painful, equally painful, or even more painful than before treatment.

Furthermore, "noise" or "variability" is not limited to the underlying sensory processes. Coppola and Gracely (1983) presented a model which incorporates decision variability as well as variability in sensory transduction. The parameter was reduced by transducer and criterion variability alike. Consequently, as they note, a "change in discrimination could represent a change in the cognitive criterion process due to increased criterion variability resulting from such factors as memory deficits or response perseveration."

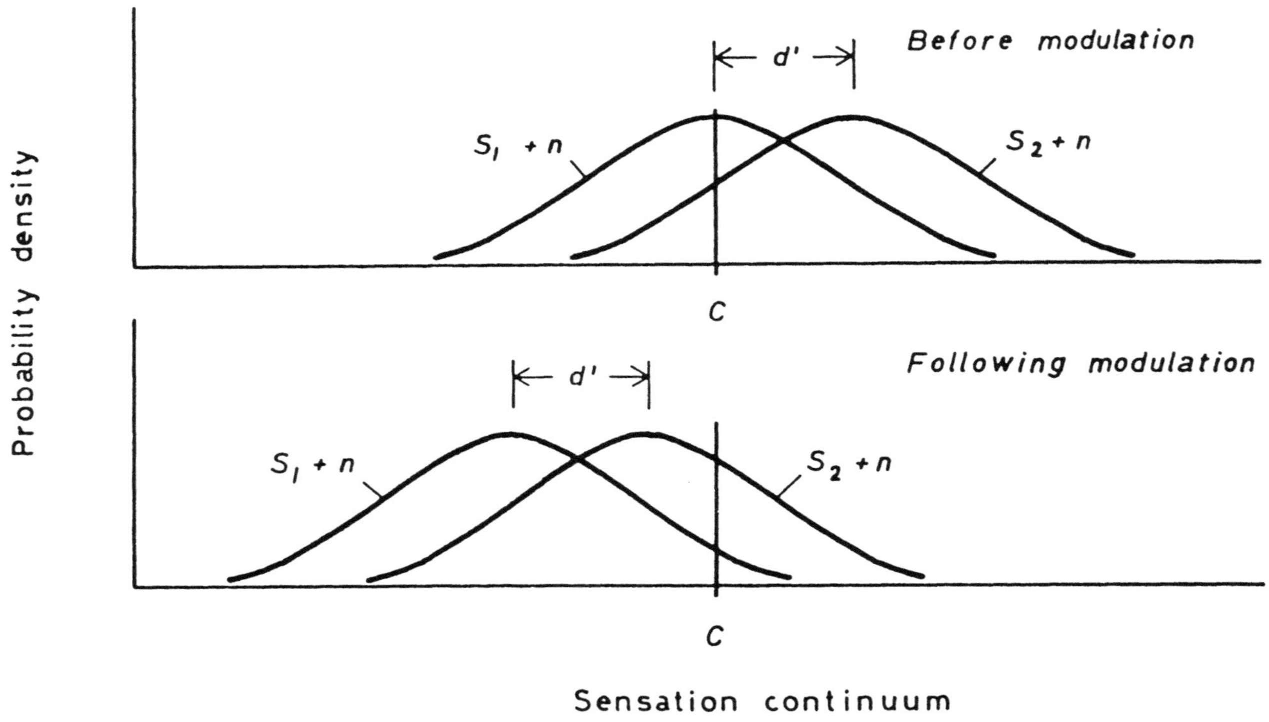

Figure 9.3: Representation of a possible change in sensory input produced by an analgesic modulation. The neural effects of noise plus both the weaker (S_1) and stronger (S_2) of two noxious stimuli are reduced, but the discrimination index remains unchanged, (from G.B. Rollman, (1977) Signal detection measurement of pain: A review and critique. *Pain*, **3**, 187-211, reprinted by permission).

SDT experiments have typically required subjects to make ratings of "painfulness" without elaboration of the component of pain which is described. Rollman (1983b) asked subjects to focus upon a specific pain dimension (intensity or unpleasantness). Other data were obtained for judgments of "pain or for discrimination capacity" (certainty that it was the stronger or the weaker member of the pair of electrocutaneous trains). For each of a number of discrimination indices, values were ordered such that the discrimination task gave the highest value, "pain" and "unpleasantness" gave approximately equal intermediate values, and intensity gave the lowest (see Figure 9.4).

This outcome suggests that discrimination of noxious stimuli is not performed on a global basis. Stimuli that can be discriminated from one another on some basis can still be equivalent in "unpleasantness." As well, stimuli equivalent in "intensity" may be unequal in "unpleasantness." This indication that intensity is less discriminable than unpleasantness also suggests that power function exponents may be steeper for unpleasantness than for intensity, a question that has received recent attention.

More recently, Irwin and Whitehead (1991) presented a model which "incorporates into the standard theory of signal detection an additional component of variance that attaches to the act of judgment itself." Their extended model includes several different kinds of criteria that determine the label, description, or identification that is assigned to a noxious stimulus. They, too, found higher sensitivity (d') scores for a resolution task (which required subjects to rate their confidence that the larger of two stimuli had been presented) than for an identification task (in which subjects attempted to identify which of 6 stimuli had occurred on that trial). A description task (in which subjects rated currents from 1 for "not painful" to 6 for "very painful") produced the worst performance.

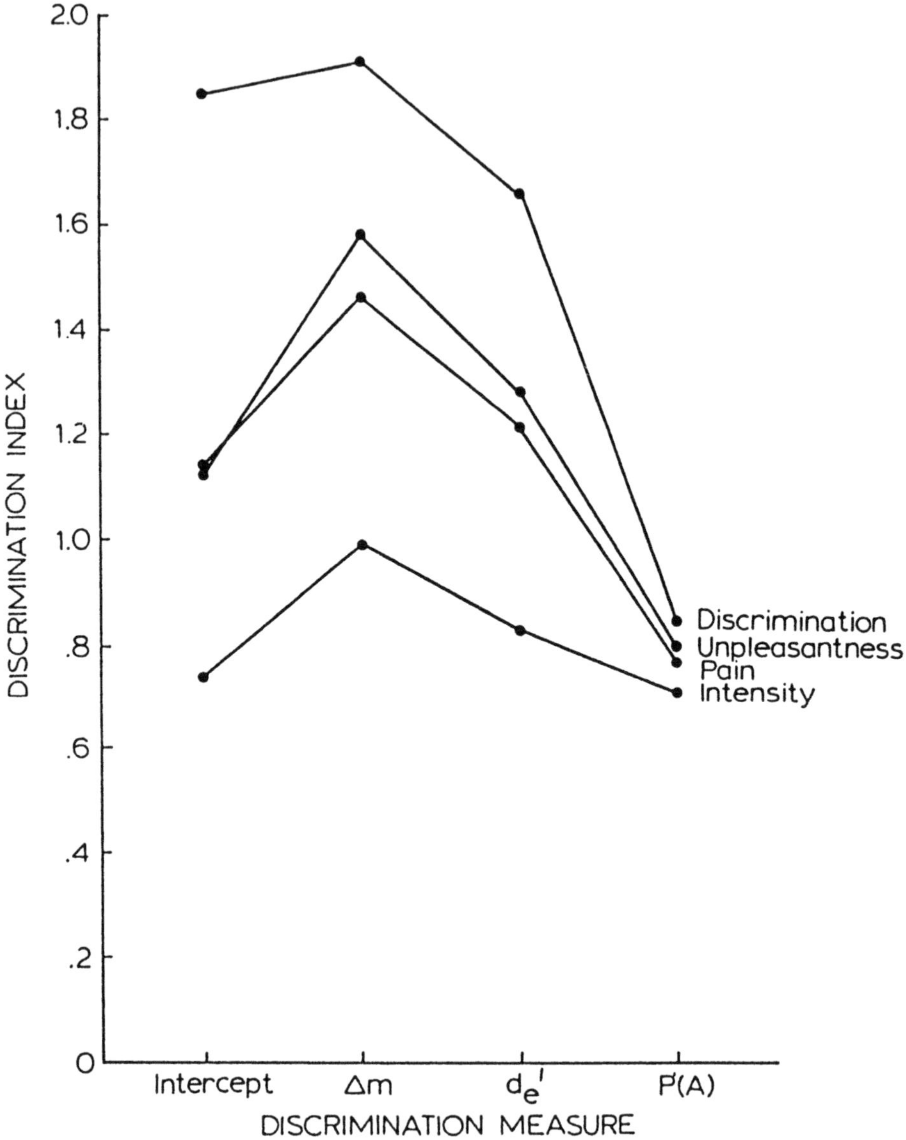

Figure 9.4: Values of several discrimination indices vary as a function of the judgmental task. (From G.B. Rollman (1983) Multiple subjective representations of experimental pain. In J.J. Bonica, U. Lindblom, & A. Iggo (Eds.), Advances in Pain Research and Therapy, Vol. 5 (pp. 865-869), reprinted by permission).

V. Verbal Scaling of Intensity and Unpleasantness

Gracely (1979) noted that most pain measures, whether using numerical scales, visual analog or graphic scales, or verbal categories, assessed pain "as if it were a simple sensation varying only in intensity." Given the considerable evidence that pain is multi-dimensional, unitary pain measures seem inadequate.

An initial approach to developing ratio scales of sensation and affect was indirect. Gracely, McGrath, and Dubner (1978a) had subjects scale the apparent magnitude of two sets of pain-descriptive adjectives: 15 sensory terms (e.g., "faint," "mild," "barely strong," and "very intense") and 15 affective ones (e.g., "distracting," "irritating," "dreadful," and "excruciating"). Subjects made magnitude estimates of these terms and of seven line lengths. They then made cross-modality matches to the adjectives and the lines using a hand dynamometer. The resulting power function between magnitude estimates and line lengths had an exponent of 0.85, while that for handgrip force and line length had an exponent of 0.48. Power functions could not be determined for the ratings of cross-modality matches to the words, since there was no suitable metric. Consequently, Gracely et al. transformed the numerical ratings and handgrip forces for each word to equivalent "line lengths" (utilizing the finding that the perceived magnitude of length has a nearly unitary relationship with actual length). A power function was determined for the relationship between the handgrip and the magnitude estimate for each of the words in a set.

The rationale for relating verbal stimuli and magnitude estimates to line length (rather than directly scaling the adjectives) was to eliminate regression bias effects. Relative magnitudes derived from handgrip and magnitude estimation showed strong agreement (Figures 9.5 & 9.6). The function for the affective words spanned a relative magnitude range of about 1 log unit (10 fold) whereas that for the sensory words spanned a nearly 2 log unit range (about 85 fold). By themselves these data do not indicate that unpleasantness grows at a faster rate than intensity, since there may be differences in the valences of the adjectives (that is, "extremely weak" and "very weak" convey a smaller magnitude than "bearable" and "distracting"), and, therefore, the "stimulus" ranges are not equivalent.

Gracely et al's (1978a) data indicate that "very weak" is about twice as intense as "extremely weak," that magnitude doubles again for "weak" and again for "mild." "Strong" is about 5 times as great as "mild" and "very intense" about twice as great as "strong." Similar comparisons can be made for affective descriptors: "distressing" is twice as unpleasant as "distracting" and "excruciating" gives twice the value of "dreadful."

Such "scaled descriptors" were then used by Gracely, McGrath, and Dubner (1978b) to study the analgesic effects of the tranquillizer diazepam (Valium). In their first experiment, subjects received trains of electrical pulses to the arm. Up to ten current levels were presented and the observers made handgrip and time duration responses proportional to the intensity or unpleasantness of the evoked sensations and chose appropriate adjectives from the lists used in the earlier study. While the exponents for time duration (1.1) and handgrip force (about 0.7) differed, equivalent functions were obtained for judgments of intensity and affect. However, when the "group mean relative magnitudes" derived from the earlier study were used to plot verbal descriptor functions relating perceived magnitude of intensity and unpleasantness as a function of current, radically different exponents were obtained, 1.6 for the sensory and 0.8 for the affective. Gracely et al. (1978b) acknowledge that the differences

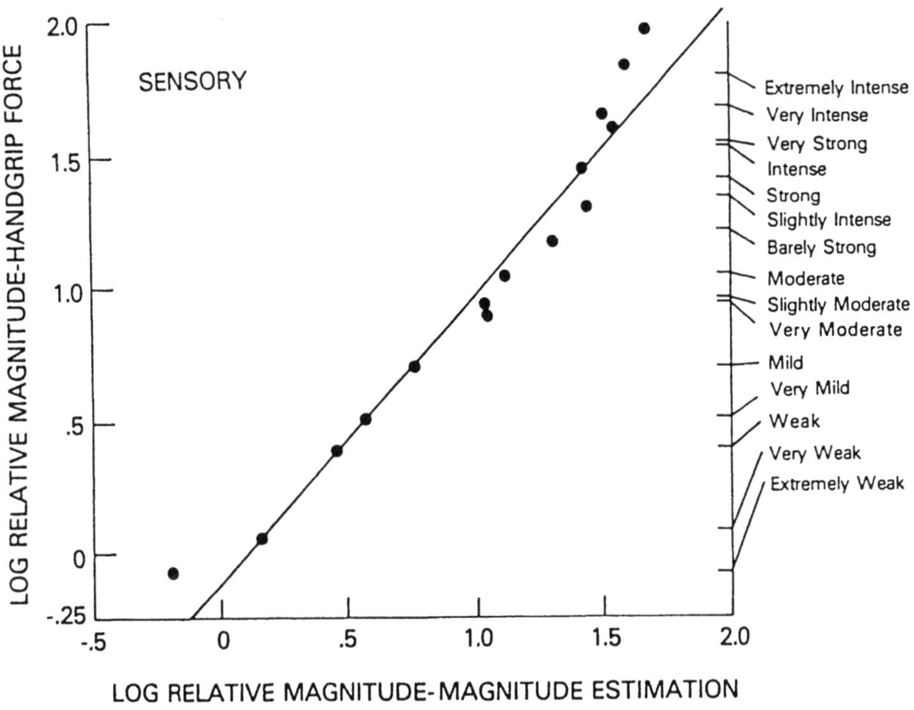

Figure 9.5: Relative handgrip force and magnitude estimation judgments for a series of adjectives describing the sensory component of the pain experience. The right ordinate shows the mean of the two magnitudes for each descriptor. (From Gracely, R.H., McGrath, P., & Dubner, R., 1978a. Ratio scales of sensory and affective verbal pain descriptors. *Pain*, **5**, 5-18, reprinted by permission).

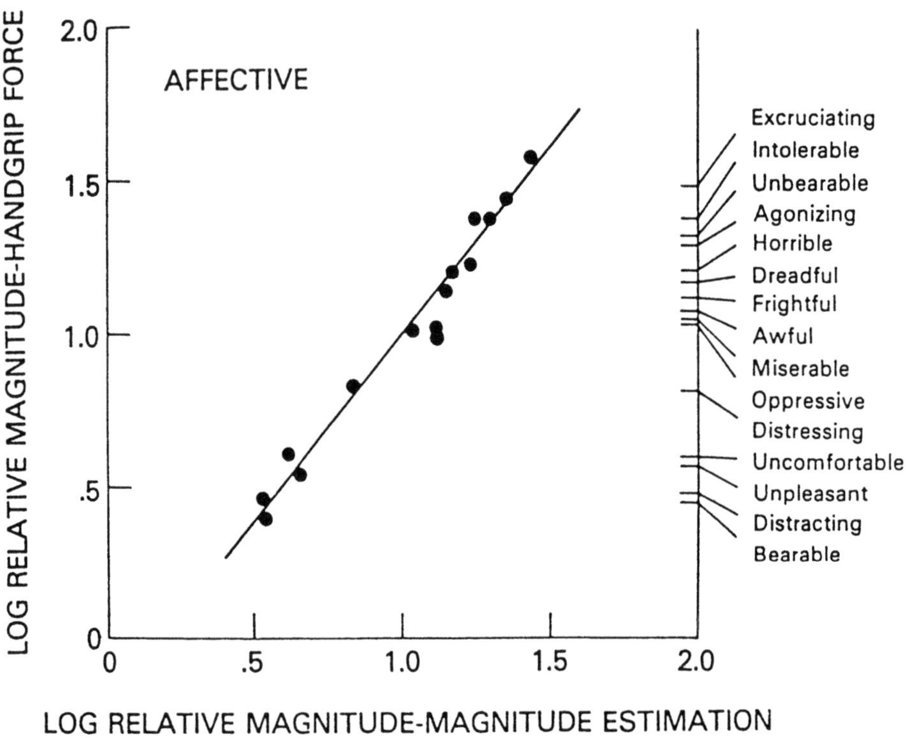

Figure 9.6: Relative handgrip force and magnitude estimation judgments for a series of adjectives describing the affective component of the pain experience. The right ordinate shows the mean of the two magnitudes for each descriptor. (From Gracely, R.H., McGrath, P., & Dubner, R., 1978b. Validity and sensitivity of ratio scales of sensory and affective verbal pain descriptors: Manipulation of affect by diazepam. *Pain*, **5**, 19-30, reprinted by permission).

may arise from "floor effects," since the affective dimension did not include adjectives with very low values, but they believe that such is not the case.

Next, a group of dental patients scheduled for oral surgery performed handgrip and verbal descriptor tasks before and after diazepam infusions. Matching handgrip force for both sensory and affective components revealed no effect of the drug. The scaled verbal descriptors for the sensory component of the pain experience associated with each level of current applied to the arm also did not change after diazepam administration, but the affective descriptors were reduced in the intermediate current range.

The authors noted that "the affective verbal descriptor and cross-modality functions were different, suggesting that one method is invalid." They believed that the former method is correct, citing similar slopes for cross modal sensory and affective functions but different slopes, even at baseline, for the verbal descriptors. Furthermore, since diazepam is an "ideal anxiety-reduction agent" and because "anxiety is assumed to be an important determinant of pain affect," the experimenters took the depression of affective verbal descriptors to be the valid outcome measure. Consequently, they concluded that "naive subjects failed to discriminate between sensory and affective dimensions on the cross-modality procedure" and that "words with affective connotations help naive subjects to discriminate between the sensory and affective qualities of the electrocutaenous stimuli."

Gracely et al. acknowledge that trained observers may more readily be able to distinguish between sensory and affective components of pain. However, naive subjects were able to consistently and differentially match handgrip force to sensory and affective words. As well, those showing a reduction in the relative magnitude of the affective descriptors were a different group than those describing the pain using sensory terms.

Any use of scaled verbal descriptors seems to require individualized determination of relative magnitudes for the adjective lists. While functions such as those shown in Figures 9.5 and 9.6 are based on group data, Gracely, Dubner, McGrath, and Heft (1978) presented individual functions relating log relative magnitude for sensory and affective terms to the current applied to tooth pulp. The individual power functions differed appreciably in both slope and intercept, but it is difficult to know whether this represents individual differences in the growth of pain functions or in the use of the adjectives. Subjects were asked to describe the intensity and unpleasantness of ethyl chloride applied to the exposed dentin of a cavity preparation by using verbal descriptors or cross-modal matches to electrical tooth pulp stimuli. The verbal descriptors were also used to describe the electrical pulses. In general, if a particular adjective was used to describe the cold pain produced by the ethyl chloride, the subject used the same adjective to describe the matching electrically-induced discomfort.

Tursky, Jamner, and Friedman (1982) developed a Pain Perception Profile which also included scaled verbal descriptors (in addition to pain threshold and tolerance determinations, magnitude estimation of electrocutaneous stimuli, and a pain diary). Their relative scale values for "intensity" (terms such as "weak," "mild," and "intense") "reaction" (e.g., "tolerable," "miserable," or "agonizing") and "sensation" (e.g., "tingling," "throbbing," and "shooting"), were derived, in part, from the McGill Pain Questionnaire. A series of descriptors were scaled using cross-modality matching to handgrip and loudness as well as direct magnitude estimation. As with the data obtained by Gracely et al. (1978a), affective terms spanned a smaller range (7 fold) than the intensity ones (28 fold). As well, subjects did not assign low numerical or matching values to the descriptors of unpleasantness.

Experimenters seem to have some difficulty deciding whether certain terms describe intensity or affect. Tursky et al. (1982) included "excruciating" in their list of intensity terms while Gracely et al. (1978a) listed it as an affective descriptor. The rank ordering of adjectives in the two studies, however, agreed very well, and, with a few exceptions, so did the relative magnitude. "Uncomfortable" and "intolerable" were on both the "intensity" and "reaction" lists used by Tursky et al. Interestingly, the intensity scale values for both descriptors were higher than the reaction values. Moreover, while "intolerable" is nearly three times as intense as "uncomfortable" it is more than four times as unpleasant.

Subjects are also aware that many of the adjectives load onto two or more dimensions. Jamner and Tursky (1987) had 21 subjects indicate whether a descriptor belonged to the intensity or affective category. While all 21 agreed that "very strong" was an intensity term, only 11 considered "very weak" to classify intensity. Numerous other terms received less than two-thirds agreement. A similar outcome occurred for the affective descriptors. All agreed that "uncomfortable" belonged in the affective category, but fewer than two thirds judged "agonizing," "intolerable," "unbearable," "tolerable," or "bearable" as describing reaction rather than intensity. Such confusion about categories raises serious questions about the claim by Gracely, McGrath, and Dubner (1978b) that discrimination between sensation and affect is "greatly facilitated in naive subjects by limiting their responses to randomized lists of verbal descriptors specific to that dimension."

Urban, Keefe, and France (1984) took a group of chronic pain patients and asked them to use the psychophysical scaling methods presented in the Pain Perception Profile developed by Tursky et al. (1982). About 10 percent failed to perform well (a correlation of at least 0.9 between stimulus and response variables) when doing magnitude estimations of line length; a somewhat higher number had difficulty in drawing lines proportional to random numbers. Patients had reasonable success in assigning numbers or line lengths to intensity descriptors ("mild," "moderate," "strong," etc.), but only 18% could reliably scale the unpleasantness words ("tolerable," "distressing," "awful," etc.). This value rose to only 50% for a group given specific training in the task.

These findings were confirmed by Morley and Hassard (1989). Using the same intensity and affective descriptors as Urban et al. (1984), and testing on two occasions, internal consistency criteria ($r \geq 0.90$) were met by 65 to 70% of their pain patients for intensity terms but only 25 to 40% for words describing unpleasantness. Analysis of regression coefficients between individual and group scale scores revealed considerable between-subject and within-subject variability. Correction for regression bias showed a strong tendency to underestimate large values on the affective scale, but still left substantial session to session variability even in the patients who were internally consistent in their response patterns.

Morley and Hassard (1989) suggested the failure of patients to consistently scale unpleasantness descriptors may suggest that the terms don't represent a single dimension. If so, they observed, unpleasantness descriptors might be located in multidimensional perceptual space rather than along a single perceptual continuum.

Morley (1989) examined this proposition. Noting that pain "might be both 'bearable' and 'distressing'," he hypothesized that affective descriptors are drawn from more than one dimension within a general affective domain. A group of subjects, consisting of both pain patients and healthy controls, sorted terms used in the Pain Perception Profile into an unrestricted number of groups with similar meaning and made similarity ratings of all possible pairings within the intensity and affect lists.

Multidimensional scaling analysis of the sorting data indicated that intensity and unpleasantness terms are not clearly separated within a 2-dimensional space. A 3-dimensional solution provided the best fit for the similarity data obtained for the affective descriptors (with the dimensions associated with tolerability, emotional reaction, and focus of attention). Intensity terms were described by a unidimensional representation.

The Relationship Between Sensation and Affect

Reduction in the sensory component of pain, as assessed by scaled verbal descriptors, is not necessarily accompanied by a reduction in affect. If the two components were truly independent, of course, such would readily be the case, but common wisdom suggests that reduction in the intensity of a noxious stimulus ought to be accompanied by reduction in its unpleasantness. Gracely, Dubner, and McGrath (1979) had subjects rate the sensory intensity and unpleasantness of electrically-evoked tooth pulp pain, using scaled descriptors, before and after the administration of saline or the synthetic narcotic fentanyl.

As can be seen in Figure 9.7, the saline placebo reduced the unpleasantness of the low and moderate stimuli, but had no effect on the intensity. Fentanyl reduced the sensory intensity, but the unpleasantness to each of the current values remained the same. The authors suggested that the dysphoria produced by the narcotic, with possible nausea and dizziness, may have countered its analgesic effects.

One interpretation of the collection of findings reviewed in the previous section is that the cognitive components of the pain experience are less amenable to psychophysical analysis than are the sensory components. That may be particularly the case for pain patients, since Morley (1989) found that headache sufferers placed greater weight on the emotional and attention diversion dimensions of the affective descriptors than did healthy volunteers. Their less

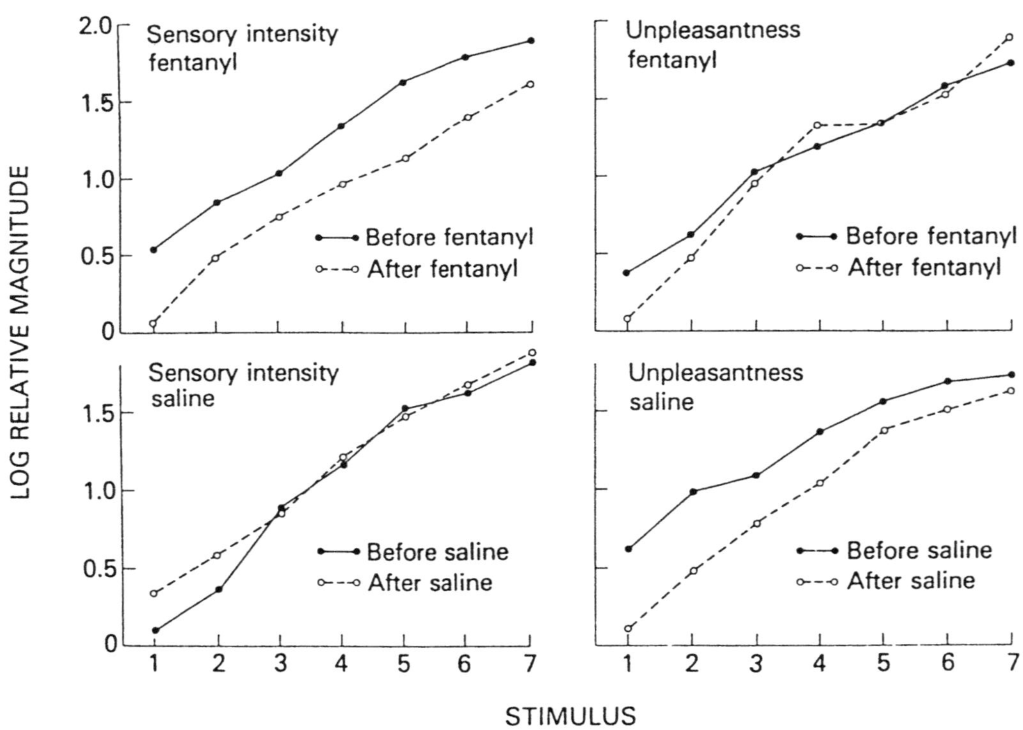

Figure 9.7: Relative magnitude of the sensory and affective (unpleasantness) components of pain induced by electrical tooth-pulp stimuli of different intensities before and after administration of saline or the synthetic narcotic, fentanyl. (From Gracely, R.H. (1979). Psychophysical assessment of human pain. In J. Bonica, J.C. Liebeskind, & D.G. Albe-Fessard (Eds.), Advances in Pain Research and Therapy, Vol. 3 (pp. 805-824), reprinted by permission.)

reliable performance may occur because they respond to different attributes on different occasions.

Support for this distinction between patients and control subjects comes from a multidimensional scaling study conducted by Clark et al. (1989). They had cancer patients and non-pain controls rate the similarity of 9 pain descriptors which dealt with pain quality (e.g., "burning" and "cramping"), intensity ("mild," "intense"), affect ("sickening") and evaluation ("annoying," "miserable," and "unbearable"). A 3-dimensional solution indicated that stimulus weights were further apart for patients than controls, that the patients found some sensory descriptors to have strong emotional qualities, and, perhaps surprisingly, that the healthy volunteers gave significantly more weight to the emotional quality dimension than did the patients.

The use of scaled verbal descriptors to establish the magnitude of sensory and cognitive components of pain clearly adds several steps to the assessment process. Its use requires lengthy sessions with multiple magnitude estimation or cross-modality matching trials and, even then, it is uncertain whether group values represent individual perception or whether magnitudes of descriptive adjectives remain constant across days.

Gracely and Dubner (1987) addressed this matter in a study which derived relative magnitudes for overall painfulness (e.g., "mildly painful," "rather painful," and "decidedly painful"). Correlations between handgrip force and matching time duration for each of the descriptors was 0.99 for the group as a whole, but ranged from 0.55 to 0.96 for individual subjects (mean = 0.85). Correlations within individuals across sessions (0.92) matched the mean correlation of the data of each subject to the list of the group (0.93). The range of such values and their absolute value rather than ordering will likely reflect considerably greater variability.

VI. Direct and Cross-modal Scaling

Notwithstanding this support for verbal descriptors, there is a sizeable body of literature on direct magnitude estimation and, more recently, on cross-modality scaling of pain, particularly using variants of matched line length procedures. Magnitude estimates of electrically-induced sensations have yielded power functions with widely different exponents, ranging from near 1.0 to beyond 3.0 (see Rollman & Harris, 1987). The differences arise, at least in part, because of the effects of stimulus parameters, regression and range effects, the painfulness of the presentations, the experience of the observers, and correction of the stimulus intensities for threshold.

Rollman and Harris (1987) determined power functions for electrical pulse trains. All stimuli were within the pain range determined for each subject. Exponents varied considerably, but the median slope of 1.73 agreed well with other data. Correction of the data for individualized pain threshold had a marked effect on exponent, reducing the median value to 0.70 and the mean to 0.83.

Bromm and Treede (1980) obtained exponents, using a visual analog scale, for nonpainful and painful ranges of current applied to the fingertip. Although there were considerable interindividual differences in perceived magnitude for each current, data spanning the full range yielded a function with a slope of 1.03 when plotted on linear-linear coordinates. When the data were transformed to logarithmic functions, a power function with a slope of 1.60 was obtained. Brown and Treede attribute this to a disproportionate influence of low intensities on the double logarithmic plot, whereas "in the linear scale the values for higher stimulus intensities, essential in measuring pain, gain in weight for the curve approximation." Correcting the "prepain" sensations for detection threshold and the "pain" sensations for pain threshold produced a pair of power functions, each with a slope of about 1.0. Bromm (1984) has suggested that if analgesic treatments increase pain threshold intensity, reliance on the baseline pain threshold will produce "fictitious" changes in the exponent of post-treatment power functions. This important point has not received the attention it deserves.

These data point to the importance of the pain threshold value as a key element in pain evaluation. In the case of functions with exponents greater than unity, the effect of threshold corrections is to sharply reduce the value. Lautenbacher, Moltner, and Strian (1991) have examined power functions for contact thermodes applied to the hand. Although Adair, Stevens, and Marks (1968) found exponents for pain induced by radiant heat to be close to unity, the work of Price (1988), with contact thermodes, points to much more expansive functions (exponents of about 2.0). Price corrected for base temperature (34 or 35° C), although the pain threshold is generally about 44 to 45° C (Watkins, 1988. Lautenbacher et al. showed that exponents are steeper in the pain range than in the heat range. Functions which span the two have exponents close to 2.0, but correction for pain threshold brings values in the pain range close to unity.

Anderson (1989) observed that the use of a zero point of 34° C by Price, McGrath, Rafii, and Buckingham (1983) suffers from a "fatal objection." "Since normal body temperature is 37° C, their result implies that a finger in the mouth would feel painfully hot." While Price et al. certainly did not intend to leave such an impression, their use of a 34° C threshold in this and later studies seems inappropriate.

Price, Barrell, and Gracely (1980) examined whether experiential factors selectively influence an affective component of pain. Noting that the division of the pain experience into two dimensions is "an oversimplification since affective responses are so critically dependent on the psychological context of the person, including such factors as the cognitive strategy with which one deals with unpleasant situations," they hypothesized that the unpleasantness of warm and noxious heat stimuli will be influenced by expectations and goals.

Affective and sensory magnitudes were expressed by drawing lines on 28 cm strips of paper and, since the exponent for the power function relating line length to a series of random numbers between 5.5 and 100 had a value close to unity, were taken as direct magnitude estimates. Overall, signalled warnings that the temperature produced at a contact thermode would shift to an intense range (45-51°C) led subjects to describe the sensation as equally "intense" as on unsignalled trials but to consider the stimuli as producing less of a "negative feeling." Further analysis showed that 4 of 7 subjects had their affective responses modified by the warning stimulus; the other three were unaffected.

A combination of a verbal descriptor and linear scaling method was developed by Gracely and Kwilosz (1988). Their Descriptor Differential Scale presents sensory and affective words at the center of a printed line, with a minus sign anchoring the left end and a plus sign anchoring the right. Patients are instructed to rate the magnitude of their pain in relation to each descriptor. If, for example, the pain is moderate, subjects might place a mark somewhere along the left side of the line when the reference word is "strong," "intense," "extremely intense," etc. and somewhere on the right for key words such as "faint," "weak," or "mild." The length of the line is described in "dash widths," so that 0 to 9 represent values to the left of the descriptor and 11 to 20 values to the right.

Gracely and Kwilosz (1988) plotted the item response score for each descriptor at one point in time (abscissa) against the scores at the later time (ordinate), finding functions that are generally linear. Downward shifts in the Y-intercept of the regression line would represent analgesic shifts in intensity or unpleasantness. Individual item correlations between periods one and two hours after removal of a molar tooth ranged from 0.61 to 0.83 (mean = 0.71) for intensity descriptors and 0.43 to 0.71 (mean = 0.59) for unpleasantness items.

The correlations between items at the two testing periods provide a useful measure of individual consistency. Most subjects performed well, but the repeated measures task permitted the identification of some who provided unreliable information and allowed an increase in overall reliability coefficients.

Visual Analog Scales

Price and his colleagues have typically had pain intensity scaled by having subjects mark a 150 mm wide visual analog scale whose endpoints are "no sensation" and "the most intense sensation imaginable" and examined pain affect by a similar scale ranging from "not bad at all" to "the most intense bad feeling possible for me."

A concern regarding this form of cross-modality matching is that the anchors restrict the scale from being open-ended and, consequently, the obtained values may not have true ratio properties. Price, McGrath, Rafii, and Buckingham (1983) addressed the first of these concerns by comparing sensory and affective VAS scales for contact thermode temperatures of 43 to 51° C with those obtained in the earlier Price, Barrell, and Gracely (1980) study that used line production as the cross-modal match. In both instances, the exponent (corrected for 34° C) for the affective function (3.87) was steeper than that for the sensory one (2.1) (thus stimuli became unpleasant much faster than they became intense), but the two methods yielded essentially identical data.

The second issue, that of ratio scale properties, was examined by having subjects adjust the temperature until it was double that evoked by a stimulus of

43 or 45° C. Subjects also used direct magnitude estimation to compare the unpleasantness of two temperature pairs. The values obtained in these tasks showed excellent agreement with the predictions based on the visual analog scale power functions.

Pain patients used visual analog scales to describe the intensity of their own chronic pain during the previous week, describing it at its minimal, usual, and maximal levels. Obviously this task places demands on memory phenomena (Erskine, Morley, & Pearce, 1990; Jamison, Sbrocco, & Parris, 1989; Hunter, Philips, & Rachman, 1979; Roche & Gijsbers, 1986), but the visual analog scale values generally well-matched the temperature values the patients selected as equalling the intensity of their chronic pain at the same three levels.

Given this evidence that visual analog scales may have ratio properties and that subjects can use them to scale at least the intensity of their clinical pain, Price's group examined whether sensory-intensive and affective dimensions can be selectively influenced. In one study (Price, Von der Gruen, Miller, Rafii, & Price, 1985), low doses of morphine reduced the affective visual analog scale responses to a range of heat pain stimuli, but did not change the sensory components. Higher doses of the narcotic reduced both. The difference in outcome from the fentanyl study conducted by Gracely et al. (1979) was explained in terms of "radically different psychological contexts" in that the subjects in the earlier experiment walked around after receiving the drug (possibly inducing adverse side effects) whereas Price et al.'s subjects lay on beds throughout the session. Alternatively, VAS affective responses may be more sensitive than the verbal descriptors (although the data of Duncan, Bushnell, & Lavigne [1989] suggest the opposite).

In a follow-up study (Price, Harkins, Rafii, & Price, 1986), intravenous administration of fentanyl to low back pain patients reduced both the intensity and affective visual analog scale responses to thermal pain as well as similar components of their clinical pain. Whereas the reductions in the two components of experimental discomfort were roughly equal, the drug produced a greater effect on the affective than the intensity component of the clinical pain.

These differential effects may reflect a steeper sensory-affective relationship for clinical pain. In particular, the cognitive-evaluative and motivational-affective components of pain are more likely to reach high levels for a chronic pain, with its potentially debilitating or disabling outcome, than for a short-acting experimental pain. As Price et al. (1986) note, morphine may have anti-anxiety or euphoric effects that are mediated at supraspinal sites and, consequently, it will have a larger effect on the non-sensory reactions produced by clinical pain than by experimental pain.

VII. Serial and Parallel Processing

In instances such as this, where intensity and affect are reduced by an analgesic, the question remains as to whether both components are directly influenced by the treatment or whether a reduction in pain intensity is the primary outcome and the reduction in affect is secondary. The first instance is described by a parallel model of information processing in nociceptive pathways; the second represents a serial or sequential model.

Melzack and Casey's (1968) conceptual model provided for a number of interacting systems. The primary paths run from the spinal gating system to separate sensory and affective modules which feed into neocortical and higher "central control processes" that evaluate the dual inputs on the basis of cognitive processes and exert descending inhibitory control over the lower systems.

If affect simply followed sensation, then, if the two were not related by a function with unitary slope, at the least they ought to have a monotonic relationship. Generally, that's the case. There are, however, differences among studies in whether intensity or affect takes on greater values. In most experiments (e.g., Price et al., 1983, 1985, 1986) affective scores are lower than sensory ones (but they generally have a greater slope).

Price, Harkins, and Baker (1987) assessed the sensory and affective components of a variety of clinical pain states (minimum, usual, maximum) as well as for experimental pain. For the latter, at each of a series of temperatures, affective scores were lower than sensory ones. For most clinical pains, however, such as back pain, causalgia (a burning pain which can follow nerve injury), and cancer pain, affective scores, particularly at usual and maximum levels, were significantly higher than intensity ones. The one exception was labor pain where, for the later three stages of the birthing process, the unpleasantness of the experience was significantly lower than its intensity. Clearly, cognitive factors shape the relative valence of pain sensation and pain affect.

The precise nature of the linkage among these components is not revealed by such experiments. Price (1988) presents a sequential processing model which challenges Melzack and Casey's parallel processing one. He suggests that nociceptive stimulation engages sensory and arousal mechanisms whose joint input influences cognitive appraisals. That is, "the evoked emotional response can be one of fear, anxiety, frustration, or anger depending upon the meanings that occur in relation to the nociceptive sensations and to the psychological context in which they occur." Attitudes, memories, and personality factors are held to influence cognitive appraisals. These, then, give rise to affective-motivational states. As Price notes, "People say that pain is unpleasant because it hurts, suddenly arouses and alarms them, and produces thoughts of concern or annoyance." It follows, then, that reductions in pain sensation will generally reduce pain affect. Pain affect, however, can be diminished by cognitive manipulations without concurrent declines in pain intensity.

Cognitive Comparison Processes

The sequential model of Price (1988) presents one formulation of a cognitive-sensory-affective interaction. Others, clearly, are possible as well. The psychological and psychophysical studies presented in this chapter make clear that pain has multiple components and that selective manipulation of each of them can be produced and can be measured.

Rollman's (1979) demonstration that noxious stimuli are not judged on an absolute basis, but within the context of the set of stimuli occurring within a session, suggests that the values assigned to equally-spaced stimuli within the usual psychophysical experiment may also be capable of contextual manipulation. The adaptation level theory of pain (Rollman, 1979) posited that pain patients use their endogenous pain level as an anchor or reference point for judging experimentally induced pain. Considerable confirmatory evidence has been gathered (Naliboff & Cohen, 1989; Rollman, 1983a, 1989) to show that pain patients suffering from various disorders have higher pain threshold or tolerance than normal controls and that these levels decline as pain diminishes. The apparent paradox of a lessened clinical pain and increased discomfort to a stimulus earlier judged as innocuous becomes understandable within such a contextual model.

Other pain disorders (Rollman, 1989; Scudds, Rollman, Harth, & McCain, 1987) are accompanied by a heightened degree of responsiveness or hypervigilance (Chapman, 1978), which leads to lower than normal pain threshold or tolerance. These shift towards higher levels with successful treatment (Scudds, McCain, Rollman, & Harth, 1989), suggesting an adjustable set point.

Such integration of clinical and experimentally-induced pain can be conceptualized within the framework of integration psychophysics (Anderson, 1970; see his chapter in this volume). Algom, Raphaeli, and Cohen-Raz (1986, 1987) have shown that multiple noxious stimuli summate in a linear manner. Further , the integration of such intense signals across modalities (e.g., strong shocks and loud tones) points to the role of higher order processes within the central nervous system. It remains to be determined whether there are different integration patterns within the functional measurement approach for sensory, affective, or cognitive judgments than for overall ratings of painfulness.

Such can be the case for stimuli that are spatially separated. Price (1988) states, "a pain sensation occurring in one part of the body does not add to the intensity of pain that occurs in another part of the body" (although this requires experimental confirmation and may well be incorrect) but "the unpleasantness of the two pains tend to combine into an overall experience."

Although integration psychophysics provides for additive combinations such as might occur in instances of hypervigilance, where internal pain may contribute to the discomfort of an externally-applied stimulus (e.g., Lautenbacher, Galfe, Karlbauer, Moltner, & Strian, 1990), it also provides (Anderson, 1989) for an averaging model which "implies that placing greater weight on one stimulus necessarily decreases the relative weight of any other stimulus." The adaptation level model of pain provides for such relative suppression effects. Frequently, pain patients will say something to the effect that "this stimulus is nothing compared to the pain within my body."

VIII. Final Observations

In the end, whether the interest is in diagnosis and evaluation of pain patients, in studying pain mechanisms in the laboratory, or in learning about the scaling of noxious signals, a behavioral response will remain the most certain measure. Although there have been some interesting developments in the use of human single peripheral nerve responses (e.g., Torebjork & Ochoa, 1984), cortical evoked potentials (e.g., Chen, Chapman, & Harkins, 1979), and magnetic resonance imaging and positron emission tomography (Talbot, Marrett, Evans, Meyer, Bushnell, & Duncan, 1991), their data can only be confirmed and validated against expressed human experience. For better or worse, numbers, words, and matches will tell us about pain.

The questions which confront psychophysicists interested in pain are the same ones which apply to other modalities (Gescheider & Bolanowski, 1991): what do subjects judge, what are the response biases, how do we deal with individual differences, what is the value of absolute magnitude estimates vs. matching tasks, do we study psychological magnitude or the judgment of psychological magnitude, is there a psychophysical law? The multiple dimensions of the pain experience, of which the cognitive has probably received the least attention (witness that only one of the 20 scales on the McGill Pain Questionnaire claims to measure the cognitive-evaluative component), provide added challenges. The importance of obtaining answers to these questions and the lively debate that punctuates that quest supply sustenance.

References

Adair, E., Stevens J.C., & Marks E.L. (1968). Thermally induced pain, the dol scale, and the psychophysical power law. *American Journal of Psychology*, **81**, 147-164.

Algom, D., Raphaeli, N., & Cohen-Raz, L. (1986). Integration of noxious stimulation across separate somatosensory communications systems: A functional theory of pain. *Journal of Experimental Psychology: Human Perception and Performance*, **12**, 92-102.

Algom, D., Raphaeli, N., & Cohen-Raz, L. (1987). Pain combines additively across different sensory systems: A further support for the functional theory of pain. *Perceptual and Motor Skills*, **65**, 619-625.

Anderson, N.H. (1970). Functional measurement and psychophysical judgement. *Psychological Review*, **77**, 153-170.

Anderson, N.H. (1989). Information integration approach to emotions and their measurement. In R. Plutchik & H. Kellerman (Eds.). *Emotion: Theory, Research and Experience* (Vol. 4) (pp. 133-186). New York: Academic Press.

Bakal, D.A., Demjen, S., & Kaganov, J.A. (1981). Cognitive behavioral treatment of chronic headache. *Headache*, **21**, 81-86.

Bandura, A. (1977). Self-efficacy: Toward a unifying theory of behavioral change. *Psychological Review*, **84**, 191-215.

Bandura, A., O'Leary, A., Taylor, C.B., Gauthier, J., & Gossard, D. (1987). Perceived self-efficacy and pain control: Opioid and nonopioid mechanisms. *Journal of Personality and Social Psychology,* **53**, 563-571.

Beecher, H.K. (1959). *Measurement of subjective response: Quantitative effects of drugs*. New York: Oxford University Press.

Bishop, G.H. (1946). Neural mechanisms of cutaneous sense. *Physiological Review*, **26**, 77-102.

Blitz, B., & Dinnerstein, A.J. (1971). Role of attentional focus in pain perception. *Journal of Abnormal Psychology*, **77**, 42-45.

Bobey, M.J., & Davidson, P.O. (1970). Psychological factors affecting pain tolerance. *Journal of Psychosomatic Research*, **14**, 371-376.

Boring, E.G. (1942). *Sensation and perception in the history of experimental psychology*. New York: Appleton-Century-Crofts.

Bradley, L.A., Young, L.D., Anderson, K.O., McDaniel, L.K., Pisko, E.J., Semble, E.L., & Morgan, T.M. (1987). Effects of psychological therapy on pain behavior of rheumatoid patients: Treatment outcome and six-month follow-up. *Arthritis and Rheumatism*, **30**, 1105-1114.

Bromm, B. (1984). The measurement of pain in man. In B. Bromm (Ed.). *Pain Measurement in Man: Neurophysiological Correlates of Pain* (pp. 3-14). New York: Elsevier.

Bromm, B., & Treede, R.-D. (1980). Withdrawal reflex, skin resistance reaction and pain ratings due to electrical stimuli in man. *Pain*, **9**, 339-354.

Brown, R.A., Fader, K. & Barber, T.X. (1973). Responsiveness to pain: Stimulus-specificity versus generality. *Psychological Record*, **23**, 1-7.

Campbell, D.T., & Fiske, D.W. (1959). Convergent and discriminant validation by the multitrait-multimethod matrix. *Psychological Bulletin*, **56**, 81-105.

Cattel, J. McK. (1943) The action and use of analgesics. *Proceedings of the Association for Research on Nervous Diseases*, **23**, 365-372.

Chapman, C.R. (1978). the perception of noxious events. In R.A. Sternbach, (Ed.). *The psychology of pain* (pp. 169-203). New York: Raven Press.

Chapman, C.R., Gehrig, J.d., & Wilson, M.E. (1975). Acupuncture compared with 33 percent nitrous oxide for dental analgesia: A sensory decision theory evaluation. *Anesthesiology*, **42**, 532-537.

Chen, A.C.N., Chapman, C.R., & Harkins, S.W. (1979). Brain evoked potentials are functional correlates of induced pain in man. *Pain*, **6**, 365-374.

Clark, W.C., Ferrer-Brechner, T., Janal, M.N., Carroll, J.D., & Yang, C. (1989). The dimensions of pain: A multidimensional scaling comparison of cancer patients and healthy volunteers. *Pain*, **37**, 23-32.

Clark, W.C., & Yang, J.C. (1974). Acupunctural analgesia? Evaluation by signal detection theory. *Science*, **184**, 1096-1098.

Colt, E.W.D., Wardlaw, S.L., & Frantz, A.G. (1981). The effects of running on beta-endorphin. *Life Sciences*, **28**, 1637-1640.

Coppola, R., & Gracely, R.H. (1983). Where is the noise in SDT pain assessment? *Pain*, **17**, 257-266.

Dadson, R.S., & King, J.H. (1952). A determination of the natural threshold of hearing and its relation to the standardization of audiometers. *Journal of Laryngology and Otology*, **66**, 326-378.

Davidson, P.O., & McDougall, C.E. (1969). The generality of pain tolerance. *Journal of Psychosomatic Research*, **13**, 82-89.

Duncan, G.H., Bushnell, M.C., & Lavigne, G.J. (1989). comparison of verbal and visual analogue scales for measuring the intensity and unpleasantness of experimental pain. *Pain*, **37**, 295-303.

Eriksson, M.B.E., Rosen, I., & Sjolund, B. (1985). Thermal sensitivity in healthy subjects is decreased by a central mechanism after TNS. *Pain*, **22**, 235-242.

Erskine, A., Morley, S., & Pearce, S. (1990). Memory for pain: A review. *Pain*, **41**, 255-266.

Gescheider, G.A., & Bolanowski, S.J. (1991). Final comments on ratio scaling of psychological magnitudes. In S.J. Bolanowski & G.A. Gescheider (Eds.). *Ratio Scaling of Psychological Magnitude* (pp. 295-312). Hillsdale, NJ: Lawrence Erlbaum Associates.

Goff, G.H., Rosner, B.S., Detre, T., & Kennard, D. (1965). Vibration perception in normal man and medical patients. *Journal of Neurology*, **28**, 503-509.

Gracely, R.H. (1979). Psychophysical assessment of human pain. In J. Bonica, J.C. Liebeskind, & D.G. Albe-Fessard (Eds.). *Advances in Pain Research and Therapy*, Vol. 3 (pp. 805-824). New York: Raven Press.

Gracely, R.H. (1989). Methods of testing pain mechanisms in normal man. In R. Melzack & P.D. Wall (Eds.). *Textbook of pain* (pp. 257-268). Edinburgh: Churchill Livingstone.

Gracely, R.H., & Dubner, R. (1987). Reliability and validity of verbal descriptor scales of painfulness. *Pain*, **29**, 175-186.

Gracely, R.H., Dubner, R., & McGrath, P.A. (1979). Narcotic analgesia: Fentanyl reduces the intensity but not the unpleasantness of painful tooth pulp sensations. *Science*, **203**, 1261-1263.

Gracely, R.H., Dubner, R., McGrath, P., & Heft, M. (1978). New methods of pain measurement and their application to pain control. *International Dental Journal,* **28**, 52-65.

Gracely, R.H., & Kwilosz, D.M. (1988). The descriptor differential scale: Applying psychophysical principles to clinical pain assessment. *Pain*, **35**, 279-288.

Gracely, R.H., McGrath, P., & Dubner, R. (1978a). Ratio scales of sensory and affective verbal pain descriptors. *Pain*, **5**, 5-18.

Gracely, R.H., McGrath, P., & Dubner, R. (1978b). Validity and sensitivity of ratio scales of sensory and affective verbal pain descriptors: Manipulation of affect by diazepam. *Pain*, **5**, 19-30.

Green, D.M., & Swets, J.A. (1966). *Signal detection theory and psychophysics*. New York: Wiley.

Harris, G. (1981). *Pain and the individual.* University of Western Ontario: Unpublished Ph.D. dissertation.

Harris, G., & Rollman, G.B. (1983). The validity of experimental pain measures. *Pain*, **17**, 369-376.

Harris, G., & Rollman, G.B. (1985). Cognitive techniques for controlling pain: Generality and individual differences. In H.L. Fields, R. Dubner, & F. Cervero (Eds.). *Advances in pain research and therapy*. (Vol. 9) (pp. 847-851). New York: Raven Press.

Hecht, S., & Mandelbaum, J. (1948). The relationship between vitamin A and dark adaptation. *Journal of the American Medical Association*, **112**, 1910-1916.

Higashiyama, A., & Rollman, G.B. (1991). Detection and localization of cathodal and anodal electrocutaneous pulses. *IEEE Transactions on Biomedical Engineering*, **38**, 679-686.

Hunter, M., Philips, C., & Rachman, S. (1979). Memory for pain. *Pain*, 6, 35-46.

Ippolitov, F.V. (1972). Interanalyser differences in the sensitivity-strength parameter for vision, hearing and the cutaneous modalities. In V.D. Nebylitsyn & J.A. Gray (Eds.). *Biological bases of individual behavior* (pp. 43-61). New York: Academic Press.

Irwin, J.R., & Whitehead, P.R. (1991). Towards an objective psychophysics of pain. *Psychological Science*, **2**, 230-235.

Jamison, R.N., Sbrocco, T., & Parris, W.C.V. (1989). The influence of physical and psychosocial factors on accuracy of memory for pain in chronic pain patients. *Pain*, **37**, 289-294.

Jamner, L.D., & Tursky, B. (1987). Discrimination between intensity and affective pain descriptors: A psychophysiological evaluation. *Pain*, **30**, 271-283.

Janal, M.N., Colt, E.W.D., Clark, W.C., & Glusman, M. (1984). Pain sensitivity, mood and plasma endocrine levels in man following long-distance running: Effects of naloxone. *Pain*, **19**, 13-26.

Lautenbacher, S., Galfe, G., Karlbauer, G., Moltner, A., & Strian, F. (1990). Effects of chronic back pain on the perception of experimental heat pain. *Perceptual and Motor Skills*, **71**, 1283-1292.

Lautenbacher, S., Moltner, A., & Strian, F. (1991). Psychophysical features of the transition from the pure heat perception to the heat pain perception. Unpublished manuscript.

Maier, S.F., Laudenslager, M.L., & Ryan, S.M. (1985). Stressor controllability, immune function and endogenous opiates. In F.R. Brush & J.B. Overmier (Eds.). *Affect, conditioning and cognition: Essays on the determinants of behavior* (pp. 183-201). Hillsdale, New Jersey: Erlbaum.

Meichenbaum, D.H. (1977). *Cognitive-behavior modification: An integrative approach*. New York: Plenum Press.

Melzack, R. (1975). The McGill Pain Questionnaire: Major properties and scoring methods. *Pain*, **1**, 277-300.

Melzack, R., & Casey, K.L. (1968). Sensory, motivational, and central determinants of pain: A new conceptual model. In D. Kenshalo (Ed.). *The skin senses* (pp. 423-443). Springfield, Illinois: Thomas.

Melzack, R., & Torgerson, W.S. (1971). On the language of pain. *Anesthesiology*, **34**, 50-59.

Melzack, R., & Wall, P.D. (1962). On the nature of cutaneous sensory mechanisms. *Brain*, **85**, 331-356.

Melzack, R., & Wall, P.D. (1965). Pain mechanisms: A new theory. *Science*, **150**, 971-979.

Melzack, R., & Wall, P.D. (1988). *The challenge of pain* (2nd ed.). London: Penguin.

Mersky, H. (1986). Classification of chronic pain: Descriptions of chronic pain syndromes and definitions of pain terms. *Pain*, Supplement 3, S1-S226.

Morley, S. (1989). The dimensionality of verbal descriptors in Tursky's pain perception profile. *Pain*, **37**, 41-50.

Morley, S., & Hassard, A. (1989). The development of self-administered psychophysical scaling method: Internal consistency and temporal stability in chronic pain patients. *Pain*, **37**, 33-40.

Naliboff, B.D., & Cohen, M.J. (1989). Psychophysical laboratory methods applied to clinical pain patients. In C.R. Chapman & J.D. Loeser (Eds.). *Advances in Pain Research and Therapy* (Vol. 12) (pp. 365-386). New York: Raven Press.

Neufeld, R.W.J., & Davidson, P.O. (1971). The effects of vicarious and cognitive rehearsal on pain tolerance. *Journal of Psychosomatic Research,* **15**, 329-335.

Price, D.D. (1988). *Psychological and neural mechanisms of pain.* New York: Raven Press.

Price, D.D., Barrell, J.J., & Gracely, R.H. (1980). A psychophysical analysis of experiential factors that selectively influence the affective dimension of pain. *Pain*, **8**, 137-150.

Price, D.D., Harkins, S.W., & Baker, C. (1987). Sensory-affective relationships among different types of clinical and experimental pain. *Pain*, **28**, 297-308.

Price, D.D., Harkins, S.W., Rafii, A., & Price, C. (1986). A simultaneous comparison of fentanyl's analgesic effects on experimental and clinical pain. *Pain*, **24**, 197-204.

Price, D.D., McGrath, P.A., Rafii, A., & Buckingham, B. (1983). The validation of visual analogue scales as ratio scale measures for chronic and experimental pain. *Pain*, **17**, 45-56.

Price, D.D., Von der Gruen, A., Miller, J., Rafii, A., & Price, C. (1985). A psychophysical analysis of morphine analgesia. *Pain*, **22**, 261-270.

Prkachin, K.M., & Cameron, R. (1990). Behavior and cognitive therapies. In E. Tunkes, A. Bellissimo, & R. Roy (Eds.). *Chronic Pain: Psychological factors in rehabilitation* (Second Ed.) (pp. 144-183). Malabar, Florida: Krieger.

Rabin, M.D., & Cain, W.S. (1986). Determinants of measured olfactory sensitivity. *Perception and Psychophysics*, **39**, 281-286.

Roche, P.A.A., & Gijsbers, K. (1986). A comparison of memory for induced ischemic pain and chronic rheumatoid pain. *Pain*, **25**, 337-344.

Rollman, G.B. (1975). Behavioral assessment of peripheral nerve function. *Neurology*, **25**, 339-342.

Rollman, G.B. (1977). Signal detection theory measurement of pain: A review and critique. *Pain*, **3**, 187-212.

Rollman, G.B. (1979). Signal detection theory pain measures: Empirical validation studies and adaptation-level effects. *Pain*, **6**, 9-22.

Rollman, G.B. (1983a). Measurement of experimental pain in chronic pain patients: Methodological and individual factors. In: R. Melzack (Ed.). *Pain measurement and assessment* (pp. 251-258). New York: Raven Press.

Rollman, G.B. (1983b). Multiple subjective representations of experimental pain. In J.J. Bonica, U. Lindblom, & A. Iggo (Eds.), *Advances in pain research and therapy*, Vol. 5 (pp. 865-869). New York: Raven Press.

Rollman, G.B. (1989). Measurement of pain in fibromyalgia in the clinic and laboratory. *Journal of Rheumatology*, **16**, 113-119.

Rollman, G.B., & Harris, G. (1987). The detectability, discriminability, and perceived magnitude of painful electrical shock. *Perception and Psychophysics*, **42**, 257-258.

Scudds, R.A., McCain, G.A., Rollman, G.B., & Harth, M. (1989). Improvements in pain responsiveness in patients with fibrositis after successful treatment with amitriptyline. *Journal of Rheumatology*, **16**, 98-103.

Scudds, R.A., Rollman, G.B., Harth, M., & McCain, G.A. (1987). Pain perception and personality measures as discriminators in the classification of fibrositis. *Journal of Rheumatology*, **14**, 563-569.

Smith, R.H., & Andrew, J.H. (1970). Gradable pain production. In: N.L. Wulfsohn & A. Sances (Eds.). *The Nervous System and Electric Currents* (pp. 89-92). New York: Plenum Press.

Stam, H.J., McGrath, P.A., & Brooke, R.J. (1984). The effects of a cognitive behavioral treatment program on temporo-mandibular pain and dysfunction syndrome. *Psychosomatic Medicine*, **46**, 534-545.

Sternbach, R.A., & Trusky, B. (1965). Ethnic differences among housewives in psychophysical and skin potential responses to electric shock. *Psychophysiology,* **1**, 241-246.

Talbot, I.D., Marret, S., Evans, A.C., Meyer, E., Bushnell, M.E., & Duncan, G.H. (1991). Multiple representations of pain in the human cerebral cortex. *Science*, **251**, 1355-1358.

Tan, S.-Y. (1982). Cognitive and cognitive-behavioral methods for pain control: A selective review. *Pain*, **12**, 201-228.

Taub, A., & Campbell, J.N. (1974). Percutaneous local electrical analgesia: Peripheral mechanisms. In J.J. Bonia (Ed.). *International Symposium on Pain, Advances in Neurology* (Vol. 4) (pp. 727-732). New York: Raven Press.

Teghtsoonian, R. (1971). On the exponents in Stevens' Law and the constant in Ekman's Law. *Psychological Review*, **78**, 71-80.

Torebjork, E., & Ochoa, J. (1984). Human skin units and sensory experience. In G. Serratrice, D. Cros, C. Desnuelle, J.-L. Gastaut, J.-F. Pellissier, J. Pouget, & A. Shiano (Eds.). *Neuromuscular Diseases* (pp. 319-322). New York: Raven Press.

Turk, D.C., & Kerns, R.D. (1983). Conceptual issues in the assessment of clinical pain. *International Journal of Psychiatry in Medicine*, **13**, 15-26.

Turk, D.C., Meichenbaum, D., & Genest, M. (1983). Pain and behavioral medicine: A cognitive-behavioral perspective. New York: Guilford Press.

Turner, J.A., & Chapman, C.R. (1982a). Psychological interventions for chronic pain: A critical review. I. Relaxation training and biofeedback. *Pain*, **12**, 1-21.

Turner, J.A., & Chapman, C.R. (1982b). Psychological interventions for chronic pain: A critical review. II. Operant conditioning, hypnosis, and cognitive-behavioral therapy. *Pain*, **12**, 23-46.

Turner, J.A., & Clancy, S. (1986). Strategies for coping with chronic low back pain: Relationship to pain and disability. *Pain*, **24**, 355-364.

Tursky, B., Jamner, L.D., & Friedman, R. (1982). The pain perception profile: A psychophysical approach to the assessment of pain report. *Behavior Therapy*, **13**, 376-394.

Urban, B.J., Keefe, F.J., & France, R.D. (1984). A study of psychophysical scaling in chronic pain patients. *Pain*, **20**, 157-168.

Vallis, T.M. (1984). A complete component analysis of stress inoculation for pain tolerance. *Cognitive Therapy and Research*, **8**, 313-329.

Wall, P.D. (1979). On the relation of injury to pain. The John J. Bonica Lecture. *Pain*, **6**, 253-264.

Watkins, L.R. (1988). Algesiometry in laboratory animals and man: Current concepts and future directions. In: C.R. Chapman & J.D. Loeser (Eds.). *Advances in Pain Research and Therapy* (Vol. 12) (pp. 249-266). New York: Raven Press.

Psychophysical Approaches to Cognition
D. Algom (Editor)

10

SENSORY, COGNITIVE AND RESPONSE FACTORS IN THE JUDGMENT OF SENSORY MAGNITUDE[1]

George A. Gescheider
Hamilton College and Institute for Sensory Research, Syracuse University
Stanley J. Bolanowski, Jr. and Ronald T. Verrillo
Institute for Sensory Research
Syracuse University

[1] This work was supported in part by Grants PO 1 DC-00380 and RO 1 DC-00098 from the National Institutes of Health, U.S. Department of Health and Human Services.

Table of Contents

I. Introduction

The role of sensory, cognitive and response factors in psychophysical judgment is clearly illustrated in research in which magnitude estimation has been used to measure the magnitude of the sensations elicited by stimuli. The numbers that subjects assign to impressions of stimuli, no doubt, are determined by sensory magnitudes, but may also be determined by cognitive factors such as concepts of the relative magnitude of the stimulus. For example, in the judgment of size, a baseball may be thought of as large relative to the size of a golf ball but relatively small in relation to the size of a basketball. Thus, the subject's concept of the size of an object must be determined, to some extent, by the sizes of other objects in the set of which the judged object is a member. It is likely that stimulus context effects observed in magnitude estimation in which a subject's judgments of a stimulus are influenced by the values of other stimuli presented in same session (e.g., Foley, et al., 1990; Gescheider & Hughson, 1991; Marks, et al, 1986; Mellers, 1983; Ward, 1987; Zwislocki & Goodman, 1980) are due, to a large extent, to this relativity of thought about the magnitudes of stimuli. It is also possible that the actual sensory impression of a stimulus is influenced by stimulus context. For example, the baseball may actually look bigger in the presence of the golf ball than in the presence of the basketball. Finally, the subject's judgments may be greatly affected by the particular strategy used for choosing numbers. For example, in magnitude estimation, if a subject were to use a fixed range of numbers independent of the position or width of the stimulus range, a response bias could emerge in which the numerical judgment of the subjective magnitude of a stimulus would depend on the numbers assigned to other stimuli (Poulton, 1979). Such response-bias tendencies, if not eliminated, would render scales of subjective magnitude meaningless.

Historically, in sensory psychophysics, the goal has been to measure properties of sensory systems with the hope that such measurements would reveal insights into underlying basic principles of sensory information processing. The measurement of sensory thresholds, particularly with modern, relatively bias-free procedures derived from the theory of signal detection, is well accepted as a means of studying sensory systems and the success of this approach is not disputed. A more controversial approach is the use of psychophysical scaling procedures to measure the sensory magnitudes of suprathreshold stimuli. The problem is that the results obtained by the various scaling methods often do not agree, suggesting that the methods may vary in their susceptibility to the influence of cognitive and response factors such that they provide measurements of sensory magnitude that are contaminated to varying degrees. This unfortunate state of affairs, however, does not diminish the importance of measuring sensory magnitude.

II. Measurement of Sensory Magnitude

The question of why it is so important to be able to measure sensory magnitudes can best be answered by considering an example. If we conceptualize a sensory system as having an environmental stimulus as its input and experienced sensation as its output, we can imagine that it has the input-output function illustrated in Figure 10.1. The absolute threshold (I_o) could be measured by determining the intensity of a stimulus that is just detectable. Likewise, intensity difference thresholds (ΔI) could be measured by determining the difference in intensity that can be discriminated. One value of ΔI at one location on the intensity axis is illustrated, but typically a number of ΔI measurements are made at various intensity values. Although knowing the absolute sensitivity and the differential sensitivity of a sensory system provides valuable information, this knowledge cannot in itself be used to describe the entire input-output function without assuming some fundamental relation between stimulus and response (e.g., Fechnerian integration of the ΔIs). A formal description of the input-output function is important because it would reveal how the nervous system operates on the continuously changing sensory information it receives, thus enhancing our understanding of the system's characteristics. As a natural outgrowth, our ability to diagnose and treat sensory disorders and to design sensory aids for individuals with sensory impairment would be greatly improved.

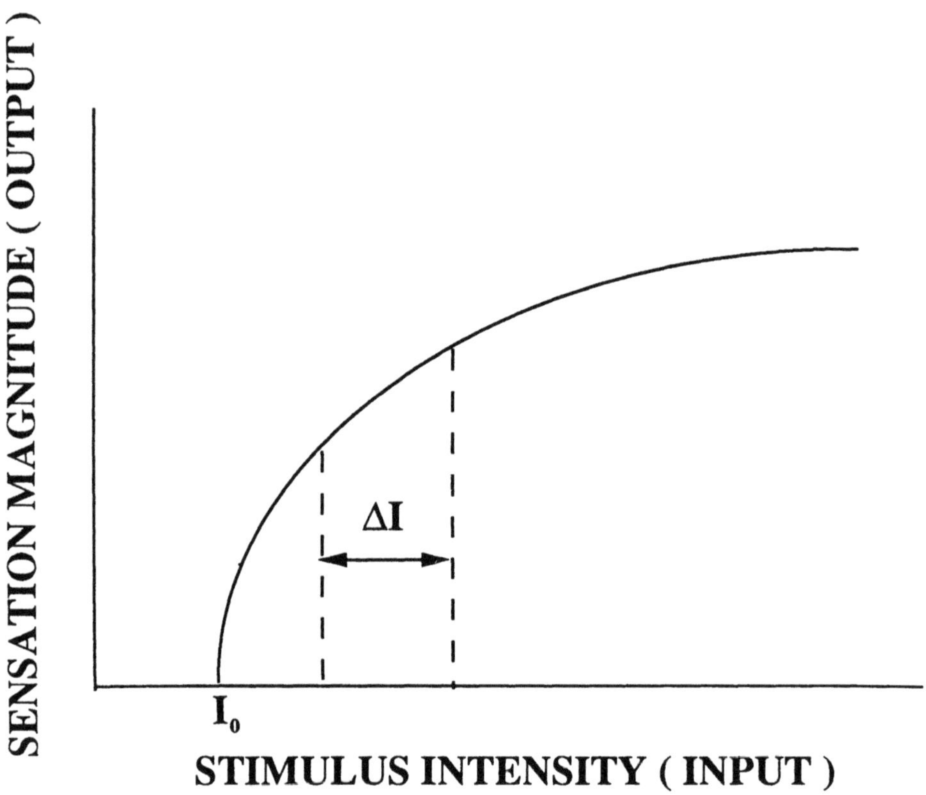

Figure 10.1: Hypothetical input-output function of a sensory system. I_o represents the absolute threshold and ΔI represents a difference threshold for intensity. From Gescheider and Bolanowski (1991).

The problem impeding progress on these matters is that there are no techniques for directly measuring the magnitudes of private sensations. The available methods are indirect, at best. The magnitude of a sensation is always inferred from the subject's response to stimuli. To redefine sensation in terms of observable neural activity does not solve the problem because to do so requires that we know the neural code for stimulus intensity, and presently no widespread agreement exists on this matter. The problem is further illustrated by the two-stage model of psychophysical scaling (e.g. Attneave, 1962; Curtis, et al., 1968; Shepard, 1981) as seen in Figure 10.2. Sensation magnitude (Υ) and its relation to stimulus intensity (ϕ), known as the psychophysical law [$\Upsilon=F_1(\phi)$], must be inferred from the relationship between the stimulus and the observable response [$R=F_3(\phi)$]. To do this, however, the relationship between the response and the sensation [$R=F_2(\Upsilon)$] must be known. Unfortunately, the relationship between response and sensation is as inaccessible to direct observation and therefore is just as elusive as the relationship between stimulus and sensation. In spite of these difficulties, psychophysical scales of sensory magnitude have been constructed and claims for their validity have been made.

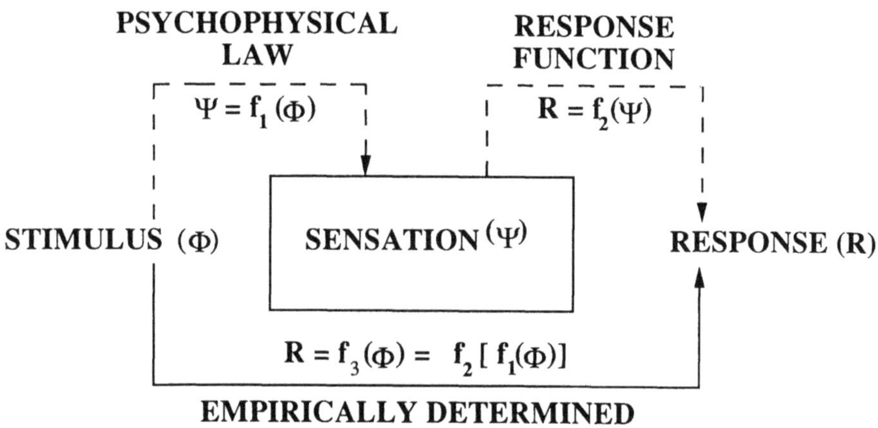

Figure 10.2: Relations among the psychophysical law (stimulus transformation function), $\Upsilon=f_1(\phi)$, the response function (response transformation function), $R=f_2(\Upsilon)$, and the empirically determined relation between stimulus intensity and response, $R=f_2(\phi)$.

It has been said that Fechner, in using intensity-discrimination measurements, indirectly measured sensory magnitude, whereas Stevens, by using the ratio-scaling methods of magnitude estimation, magnitude production, ratio estimation, and ratio production, measured it directly. Most psychophysicists today, however, agree that any observed relationship between judgments of sensory magnitude and the intensity of the stimulus provide, at best, only an indirect estimation of the relationship between sensory magnitude and stimulus intensity. Whether the proposed psychophysical law is Fechner's logarithmic function, Stevens' power function, or some entirely different function, the relationship between sensory magnitude and stimulus intensity must be inferred from the observable responses of subjects. The problem is that the subject's responses can easily be biased. Some of the bias may originate in the conditions of the experiment and some may be the product of the subject's past experiences. Whatever the source of bias may be, there is wide agreement among sensory psychophysicists that the goal should be to develop and refine methods that minimize bias so that true sensory magnitude functions can be ascertained. One of many such efforts has been the development of the method of absolute magnitude estimation (Hellman & Zwislocki, 1961, 1963; Zwislocki, 1978; Zwislocki & Goodman, 1980) as a way of minimizing biases in magnitude-estimation experiments.

III. Absolute Magnitude Estimation

An important question recently asked is whether or not there is anything absolute about absolute magnitude estimation (Gescheider & Bolanowski, 1991). The answer has a long history and is rooted in the problem of controlling bias in magnitude-estimation experiments created through the use of a standard stimulus. Absolute magnitude estimation (AME) requires subjects to match their subjective impression of the size of a number to their impression of the intensity of a stimulus, and to do so independently of prior matches. The method is based upon the hypothesis that, at a particular time and in a particular setting, a subject has a strong tendency to assign a number to a stimulus in such a way that their psychological magnitudes match. Forcing the subject to use an arbitrary modulus associated with a particular standard stimulus can violate the tendency to match psychological magnitudes -- thus resulting in bias. According to the AME hypothesis, subjects are capable of making unbiased numerical judgments of sensory magnitudes only when they are permitted to use their own natural units (Zwislocki & Goodman, 1980).

Evidence that subjects tend to judge sensory magnitude on an absolute rather than a ratio scale comes from findings on the effects of the values of the standard stimulus and the associated modulus on magnitude estimations. In accordance with the definition of a ratio scale (Stevens, 1951), a subject's numerical estimations of sensory magnitudes should be invariant to within a multiplicative transformation when the value of the modulus and/or standard stimulus is changed. Thus, it should be possible to make valid judgments of the sensation magnitudes of all stimuli in proportion to a modulus consisting of an arbitrary numerical value designated by the experimenter to represent the sensation magnitude of the standard stimulus. The work of Stevens (1956) and Hellman and Zwislocki (1961) on loudness scaling, in which the effects of using a standard stimulus with a particular modulus as a reference were investigated, casts serious doubt on the hypothesis that subjects, using an arbitrary unit, are capable of assigning numbers in proportion to the ratios of their sensations. The consequences of using a standard stimulus of 40 or 90 dB above threshold are seen in Figure 10.3. Subjects estimated the loudness of tones presented to both

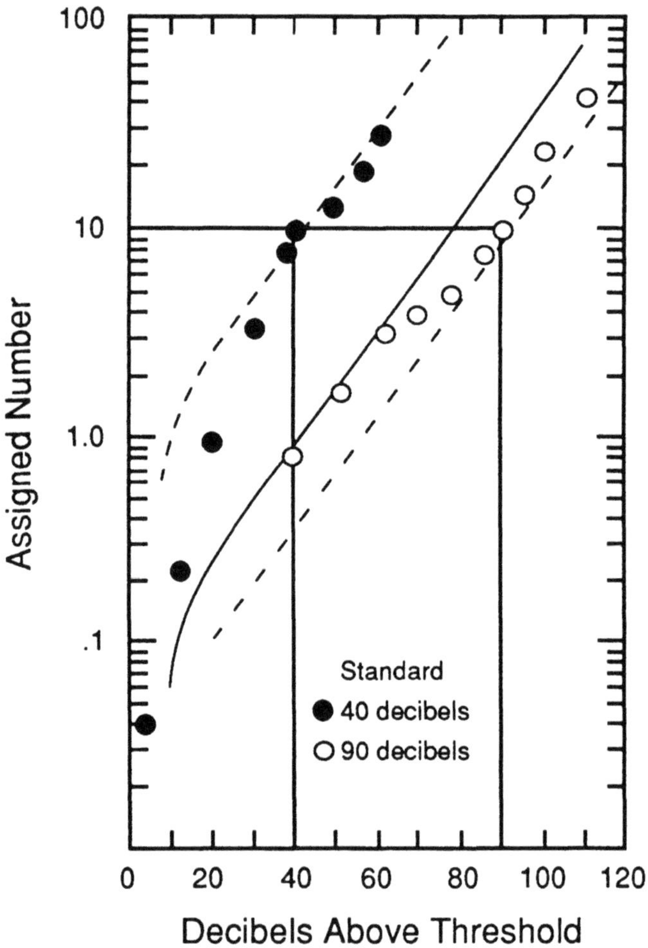

Figure 10.3: Magnitude estimation of loudness as a function of sound intensity for standard stimuli of 40 and 90 dB SL.

ears through earphones. They were told to judge the loudness of each tone relative to the loudness of 10 (the modulus) arbitrarily assigned to the standard stimulus. If the subjects had been able to make ratio judgments of loudness, the intensity of the standard stimulus would have had no effect on the form of the loudness scale, other than shifting all magnitude estimations by a constant ratio. Thus, ratio scaling would have produced a vertical shift of the entire curve by a constant distance when magnitude estimations were plotted on a logarithmic axis. Under these conditions, the ratio of the magnitude estimation values for various stimuli would remain the same even though changing the standard stimulus would force the subject to assign higher or lower numbers.

It can be seen clearly in Figure 10.3 that when the standard stimulus was 40 and 90 dB above threshold, the resulting loudness scales were not parallel over the entire range of stimulus intensities. Only within a narrow range near the value of the standard stimulus did the curves approach being parallel. The solid curve is the binaural loudness scale derived from absolute magnitude estimation (Zwislocki & Goodman, 1980). The dashed curves are parallel to the absolute magnitude estimation curve. It is evident from examination of Figure 10.3 that when a standard stimulus is used, magnitude estimations of stimuli distant from the value of the standard tend to converge on the curve derived from absolute magnitude estimation. The finding that the loudness scales obtained with 40 and 90 dB standards are reasonably parallel within the intensity range of the standard stimulus suggests that, within this limited range, subjects are capable of making ratio judgments of sensation magnitude. On the other hand, outside this range, their responses tend to drift toward what may be interpreted as a natural absolute scale.

The standard stimulus seems to bias the psychophysical scale only where the experimenter has arbitrarily assigned to it a subjective value different from that which the subject would assign in absolute scaling. When making absolute magnitude estimations, subjects assigned a tone of 76 dB a value of 10. It can be seen in Figure 10.4 that using a standard stimulus of 80 dB to which the experimenter assigns a modulus value of 10, yielded almost the same loudness scale that resulted from absolute magnitude estimation. Since the 80 dB tone has an absolute subjective loudness value near 10, the subjective values assigned by the experimenter and the subject are almost the same, and, consequently, the use of the standard has a minimal biasing effect on the scale. Presumably, using a 76 dB standard stimulus with a modulus of 10 would have totally eliminated this bias. Under these circumstances, the subjective value assigned by the experimenter and by the subjects in absolute magnitude estimation would be identical.

The hypothesis that subjects tend to assign numbers to sensations on a natural absolute scale is also suggested by the work of Ward (1973), who had subjects make magnitude estimations of the loudness of 1000-Hz tones. At the start of an experimental session, the subject was presented with a standard stimulus of 56 dB above threshold, and was told that this tone had a subjective value of 10. This and other stimuli were presented many times throughout the session, but no further statements were made by the experimenter of the subjective value of the standard stimulus. By the end of the session, the average value assigned to the standard by the subjects was not 10, but instead was 2.08. Zwislocki and Goodman (1980) have pointed out that 2.08 is almost exactly what subjects assign to this stimulus by absolute magnitude estimation. It appears that unless observers are repeatedly reminded of the arbitrary subjective value of a standard stimulus, they will eventually use their own natural numbers. It is this tendency of subjects to use their own natural numbers in judging psychological magnitudes, and the inability of subjects to judge the ratios of their sensations in arbitrary units that best characterizes what is absolute in absolute magnitude estimation.

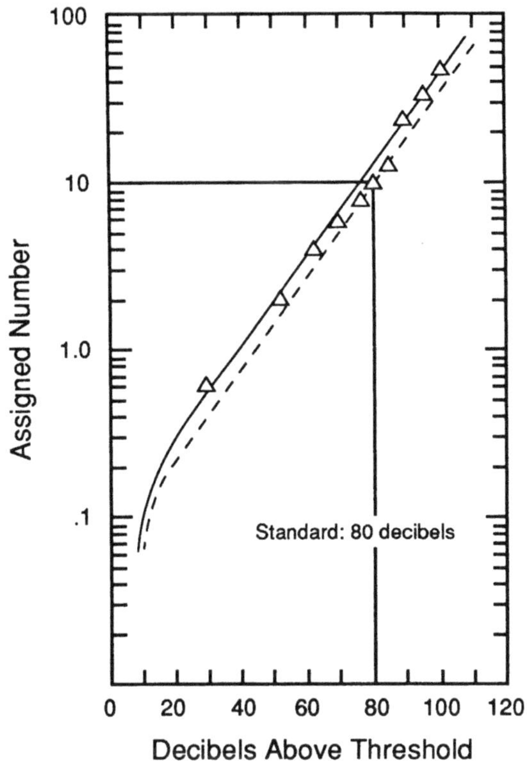

Figure 10.4: Magnitude estimation of loudness as a function of sound intensity when the standard stimulus was 80 dB SL.

The psychophysical scale resulting from AME is absolute in the sense that the unit of measurement employed by the subject in judging sensation magnitude in a particular context is fixed. Forcing the subject to change the unit produces bias. It should be made clear that the absolute in AME does *not* mean that the subject will give the same number to a stimulus on all occasions or in differing stimulus contexts. Misunderstanding of this last point has given rise to false claims against the absolute magnitude estimation hypothesis (Foley, et al., 1990; Mellers, 1983). Demonstrations that AME judgments can be influenced by the values of other stimuli presented in the session (Mellers, 1983) or on the values of stimuli presented in prior sessions (Foley, et al., 1990) do not constitute evidence against the hypothesis. In his response to Mellers' paper, Zwislocki (1983b), one of the originators of AME, pointed out that a scale is called "absolute" not because it cannot be biased, but instead because it has the formal mathematical property of having a fixed unit.

IV. Scales of Measurement

S.S. Stevens provided us with a very useful system for classifying scales of measurement in terms of permissible mathematical transformations that leave a scale invariant (i.e., transformations that do not change its essential mathematical properties). We have recently added the absolute scale to Stevens' system (Gescheider & Bolanowski, 1991). Listed in Table 10.1 are the basic operations, mathematical group structures (transformation that leaves the scale invariant), the permissible statistics, and examples. In the nominal scale, any one-to-one substitution of numbers will preserve the identity of the measurements. Any monotonic transformation of the numbers of an ordinal scale will preserve the order of the scale values and this is, therefore, permissible. An interval scale, designed to determine the differences between magnitudes, is invariant to any linear transformation in which the slope and intercept are free to vary, whereas in the ratio scale the only permissible transformation is multiplication by a constant. Thus, the ratio scale has a variable unit size and an absolute zero. The absolute scale cannot be mathematically transformed without violating the properties of the scale, and therefore the scale consists of a special instance of a ratio scale in which the unit is fixed (e.g., numerosity). It is our opinion that, as well as having a fixed unit, the absolute scale in psychophysics is one that has the properties of transitivity and additivity characteristic of ratio scales. The fixed unit is implied by the results of Hellman and Zwislocki (1961), but the results of other experiments are pertinent to the issues of transitivity and additivity of AME scales. Let us consider the requirement of transitivity.

Table 10.1
Scales of Measurement. Adapted from Stevens (1951). From Gescheider & Bolanowski (1991)

Scale	Basic Empirical Operations	Mathematical Group Structure	Permissive Statistics	Examples
Nominal	Determination of Equality	Permutation group x'=f(x). f(x) means any one-to-one substitution	Number of cases. Mode Contingency correlations	Numbering of ballplayers Assignment of type or model to classes
Ordinal	Determination of greater or less	Isotonic Group x'=f(x). f(x) means any increasing monotonic function	Median, Percentiles Order correlation (type O)	Hardness of minerals Quality of items Pleasantness of odors
Interval	Determination of equality of intervals or differences	General linear group x'=ax+b	Mean Standard deviation Order correlation (type 1) Product-moment correlation	Temperature (Fahrenheit Centigrade) Energy Calendar dates
Ratio	Determination of equality of ratios	Similarity group x'=ax	Geometric means Coefficient of variation Decibel transformation	Length, weight, density, etc. Pitch scale? Loudness scale?
Absolute	Determination of matches	Identity x'=x Special instance of ratio scale	Geometric means Coefficient of variation Decibel transformation	Numerosity Pitch scale? Loudness scale?

Note: The basic operation needed to create various scales are shown in the second column. the third column indicates the mathematical transformation that leaves the scale invariant (i.e., numeral x can be replaced by another numeral x' under the given functional relation). The fourth column shows some of the statistics that show invariance under the permissible transformation.

V. Transitivity of AME Judgments

In addition to the findings on the effects of using a standard stimulus on magnitude-estimation judgments, recent work on the prediction of cross-modality matches from AME judgments also supports the hypothesis that absolute scales can be achieved in AME. If subjects assign numbers to their sensations on an absolute scale, then stimuli in two different modalities are equal in sensation magnitude when the stimuli are given the same number in magnitude estimation. It should, therefore, be possible to demonstrate the transitivity of scales by predicting the absolute values of cross-modality matches. The prediction is that stimuli from the two modalities that have been assigned the same number in magnitude estimation will be judged to be psychologically equal in cross-modality matching. If this prediction were confirmed, it would imply that the size of the numbers used in magnitude estimation are not arbitrary and thus result in psychophysical scales in which the unit of measurement is fixed. The prediction of cross-modality matches from absolute scales is based on the assumptions that, (a) subjects are capable of making psychophysical matches between their impressions of the size of numbers and impressions of sensory stimuli and, (b) that subjects are capable of making psychophysical matches between their impressions of sensory stimuli.

How reasonable is it to assume that subjects have the ability to make matches of psychological magnitudes? The viewpoint that matching is the fundamental operation underlying all physical and psychophysical measurement was recently expressed by Zwislocki (1991) who stated that "measurement consists of matching common attributes of things and events" and "when a standard unit is involved, numbers come in to express the sum of the units required for a match." Zwislocki also pointed out that matching is natural because it is something we all do every day in interacting with our environments. For example, the single act of picking up an object requires that a match be made between the impression of the object's mass and the impression of the needed effort to accomplish the task. Thus, that the matching operation is performed with a fairly high degree of accuracy is attested to by our survival. Moreover, a good reason to expect that we should be skilled at such a task is its simplicity. According to Zwislocki, the matching operation underlying measurement is performed on an ordinal scale (see Table 10.1), and this is true whether or not numbers are involved. The question in matching is simply, which one of the items being matched is the greater, without a specification of how much. Thus, absolute magnitude estimation, requires none of the complex judgments, such as ratio judgments or difference judgments, that other psychophysical scaling procedures are so dependent upon. Instead, in absolute magnitude estimation, the subject is required, through ordinal judgments, to establish a match between the psychological magnitudes of numbers and the stimuli. Whether the subject is performing magnitude estimation or cross-modality matching, the task is essentially the same -- to judge whether one psychological magnitude located on one continuum is less than, greater than, or equal to a psychological magnitude located on another continuum. A match is made when the psychological magnitudes are judged to be equal. At this point, the two corresponding stimulus values are recorded by the experimenter. In AME, the two values that are recorded are the number selected by the subject and the physical value of the relevant dimension of the sensory stimulus (e.g., intensity, frequency, wavelength, etc.). In cross-modality matching, the physical values of the stimuli that are judged to be equal in sensory magnitude are recorded. Stevens (1975) also emphasized the fundamental nature of the matching operation in magnitude estimation and cross-modality matching.

Performance in psychophysical matching by adults and children (age range 4-7 years) was the topic of investigation by Collins and Gescheider (1989) who required subjects to match their impression of number size to their impressions of line length and to the loudness of 1000-Hz tones. In the second phase of the experiment, these same subjects were required to match their impressions of line length to the loudness of the tones. The results of one adult subject are seen in Figure 10.5. The subjective line-length scale and the loudness scale were both power functions with exponents of .93 and .27 respectively. The equations describing the best fitting power functions for subjective line length and loudness were used to predict the cross-modality matching function (see Collins and Gescheider for details). The solid line of the cross-modality matching function was predicted from the subjective line length and loudness functions. It is clear that, for this subject, the actual matches, as indicated by the data points, are in reasonably close agreement with the predicted function. The dashed lines in the figure illustrate the prediction of a single point on the cross-modality matching function where a magnitude estimation value of 2.0 corresponds to a line length of 20 cm and a tone of 40 dB sensation level. The results presented in Figure 10.5 and those of most of the other subjects supported the hypothesis that, with proper instructions, both children and adults can judge stimuli on an absolute scale. Specifically, for 9 out of 12 adults and 9 out of 11 children, lines and tones assigned the same number in absolute magnitude estimation were judged to be subjectively equal in cross-modality matching. Similar results recently have been reported in which subjects made AME judgments and cross-modality matches for brightness, loudness, the subjective magnitudes of vibration and subjective line length (Bolanowski, Zwislocki & Gescheider, 1991). In all of the experiments of this study, except for three subjects, the equality of assigned numbers in magnitude estimation fairly accurately predicted the results of cross-modality matches. It is significant that this principle also applied to a situation in which the response measure of applied pressure by the subject's fingertip was substituted for the AME response measure. Results for a single representative subject are shown in Figure 10.6. The squares are data points for cross-modality matching of loudness to the subjective magnitude of vibration. The open circles indicate the matches predicted from AME judgments of loudness and the subjective magnitude

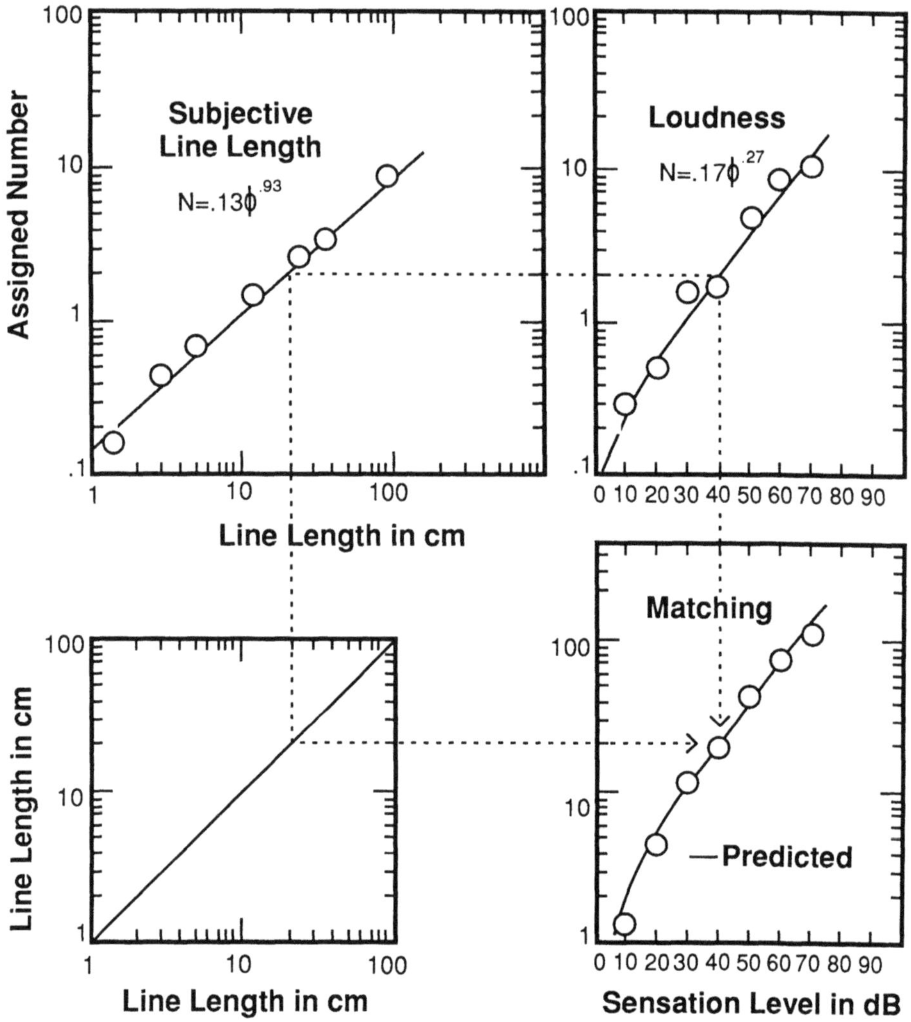

Figure 10.5: AME judgments of subjective line length and loudness as functions of line length in cm and the sensation level in dB of a 1000 Hz tone, respectively. The loudness exponent was determined over the range of 20-70 dB SL. In the lower part of the figure are seen the predicted cross-modality matches of subjective line length to loudness (solid line) and the data for this task. The dashed lines illustrate the prediction of one cross-modality match when the AME value was 2.0 for both subjective line length and loudness. Data for a single subject from Collins and Gescheider (1989).

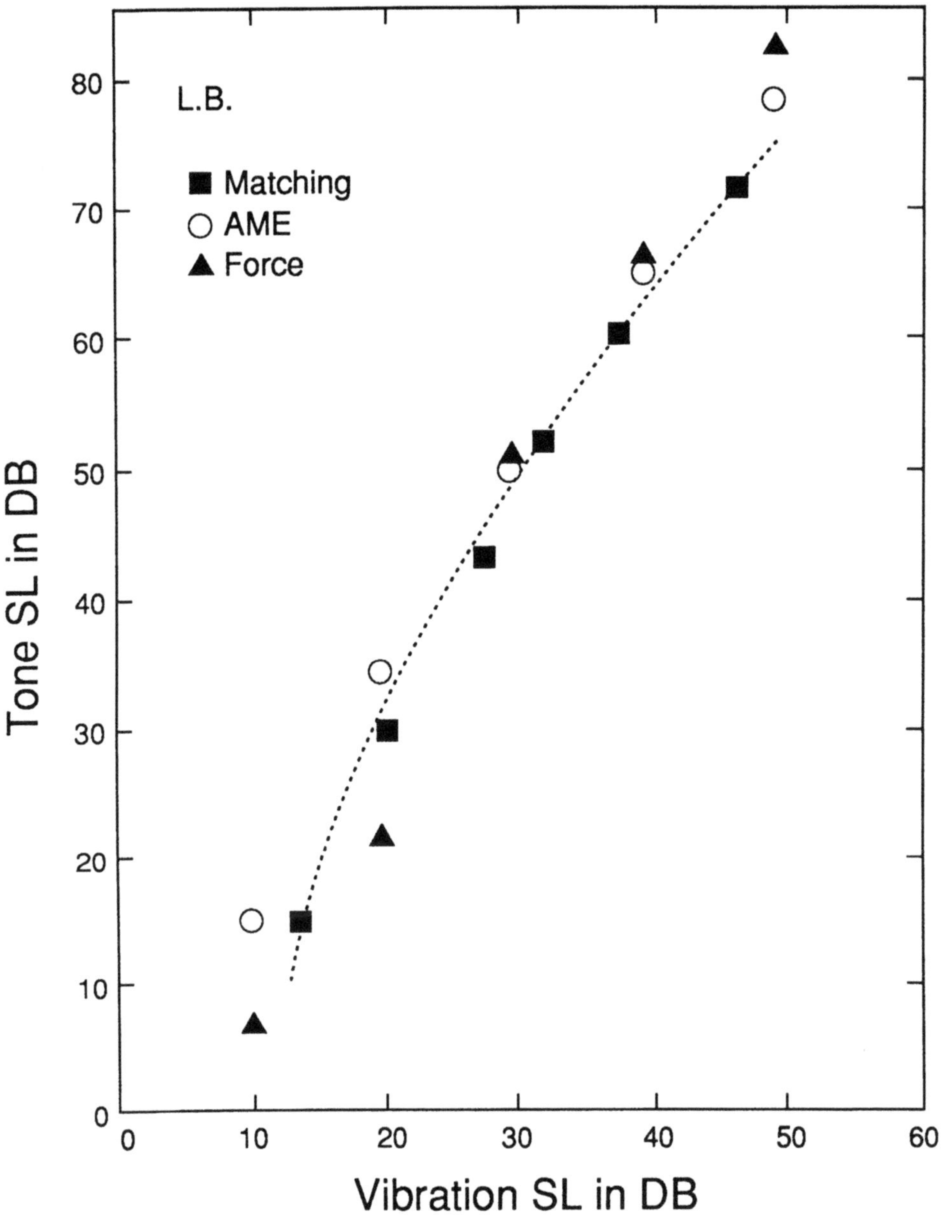

Figure 10.6: Sensation levels of the tone and vibration producing equal sensation magnitudes. The solid line is fitted to the matching data (squares). The circles show the data derived from AME and the triangles show the data derived from matching subjective pressure. From Bolanowski, Zwislocki and Gescheider (1991).

of vibration. The open circles indicate the matches predicted from AME judgments of loudness and the subjective magnitude of vibration. It is clear that the cross-modality matches were in fairly close agreement with matches derived from AME. The third set of data in Figure 10.6 represented as triangles are based on judgments in which the subject matched applied pressure from the fingertip to loudness and to the subjective magnitude of vibration. In this part of the experiment, the subject pressed a knob so that the subjective magnitude of pressure was equal to the subjective magnitude of either the sound or the vibratory stimulus. From the relationships between applied pressure and sound intensity and between applied pressure and vibration intensity, it was possible to predict cross-modality matches of loudness to the subjective magnitude of vibration. As seen in Figure 10.6, these predicted cross-modality matches are in close agreement with the actual matches performed by the subject and with those predicted from AME. Clearly, all the data sets are in approximate agreement, indicating once again that equal assigned numbers in AME represent approximately equal sensation magnitudes.

The transitivity of AME scales demonstrated in these cross-modality matching experiments has also been demonstrated in studies in which subjects made intramodality matches of the loudness of tones of different frequencies (Hellman, 1976), the loudness of tones presented in the presence of and in the absence of noise (Hellman & Zwislocki, 1964), and the subjective magnitude of vibrotactile stimuli of different frequencies (Verrillo et al., 1969). In these studies, the values of intramodality matches of the psychological magnitude of qualitatively different stimuli were accurately predicted from AME judgments.

VI. Individual Differences and Response Transformation Functions

An examination of exponents and the size of numbers used by individuals has revealed large individual differences, but a high degree of stability of responding over sessions, indicating that the subjects in AME experiments have individual ways of assigning numbers to sensations that tend to persist over time (Collins & Gescheider, 1989). Teghtsoonian and Teghtsoonian (1983) favor the view that consistency in response over sessions is due to memory of specific responses made in earlier sessions. It is doubtful that subjects would remember their judgments over the 5-14 days between sessions in the Collins and Gescheider study, or over 1 to 2 years, as in a study by Verrillo (1983) in which he found a high degree of reliability of responding in AME over these very long time intervals. Rather, it seems that subjects prefer to use certain numbers because of enduring modes of responding that are characteristically different for individual subjects. Because the individual subject's responses tend to be stable over time, there is the possibility that the individual's response mode can be identified.

As illustrated in Figure 10.2, the stimulus transformation function (psychophysical law) that describes the relationship between sensations and stimuli cannot easily be known from the subject's judgments. It is not possible to establish the relationship between stimulus intensity and sensation magnitude from experimental data without knowing the response transformation function describing the relationship between sensation magnitude and the subject's response. Zwislocki (1983b) has demonstrated that the AME exponent for subjective line length can provide a direct measure of the exponent for the generalized response-transformation function that applies to other sensory continua. According to Zwislocki, since the perception of line length is veridical, any deviation of the exponent of the subjective line-length function from 1.0 is a reflection of bias (nonlinearity) in the response transformation function. Assuming that the response bias generalizes across modalities, this response-transformation function can be used to correct exponents obtained for other sensory dimensions. This is done simply by dividing the exponent in question by the subjective line-length exponent obtained from the same subject (see Zwislocki, 1983a and Collins & Gescheider, 1989 for the formal logic).

What is the evidence that response transformation functions generalize across modalities? Zwislocki (1983a) estimated the response-transformation function in two ways for the same subjects in an experiment on loudness summation. In this study, the subjects made AME judgments of the overall loudness of two brief tones presented in rapid succession. The frequencies of the tones were in different critical bands and therefore loudness summation was expected. Consistent with the hypothesis that loudness summates linearly in the nervous system and that subjects are capable of making valid judgments of loudness, AME judgments of the tone pair were equal to the sum of the AME judgments of the individual tones. Although this additivity was evident in the average data for the group of subjects, it was absent in the data of some of the individual subjects. In the subjects where additivity was absent, either loudness summation was nonlinear, the response transformation function in which loudness is transformed to magnitude-estimation responses was nonlinear, or there existed some combination of the two nonlinear functions. If it is assumed that loudness summation is linear, it is possible to determine the nonlinear response transformations that are responsible for the lack of additivity of the magnitude estimations. Using this approach, Zwislocki determined the response transformation functions of individual subjects and found them to be power functions with exponents ranging from .83 to 1.33 with a mean of 1.08. A power functions with an exponent of 1.0 is a linear function and thus, the average data indicated a nearly perfect linear response transformation function for the group. It is clear, however, that the data of individuals indicates that some subjects deviated somewhat from this ideal. The second and independent estimation of the response transformation functions of Zwislocki's subjects was obtained by having them estimate the subjective lengths of lines. Again the average exponent of the group for this function was close to 1.0, but the exponents of some individual subjects varied considerably from this value. This finding suggests that the response transformation functions of individual subjects for judging subjective line length are sometimes nonlinear. Perhaps the most important finding of the study was the high correlation (r=.95) between the exponents for subjective line length and the theoretical response transformation exponents calculated from the loudness summation data. Thus, similar estimates of the response transformation function from line-length estimations indicate that systematic errors in assigning numbers to sensation magnitudes carry over from one modality to another.

The finding of Zwislocki that it is possible to estimate a generalized response transformation function from an individual subject's AME judgments of line length opens the possibility of using such estimations of the response transformation function to obtain unbiased estimations of the stimulus transformation (the psychophysical law). Collins and Gescheider (1989) used Zwislocki's correction procedure to correct loudness exponents of individual subjects. In this study, it was found that the intersubject variance of exponents for loudness was substantially reduced by dividing each individual loudness exponent by the line-length exponent of the same subject. The results are seen in Figure 10.7. The line in Figure 10.7(a) predicts the exponent for loudness from exponents of subjective line length under the assumptions that line-length exponents provide the exponents for the generalized response transformation function and that the true loudness function exponent is 0.3 for every subject. Deviations of measured exponents from the prediction may reflect variability among the true loudness exponents of subjects. It is clear that the loudness

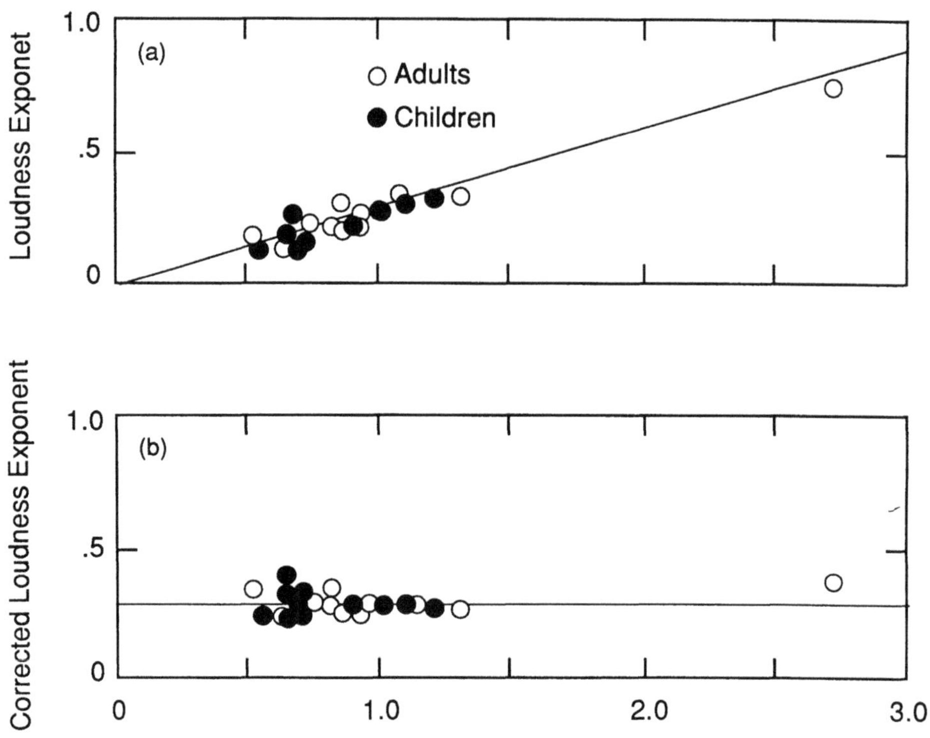

Figure 10.7: Uncorrected (a) and corrected (b) loudness exponents for each individual as a function of his/her subjective line length exponent. From Collins and Gescheider (1989).

exponents of individual subjects varied greatly and were highly correlated with their subjective line length exponents. In Figure 10.7(b) are plotted the corrected exponents for loudness as a function of the exponents for line length. The horizontal line represents the predicted function under the assumptions that the correction procedure works perfectly and that the true loudness exponent is 0.3 for every subject. One can see that, after correction, most of the loudness exponents clustered near the mean value of .3. This reduction in intersubject variability was interpreted as an indication that the correction procedure had removed a source of variability in the loudness exponents attributable to differences in the response transformation functions of individual subjects. Algom and Marks (1984), in their study of binaural summation, using conventional magnitude-estimation procedures, also attributed most of the individual differences in exponents to differences in the ways people assign numbers to sensations rather than to differences in sensory processes. It should be noted that the method of magnitude matching developed by Stevens and Marks (1980) has also been used to correct for idiosyncratic ways individual subjects use numbers in conventional magnitude estimation.

The substantial individual differences in response transformation functions might lead one to distrust the results of studies in which this potential source of error was not taken into account. Fortunately, exponents for subjective line length typically average close to 1.0 (Collins & Gescheider, 1989; Stevens & Guirao, 1963; Teghtsoonian, 1965; Verrillo, 1981, 1983; Zwislocki, 1983a; Zwislocki & Goodman, 1980), indicating linearity of the average response transformation function. Thus, exponents for other sensory attributes, such as loudness calculated from averaged magnitude-estimation data, probably represent reasonably accurate estimations of the average exponents of the underlying stimulus transformation function. This conclusion is also suggested by group magnitude-estimation data in which additivity of measurements is observed (e.g. Bolanowski, 1987; Hellman & Zwislocki, 1963; Zwislocki, 1983a). Analysis of individual differences in responding, however, demonstrates the importance of determining the response transformation function of an individual subject. Without knowing the individual's response transformation function, the form of the underlying stimulus transformation function for that subject is indeterminate from his or her magnitude estimations of the subjective magnitudes of stimuli.

VII. The Effects of Stimulus Context

Do absolute magnitude estimations depend on stimulus context? Although there are those who interpret stimulus-context effects, in which AME judgments of a stimulus depend on the values of other stimuli presented in the session (e.g. Mellers, 1983), or on the values of stimuli presented in earlier sessions (Foley et al., 1990) as evidence against the AME hypothesis, there are others who have argued that their experiments were irrelevant to this issue (Gescheider, 1988; Gescheider & Hughson, 1991; Zwislocki, 1983b). Nevertheless, if AME is to be useful as an experimental technique for measuring psychological magnitude, it is important to assess the degree to which results produced by the method are affected by stimulus context. Thus far, the findings on this issue are ambiguous with regard to the magnitude of context effects for AME. In the judgment of loudness, Zwislocki and Goodman (1980) found AME judgments to be fairly free from stimulus-context effects. Gescheider and Hughson (1991) also found context effects in AME judgments of loudness to be small for group data, as well as for the data of most of the individual subjects tested. Ellermeier, Westphal and Heidenfelder (1991) found no significant effects of stimulus context on AME type judgments or on verbally anchored category judgments of pain intensity. Ward (1987) reported context effects for several scaling methods, including AME, but they were smaller for AME and ratio magnitude estimation than for category rating. On the other hand, Mellers (1983) found substantial context effects in AME judgments. In her experiment, dot patterns of varied density were presented together and subjects made AME judgments of their apparent densities. It was found that the judgment of a particular stimulus was substantially affected by the density values of other stimuli presented at the same time. It is not known, however, whether such context effects would have been found if these stimuli had been presented one at a time.

The issue of whether judgments are affected by whether stimuli are presented singly, one at a time, or simultaneously has recently been considered in a study of the judged stressfulness of life events (Palfai, Carnrike & Gescheider, 1991). As seen in Figure 10.8, AME judgments of the stressfulness of life events were not affected by whether subjects had previously judged subjective line length by AME or by a 100-point category scale when the life-event items were presented in the single-presentation mode. When the responses of a group of subjects that had prior experience with category judgments of subjective line length were plotted as a function of the responses of a group that had prior experience with AME judgments of subjective line length, the function was nearly linear. Thus, prior experience in judging subjective line length had no effect on AME judgments of the life-event items when each item was presented alone. On the other hand, the effect of prior experience in judging subjective line length was substantial when the life-event items were presented together. In this case, the AME judgments of life-event items for a group of subjects with prior experience with category judgements of subjective line length were nonlinearly related to the judgments of a group of subjects with prior experience with AME judgments of subjective line length. The exponent of the power function fitted to the data was .54 which represents a substantial deviation from linearity. The results of this experiment clearly indicate that the magnitude or context effects in AME judgments are greatly affected by the mode of presentation of the stimulus items.

The single-presentation mode of stimulus presentation was recently employed by Gescheider and Hughson (1991) in a study of stimulus-context effects in which it was determined whether AME judgments of the loudness of a tone are influenced by the intensities of other tones presented within the same

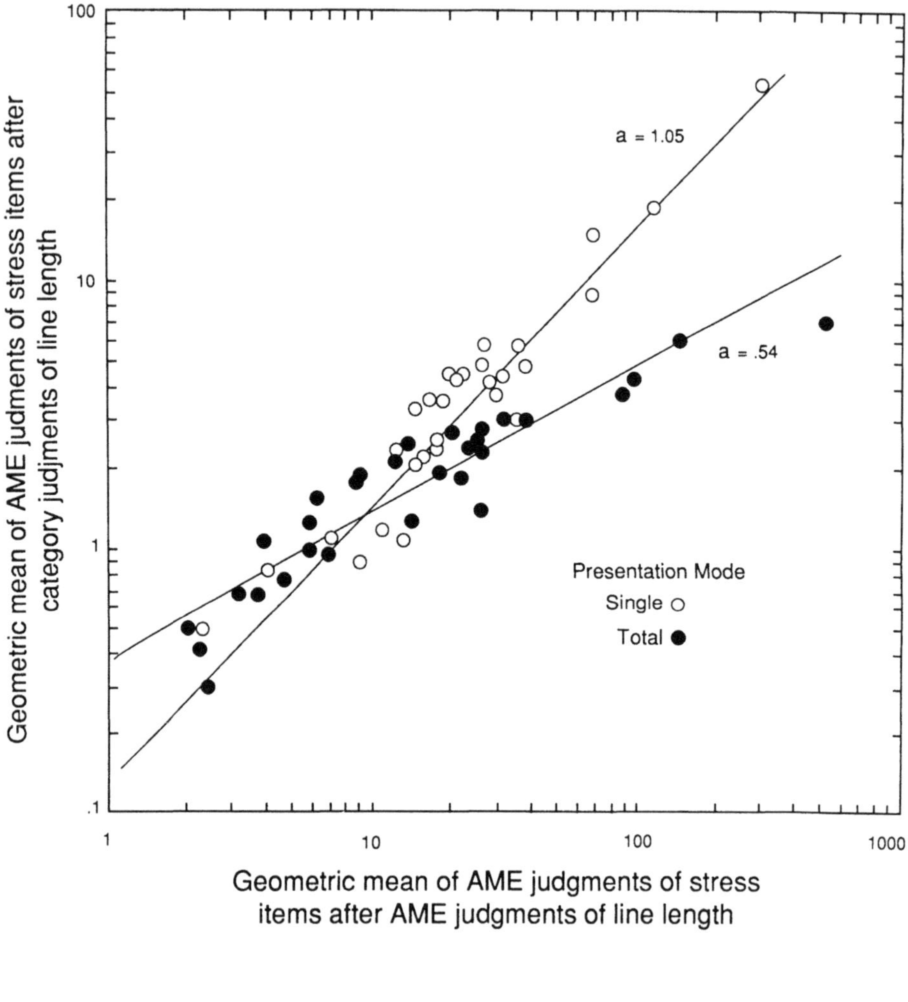

Figure 10.8: AME judgments of a group of subjects with prior experience with category judgments of subjective line length as a function of AME judgments of a group of subjects with prior experience with AME judgments of subjective line length. The mode of presentation of the stressful life event items was either single or total. From Palfai, Carnrike and Gescheider (1991).

session. In one experiment, a group of 18 subjects was tested in separate sessions in which judgments were made of the loudness of stimuli within either a low (10-60 dB SL) or high (40-90 dB SL) range of intensities. Examination of the results of individual subjects revealed that judgments of stimuli common to the two ranges (40, 50 and 60 dB SL) were, in most subjects, unaffected or only slightly affected by the position of the range. The data in Figure 10.9 indicate that in the case of 10 subjects, subjects 1 through 5 and 9 through 13, there was very little tendency for AME values for the 40, 50 and 60 dB SL tones to be systematically influenced by the location of the range. In the case of the other six subjects, subjects 6 through 8 and 14 through 16, AME judgments of the loudness of the 40, 50 and 60 dB SL tones tended to be higher when these stimuli were presented in the context of the low range than when they were presented in the context of the high range. Of these 6 subjects whose judgments were clearly affected by stimulus context, the loudness functions for the low and high range were separated on the intensity axis by no more than 5 to 10 dB. Thus, it seems that the results of the 16 subjects presented in Figure 10.9 were predominately determined by a tendency of the subject to match impressions of number size to the subjective magnitude of the stimulus, with little, if any, influence of the subjective magnitudes of other stimuli presented in the same session. It appears that in most subjects, this tendency was so strong as to override any tendencies that might have existed to judge stimuli relative to one another. About one third of the subjects in this study, however, did show some tendency to be influenced by context, but even in these cases, this tendency did not dominate the subject's judgments which were substantially more affected by changes in the intensity of the stimuli. Marks et al. (1986), using instructions that were essentially the same as those used in AME, also found large individual differences in the degree to which context affected judgments. As in the Gescheider and Hughson study, some subjects were virtually unaffected by context while others appeared to be substantially influenced.

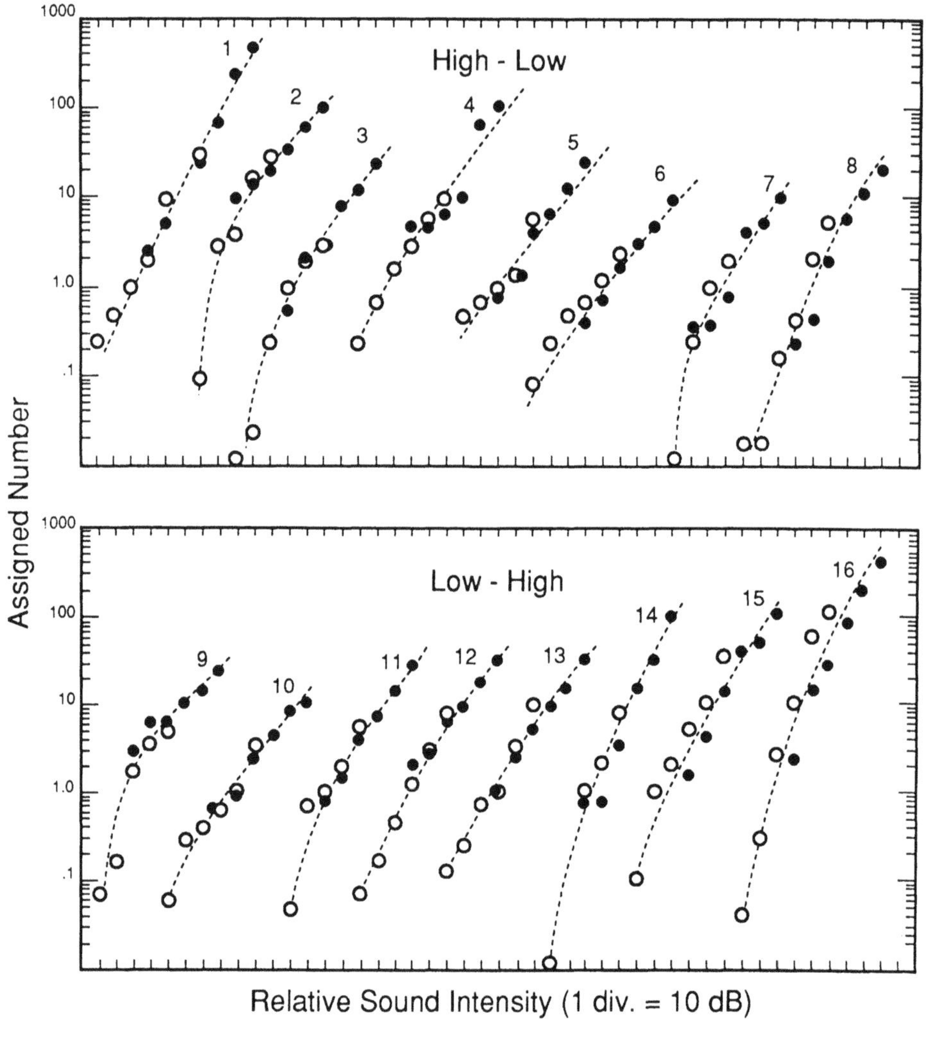

Figure 10.9: AME judgments of individual subjects as a function of relative sound intensity in dB. Subjects 1-8 received the high range first followed by the low range. Subjects 9-16 received the low range first followed by the high range. From Collins and Gescheider (1989).

It is possible that the effects of context are not due to relative judgments at all but are instead the result of sensory contrast in which a tone is perceived as louder in the context of weaker than in the context of stronger tones. It is well established that such perceptual contrast effects occur in all sensory modalities and the results of Gescheider and Hughson may be simply another example of the phenomenon. Results relevant to this hypothesis have been obtained by Ward (1982, 1985, 1986 and 1990) who has argued that sequential dependencies in magnitude estimation are based on sensory processes when the subject's response contrasts with the value of the previous stimulus. In loudness judgments, for example, a tone is judged to be louder if heard after presentation of a weaker tone than after presentation of a stronger one. This contrast effect seems to be sensory as indicated by Ward's (1990) finding that the effect is not observed when subjects judge the loudness of tones of two different frequencies except when the frequencies fall within the same critical band. The hypothesis that context affects loudness is also supported by the work of Schneider and Parker (1990) whose procedures did not require subjects to make numerical judgments and by the work of Algom and Marks (1990) who found that context affects loudness summation, a process assumed to be purely sensory, as well as the loudness function, the form of which may be influenced by both sensory processes and response bias.

At the end of the second experimental session of the Gescheider and Hughson (1991) study, to ascertain whether subjects had followed the AME instructions, subjects were asked to write a brief description of how they performed the task. Most subjects reported that, as instructed, they tried to match their impression of number size to the loudness of the tone. A few reported assigning numbers proportionally so that small ones went with weak sounds and large ones went with loud sounds. The two subjects whose data are presented in Figure 10.10, however, reported judging loudness in terms of categories. Subject 17 reported limiting the range of numbers to 1 to 30 with the exception that very weak sounds were given numbers less than 1.0. Subject 18 reported using a 0 to 10 scale with the exception that the loudest sound was given a value of 20. It is interesting that in these two cases in which the subject clearly failed to follow the AME instructions, very large biases occurred. The loudness functions obtained for the low and high stimulus ranges were separated by nearly 30 dB, indicating that nearly the same range of numbers were used for both stimulus ranges. This observation clearly indicates that, to minimize bias, it is essential that subjects carefully follow instructions in AME experiments.

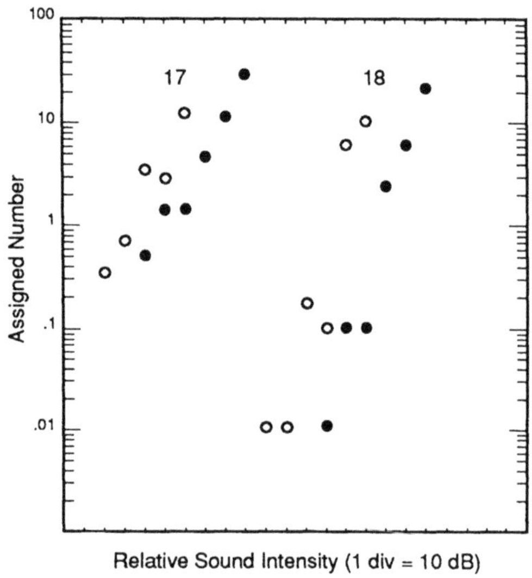

Figure 10.10: AME judgments as functions of relative sound intensity for two subjects who admitted using category scales in their judgments. From Collins and Gescheider (1989).

The AME instructions, in which the subject is told to match impressions of number size to impressions of sensation magnitude independently for each stimulus, essentially instruct the subject to produce an absolute scale (see Zwislocki, 1991). Thus, the question is whether or not the subjects can follow these instructions. Only one number has exactly the same subjective magnitude as that of the stimulus. There should be nothing arbitrary about the subject's choice of the number. Compliance with instructions should produce judgments that form the basis of an absolute scale with its fixed unit.

To determine the extent to which instructions in magnitude estimation influence the size of context effects, Gescheider and McDonnell (1991) compared results obtained using AME instructions with those obtained using more conventional magnitude estimation (ME) instructions. In this study, the following conventional magnitude instructions were given:

> Your task is to assign numbers to stand for the loudness of tones. Assign any number that you think is appropriate for the first tone you hear. Then, assign numbers to succeeding tones in proportion to your first judgment. You are free to use any positive numbers. You can use decimals or fractions if you feel they are appropriate.

These instructions can be contrasted with the AME instructions used by Gescheider and Hughson (1991) which stated the following:

> You have impressions of quiet, moderately loud and loud sounds. You also have impressions of what is a small, medium and large size number. When I present a tone, I would like you to assign a number to it so that your impression of the size of the number matches your impression of the loudness of the tone. Do not worry about comparing tones. Just listen to each tone and say a number that seems right for it. You can use any positive number that you want to. You can use decimals or fractions if you feel they are appropriate.

The procedures employed by Gescheider and McDonnell were virtually identical to those used by Gescheider and Hughson which even included having the same person give the instructions in both studies. The only difference was in the instructions given to the subjects. Seen in Figure 10.11 are the geometric means of the data of the 16 subjects who followed the AME instructions and the data of 20 subjects who were given conventional magnitude-estimation instructions. In both AME and ME conditions, shifting form one stimulus range to another significantly affected the loudness judgments of the 40, 50 and 60 dB SL tones common to both ranges. In both cases, the assigned numbers were higher for these stimuli when presented in the context of the tones of lower than higher sensation level. The magnitude of this context effect, however, was significantly greater for ME than for AME instructions. Furthermore, the data of only 3 of the 20 ME subjects exhibited insensitivity to context whereas, it should be recalled, the data of 10 of 16 AME subjects showed no context effects.

Why do stimulus-context effects in AME tend to be small or nonexistent (also see Ward, 1987 and Zwislocki & Goodman, 1980) but substantial for conventional magnitude estimation? The results of Gescheider and Hughson and Gescheider and McDonnell suggest that the answer is attributable to the difference in instructions used in the two methods. Although in both methods the subject is free to choose any numbers that seem appropriate, in conventional magnitude estimation there is no requirement that the subjective magnitudes of numbers and of the stimuli match. Instead, the subject is instructed to assign any number to the sensation magnitude of the first stimulus and to assign numbers proportional to the sensation magnitudes of all subsequently presented stimuli. If subjects interpret these instructions to mean that they can assign an arbitrary number to the first stimulus of the session, then they may have a tendency to work with the same set of numbers for different stimulus ranges. The consequence of this tendency would be to assign a new number to a stimulus when it is presented in the context of a new stimulus range.

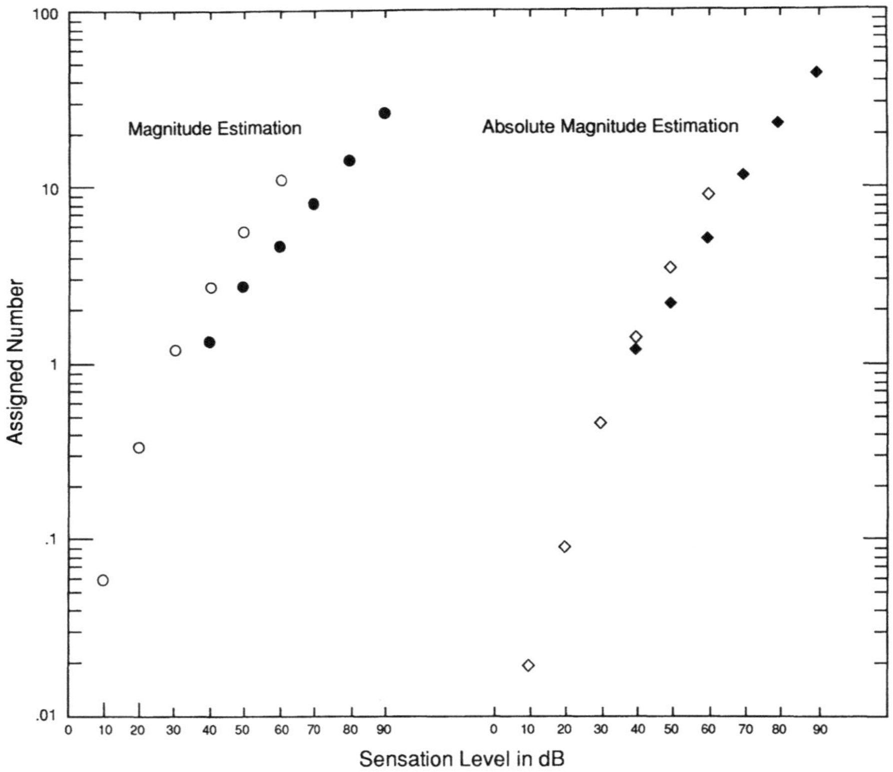

Figure 10.11: AME and ME judgments of loudness as a function of the sensation level of a 1000 Hz tones. Data are presented for a low (10-60 dB SL) and high (40-90 dB SL) stimulus range. AME data from Gescheider and Hughson (1991).

It should be pointed out that such a tendency in conventional magnitude estimation does not always dominate the subject's judgments, as indicated by individual differences in the magnitude of context effects when the position of the stimulus range is varied. Finally, it must be said that the use of AME instructions does not always eliminate this tendency in subjects' responses as indicated by the existence of context effects in the AME judgments of some of the subjects. In extreme cases, such as subjects 17 and 18 in the Gescheider and Hughson (1991) study, the results may indicate a failure to follow instructions.

The effects of the width of the stimulus range have also been examined (Gescheider & Hughson, 1991 and Gescheider & McDonnell, 1991). In the wide range, the sensation levels of the tones were 20, 30, 40, 50, 60, 70 and 80 dB whereas the narrow range consisted of tones with sensation levels of 35, 40, 45, 50, 55, 60 and 65 dB. The center of both the 60 dB and the 30 dB range was the same 50-dB SL tone. As in the experiments on the position of the stimulus range, the important question was whether the subject's judgments of the stimuli common to both the narrow and wide range (40, 50 and 60 dB SL) were significantly different, and whether prior experience with one range influenced judgments of the loudness of stimuli in the other. As seen in Figure 10.12, Gescheider and Hughson (1991) found that AME judgments were not significantly affected by the size of the stimulus range. Furthermore, the mean power-function exponents of individual subjects fitted to overlapping portions of the two ranges were essentially identical for the narrow (mean exponent, .359) and the wide (mean exponent, .357) range. In the case of nearly every subject, the exponents of the power functions fitted to the data were essentially the same for the two ranges. This, however, was not the case in the study of Gescheider and McDonnell (1991) in which this experiment was repeated with conventional magnitude estimation instructions. The judgments of many of the subjects in this experiment were affected by the size of the stimulus range and these context effects are clearly manifested in the average data for the group of 20 subjects seen in Figure 10.12. The mean exponents for the narrow and wide ranges were .352 and .241, respectively. This range effect, in which the slope of the sensation-magnitude function is inversely related to the width of the stimulus range, has also been reported in other studies using conventional magnitude-estimation instructions (e.g., Foley, et al., 1983; Frederiksen, 1975; Montgomery, 1975; Teghtsoonian, 1973; Teghtsoonian & Teghtsoonian, 1978). The results seen in Figure 10.12 indicate that there is no evidence that subjects, in performing AME, commit what Poulton (1979) has identified in magnitude estimation as the stimulus-range equalizing bias in which the subject uses much the same range of numbers, regardless of the size of the stimulus range. This, however, does not seem to be the case in conventional magnitude estimation where this bias may be substantial. That some subjects in conventional magnitude estimation tend to use the same response range when the stimulus range is changed might result from how the task is interpreted. Many of the subjects tested by Gescheider and McDonnell (1991) reported that they choose a scale at the start of the experiment and spread their responses over the entire range. When such subjects decide on their response ranges before experiencing the stimuli, one would expect that their responses would be fairly insensitive to changes in the width of the stimulus range. One consequence of this strategy would be the observed change in the slope of the sensation-magnitude function determined by ME when the size of the stimulus range is changed.

The results of Gescheider and McDonnell (1991) suggest that response bias associated with subjects setting scales for themselves in advance of the presentation of the stimuli may frequently result from giving subjects ME rather than AME instructions. Thus, in experiments where the width of the stimulus range could artifactually influence the results, it is highly recommended that appropriate means be taken to eliminate this source of bias in ME or, alternatively, the relatively bias free AME instructions be used.

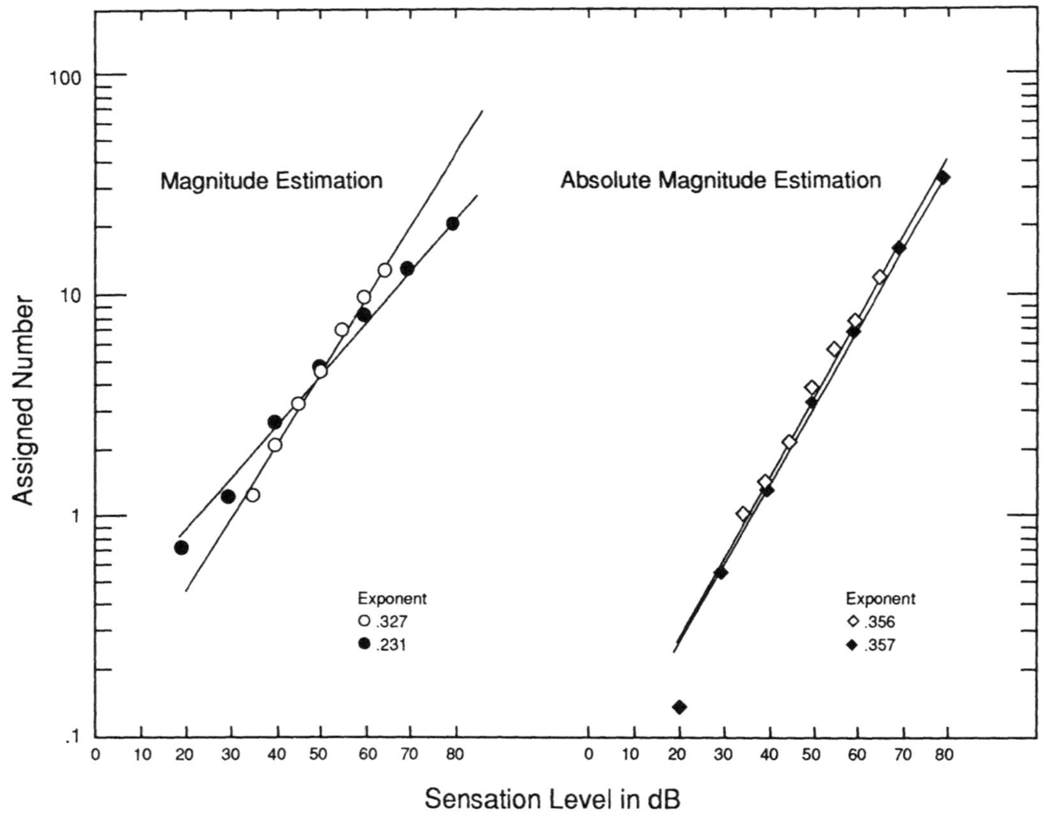

Figure 10.12: AME and ME judgments of loudness as a function of the sensation level of a 1000 Hz tone. Data are presented for a narrow (30 dB) and wide (60 dB) range. AME data from Gescheider and Hughson (1991).

VIII. Conclusion

Context effects in psychophysical scaling, such as those described in this chapter, can be found with the use of virtually every psychophysical-scaling procedure, although some methods are more susceptible to them than are others. Whichever method is chosen, the sensory scientist in pursuit of pure sensory functions has attempted to eliminate context from the measurement situation. We have discussed, in detail, one such attempt. In this case, we considered the method of absolute magnitude estimation as it has been used to reduce response bias associated with stimulus context. It appears that AME scales are less affected by such context effects than are scales determined by conventional magnitude estimation procedures. Although tests of transitivity and additivity support the conclusion that AME scales derived from group data are valid, problems do arise with the scales of individual subjects when they are affected by the nonlinear use of numbers. Therefore, we strongly recommend that such nonlinear response transformation functions be determined for individual subjects and that the results be corrected accordingly so that the true stimulus transformation function, uncontaminated by bias, can be established. In this regard, the procedure developed by Zwislocki (1983a) in which the response transformation function is estimated from the subject's judgments of the subjective lengths of lines has been successfully used.

Although it is the goal of the sensory scientist, using scaling methods, to eliminate stimulus context effects attributable to response bias, other stimulus context effects may be of great interest. These context effects do not affect the subject's responses through biasing judgments but instead affect responses by affecting the sensory experience itself. Lateral inhibition, masking and summation are examples of phenomena in which the sensation produced by a stimulus is affected by the presence of other stimuli in the situation. Clearly, the study of such context effects has enhanced our understanding of sensory systems.

In addition to response bias and sensory mechanisms, context effects may be attributable to cognitive factors such as the subject's concept of the relative magnitudes of stimuli within a set of stimuli. When encouraged to judge the sensory magnitudes of stimuli relative to one another, the subject's concept of the relative magnitude of a particular stimulus may be very different when it is presented within the context of different sets of stimuli, even though the sensory magnitude of the stimulus is unchanged. Indeed, this is probably the way judgments are made of most stimuli in real-world situations. Although such effects of context on judgment may be of great interest to those studying cognition, they present serious problems when scaling methods in which subjects must estimate sensory magnitudes are used to study sensory processes. The method of absolute magnitude estimation is a technique designed to solve this problem. In AME, the subject is specifically instructed *not* to compare stimuli but instead to match an impression of number size to an impression of the sensory stimulus without thinking about prior matches. Thus far, the method has produced results that are consistent with those produced by other methods such as matching of sensory stimuli, both within and across modalities, and with the hypothesis of additivity of sensory magnitudes in the modalities of vision and audition.

References

Algom, D. & Marks, L.E. (1984). Individual differences in loudness processing and loudness scales. *Journal of Experimental Psychology: General*, **113**, 571-593.

Algom, D. & Marks, L.E. (1990). Range and regression, loudness scales, and loudness processing: Toward a context bound psychophysics. *Journal of Experimental Psychology: Human Perception and Performance*, **16**, 706-727.

Attneave, F. (1962). Perception and related areas. In S. Koch (Ed.), *Psychology: A Study of a science,* **4** (pp. 619-659). New York: McGraw-Hill.

Bolanowski, S.J., Jr. (1987). Contourless stimuli produce binocular brightness summation. *Vision Research*, **27**, 1943-1951.

Bolanowski, S.J., Jr., Zwislocki, J.J. & Gescheider, G.A. (1991). Intersensory generality and psychological units. In S.J. Bolanowski, Jr., & G.A. Gescheider. Ratio Scaling of Psychological Magnitude: A Tribute to the Memory of S.S. Stevens (pp. 277-293). Hillsdale: Lawrence Erlbaum Associates.

Collins, A.A. & Gescheider, G.A. (1989). The measurement of loudness in children and adults by absolute magnitude estimation and cross-modality matching. *Journal of the Acoustical Society of America*, **85**, 2012-2021.

Curtis, D.W., Attneave, F., & Harrington, T.L. (1968). A test of a two-stage model of magnitude judgment. *Perception & Psychophysics*, **3**, 25-31.

Ellermeier, W., Westphal, W. & Heidenfelder, M. (1991). On the "absoluteness" of category and magnitude scales of pain. *Perception & Psychophysics*, **49**, 159-166.

Foley, H.J., Cross, D.V., Foley, M.A. & Reeder, R. (1983). Stimulus range, number of categories and the "virtual" exponent. *Perception & Psychophysics*, **34**, 505-512.

Foley, H.J., Cross, D.V. & O'Reilly, J.A. (1990). Pervasiveness and magnitude of context effects: Evidence for the relativity of absolute magnitude estimation. *Perception & Psychophysics*, **48**, 551-558.

Frederiksen, J.R. (1975). Two models for psychological judgment: scale invariance with changes in stimulus range. *Perception & Psychophysics,* **17**, 147-157.

Gescheider, G.A. (1988). Psychophysical Scaling. *Annual Review of Psychology* **39**, 169-200.

Gescheider, G.A. & Bolanowski, S.J., Jr. (1991). Introduction to Conference on Ratio Scaling of Psychological Magnitudes. In S.W. Bolanowski, Jr. & G.A. Gescheider (Eds.), *Ratio Scaling of Psychological Magnitude: Attribute to the Memory of S.S. Stevens* (pp. 1-7). Hillsdale: Lawrence Erlbaum Associates.

Gescheider, G.A. & Bolanowski, S.J., Jr. (1991). Final comments on ratio scaling of psychological magnitude. In S.J. Bolanowski, Jr., & G.A. Gescheider (Eds.), *Ratio Scaling of Psychological Magnitude: A tribute to the Memory of S.S. Stevens* (pp. 1-7). Hillsdale: Lawrence Erlbaum Associates.

Gescheider, G.A. & Hughson, B.A. (1991). Stimulus context and absolute magnitude estimation: A study of individual differences. *Perception & Psychophysics*, **50**, 45-57.

Gescheider, G.A. & McDonnell, K. (unpublished manuscript). The effects of stimulus context on magnitude estimation: The importance of instructions.

Hellman, R.P. (1976). Growth of loudness at 1000 and 3000 Hz. *Journal of the Acoustical Society of America*, **60**, 672-679.

Hellman, R.P. & Zwislocki, J.J. (1961). Some factors affecting the estimation of loudness. *Journal of the Acoustical Society of America*, **33**, 687-694.

Hellman, R.P., & Zwislocki, J.J. (1963). Monaural loudness function at 1000 cps and interaural summation. *Journal of the Acoustical Society of America,* **35**, 856-865.

Hellman, R.P. & Zwislocki, J.J (1964). Loudness function of a 1000 cps tone in the presence of a masking noise. *Journal of the Acoustical Society of America*, **36**, 1618-1627.

Marks, L.E., Szczesiul, R. & Ohlott, P. (1986). On the cross-modality perception of intensity. *Journal of Experimental Psychology: Human Perception and Performance*, **12**, 517-534.

Mellers, B.A. (1983). Evidence against "absolute" scaling. *Perception & Psychophysics*, **33**, 523-526.

Montgomery, H. (1975). Direct estimation: effect of methodological factors on scale type. *Scandinavian Journal of Psychology*, **16**, 19-29.

Palfai, T., Carnricke, C.L.M. & Gescheider, G.A. Absolute magnitude estimation and category scaling of the perceived stressfulness of live events (submitted).

Poulton, E.C. (1979). Models for biases in judging sensory magnitude. *Psychological Bulletin*, **86**, 777-803.

Schneider, B. & Parker, S. (1990). Does stimulus context affect loudness or only loudness judgments? *Perception & Psychophysics*, **48**, 409-418.

Shepard, R.N. (1981). Psychological relations and psychophysical scales: on the status of "direct" psychophysical measurement. *Journal of Mathematical Psychology*, **24**, 21-57.

Stevens, J.C., & Marks, L.E. (1980). Cross-modality-matching functions generated by magnitude estimation. *Perception & Psychophysics*, **27**, 379-389.

Stevens, S.S. (1951). Mathematics, measurement and psychophysics. In *Handbook of Experimental Psychology* ed. S.S. Stevens, pp. 1-49. New York: Wiley.

Stevens, S.S. (1956). The direct estimation of sensory magnitude: loudness. *American Journal of Psychology*, **69**, 1-25.

Stevens, S.S., & Guirao, M. (1963). Subjective scaling of length and area and the matching of length to loudness and brightness. *Journal of Experimental Psychology*, **66**, 177-186.

Teghtsoonian, M. (1965). The judgment of size. *American Journal of Psychology* **78**, 392-402.

Teghtsoonian, M., and Teghtsoonian, R. (1983). Constancy of individual exponents in cross-modality matching. *Perception & Psychophysics*, **33**, 203-214.

Teghtsoonian, R. (1973). Range effects in psychophysical scaling and a revision of Stevens' Law. *American Journal of Psychology*, **86**, 3-27.

Teghtsoonian, R. & Teghtsoonian, M. (1978). Range and regression effects in magnitude scaling. *Perception & Psychophysics*, **24**, 305-314.

Verrillo, R.T. (1981). Absolute estimation of line length in three age groups. *Journal of Gerontology*, **36**, 625-627.

Verrillo, R.T. (1983). Stability of line-length estimates using the method of absolute magnitude estimation. *Perception & Psychophysics*, **33**, 261-265.

Verrillo, R.T., Fraioli, A.J. & Smith, R.L. (1969). Sensory magnitude of vibrotactile stimuli. *Perception & Psychophysics*, **6**, 366-372.

Ward, L.M. (1973). Repeated magnitude estimations with a variable standard: sequential effects and other properties. *Perception & Psychophysics*, **13**, 193-200.

Ward, L.M. (1982). Mixed-modality psychophysical scaling: Sequential dependencies and other properties. *Perception & Psychophysics*, **31**, 53-62.

Ward, L.M. (1985). Mixed-modality psychophysical scaling: Inter- and intramodality sequential dependencies as a function of lag. *Perception & Psychophysics*, **38**, 512-522.

Ward, L.M. (1986). Mixed-modality psychophysical scaling: Double cross-modality matching for "difficult" continua. *Perception & Psychophysics*, **39**, 407-417.

Ward, L.M. (1987). Remembrance of sounds past: memory and psychophysical scaling. *Journal of Experimental Psychology: Human Perception and Performance*, **13**, 216-227.

Ward, L.M. (1990). Critical bands and mixed-frequency scaling: Sequential dependencies, equal-loudness contours, and power function exponents. *Perception & Psychophysics*, **47**, 551-562.

Zwislocki, J.J. (1978). Absolute scaling. *Journal of the Acoustical Society of America*, **63**, 516 (Abstract).

Zwislocki, J.J. (1983a). Group and individual relations between sensation magnitudes and their numerical estimates. *Perception & Psychophysics*, **33**, 460-468.

Zwislocki, J.J. (1983b). Absolute and other scales: question of validity. *Perception & Psychophysics*, **33**, 593-594.

Zwislocki, J.J. (1991). Natural measurement. In S.J. Bolanowski, Jr. & G.A. Gescheider, (Eds.), *Ratio Scaling of Psychological Magnitude: A Tribute to the memory of S.S. Stevens*. Hillsdale: Lawrence Erlbaum Associates.

Zwislocki, J.J. & Goodman, D.A. (1980). Absolute scaling of sensory magnitude: a validation. *Perception & Psychophysics*, **28**, 28-38.

SUBJECT INDEX

J

L

M

O

P

Q

R

S

T

U

V

W

www.ingramcontent.com/pod-product-compliance
Ingram Content Group UK Ltd.
Pitfield, Milton Keynes, MK11 3LW, UK
UKHW020224290926
15470UKWH00001B/362

9 780444 889782